Bioactive Compounds from Functional Foods, 2nd Edition

Bioactive Compounds from Functional Foods, 2nd Edition

Guest Editors

Michał Halagarda
Sascha Rohn

MDPI

Basel • Beijing • Wuhan • Barcelona • Belgrade • Novi Sad • Cluj • Manchester

Guest Editors

Michał Halagarda
Department of Food Product Quality
Krakow University of Economics
Kraków
Poland

Sascha Rohn
Department of Food Chemistry and Analysis
Technische Universität Berlin
Berlin
Germany

Editorial Office
MDPI AG
Grosspeteranlage 5
4052 Basel, Switzerland

This is a reprint of the Special Issue, published open access by the journal *Molecules* (ISSN 1420-3049), freely accessible at: https://www.mdpi.com/journal/molecules/special_issues/9Q19EQOJBS.

For citation purposes, cite each article independently as indicated on the article page online and as indicated below:

Lastname, A.A.; Lastname, B.B. Article Title. *Journal Name* **Year**, *Volume Number*, Page Range.

ISBN 978-3-7258-7777-5 (Hbk)
ISBN 978-3-7258-7778-2 (PDF)
https://doi.org/10.3390/books978-3-7258-7778-2

Contents

About the Editors

Michał Halagarda

Michał Halagarda, born 1984, is an associate professor and the Head of the Department of Food Product Quality at the Krakow University of Economics (Poland). He graduated from the University of Abertay in Dundee, Scotland (BSc in Food Product Design, 2007), and the Krakow University of Economics (MSc in Commodity Science, specialty: Product Quality Management, 2008). In 2014, he obtained his Ph.D. in Commodity Science from the Faculty of Commodity Science at the Krakow University of Economics, Poland, with a dissertation focused on modeling new food product development processes based on bakery industry products. In 2019, he completed his habilitation at the Faculty of Commodity Science and Product Management of the Krakow University of Economics. He completed research internships at the Institute of Food Chemistry (University of Hamburg, Germany), the Department of Chemical Engineering (Food Technology area) at the University of Vigo (Spain), the Department of Grain Processing and Baking Technologies at the Institute of Agricultural and Food Biotechnology in Warsaw (Poland), and the Seidman College of Business at Grand Valley State University (USA). He is a member of the Polish Commodity Science Society, the International Society of Commodity Science and Technology (IGWT), and the Honey Platform—an expert group established by the European Commission bringing together stakeholders, researchers, and specialists to support the development of harmonized methods for honey authenticity, traceability, and quality control, and to combat food fraud. His research mainly covers Food Science and Consumer Economics. His scientific interests include authentication of traditional, regional and organic food products, bioactive compounds in foods, food product quality development and assessment, consumer market behavior.

Sascha Rohn

Sascha Rohn, born 1973, is a full professor for Food Chemistry at the Technische Universität Berlin, Germany. He graduated from the University of Frankfurt/Main, Germany, with the first and second state examination in Food Chemistry, 1999. In 2002, he obtained his Ph.D. in Food Chemistry from the Institute of Nutritional Science, University of Potsdam, Germany, working on interactions of polyphenols with food proteins. After two years as a postdoc, he left Potsdam towards Berlin, where he was an assistant professor at the Institute of Food Technology and Food Chemistry of the Technische Universität Berlin. From October 2009 to October 2020, he was a full professor at the Institute of Food Chemistry, University of Hamburg, Germany. His group deals with the analysis of bioactive food compounds. In particular, they characterize the reactivity and stability of bioactive compounds. The aim is to identify degradation products that serve as quality parameters, as process markers during food/feed processing, or as biomarkers in nutritional physiology. Results of their work have been presented in more than 300 publications so far (Scopus h index is 70 and more than 15,000 citations). More than 30 well-known scientific journals regularly ask Prof. Rohn to review scientific manuscripts. From 2006 to 2012, he was chairman of the Northeastern branch of the German Food Chemical Society (LChG). He is a member of the board of the German Nutrition Society (DGE) and chair of the scientific advisory board of the Max Rubner-Institut (MRI), Germany.

Preface

The growing interest in functional foods and their health-promoting potential continuously stimulates intensive scientific research. From a chemical in-depth view, bioactive compounds remain at the core of this field, contributing to physiological benefits and playing an important role in advancing research in food science, nutrition, and further related disciplines. In this context, ongoing research efforts continue to broaden understanding of the diversity of bioactive compounds, their mechanisms of action, and their relevance within biological systems and food matrices.

The second edition of "Bioactive Compounds from Functional Foods" reflects these developments and emphasizes the increasing depth and interdisciplinarity of current research. Particular attention is given to the molecular mechanisms underlying bioactivity, including interactions with the gut–brain axis, modulation of immune responses, and regulation of inflammatory and metabolic pathways. Recent studies indicate that compounds such as omega-3 fatty acids may influence neurophysiological processes and microbiota composition, demonstrating their systemic importance and multifunctional character. At the same time, experimental approaches, including in vivo models, provide further insight into immunomodulatory effects and the biological relevance of functional ingredients.

This Special Issue presents a broad spectrum of sources of bioactive compounds, extending beyond traditional plant-derived metabolites. Contributions include phytochemicals from medicinal plants, polysaccharides, and other metabolites from fungi and marine organisms, as well as protein- and lipid-derived bioactives, originating from animal-based raw materials such as milk and eggs. Particular emphasis is given on bioactive peptides generated through enzymatic hydrolysis, with selected studies highlighting the role of protein structure, genotype, and processing in shaping bioactivity. These studies demonstrate the diversity of matrices and the importance of structure–function relationships in determining the biological potential of food-derived compounds.

In addition to experimental studies, this edition highlights the growing importance of analytical and computational approaches. Advanced analytical techniques, such as LC-MS-based approaches, enable the identification and quantification of bioactive compounds, including compounds with beneficial and, in some cases, potentially adverse health implications. At the same time, in silico analyses support the prediction of bioactivity and the exploration of complex peptide and metabolite profiles, complementing laboratory-based research.

Technological aspects and food processing remain central to the discussion, as they significantly influence the stability, bioavailability, and functionality of bioactive compounds. Contributions address the effects of thermal processing, as well as innovative strategies such as enrichment, modification, and impregnation of food matrices to enhance functional properties. These studies underline that the final biological effect of a compound is not only dependent on its intrinsic properties but also on the structure of the food matrix and the conditions during processing and subsequent stages that affect food quality and functionality.

An important aspect emphasized in this edition is the dual and sometimes controversial nature of bioactive compounds. While many exhibit antioxidant, anti-inflammatory, or immunomodulatory effects, others may also be associated with context-dependent or potentially adverse health outcomes. The example of trimethylamine-N-oxide in fish oil illustrates the necessity for careful analytical evaluation and critical interpretation of health-related claims. This underscores the need for a balanced, evidence-based approach in the development and application of functional foods.

Overall, this Special Issue brings together a diverse collection of review articles and original research papers that address selected key aspects of bioactive compounds, including their sources, chemical characterization, biological activity, and technological application. The contributions reflect the complexity of this field and suggest future research directions, integrating experimental and computational methods, the development of novel functional ingredients, and the advancement of personalized nutrition strategies.

We would like to express our sincere appreciation to all authors for their valuable contributions and to the reviewers for their critical and constructive feedback. Their efforts have made it possible to compile this comprehensive and up-to-date collection, which we hope will serve as a valuable resource and inspiration for further research in the field of functional foods and bioactive compounds.

Michał Halagarda and Sascha Rohn
Guest Editors

molecules

MDPI

Article

Chemical Exploration of Polysaccharides, Fatty Acids, and Antioxidants as Functional Ingredients from Colombian Macroalgae *Acanthophora spicifera*, *Sargassum ramifolium*, and *Sargassum fluitans*

Jhonny Colorado-Ríos [1,2,*], Diana C. Restrepo-Espinosa [1], Yuli Restrepo-Moná [1], Juan David Monsalve [1], Diana M. Márquez-Fernández [1], Leonardo Castellanos [3] and Alejandro Martínez-Martínez [1]

1 Grupo Productos Naturales Marinos, Facultad de Ciencias Farmacéuticas y Alimentarias, Universidad de Antioquia, Calle 70 No. 52-21, Medellín 050010, Colombia; diana.restrepoe@udea.edu.co (D.C.R.-E.); millerlay.restrepo@udea.edu.co (Y.R.-M.); juanmonsalve.mgvc@gmail.com (J.D.M.); diana.marquez@udea.edu.co (D.M.M.-F.); alejandro.martinez@udea.edu.co (A.M.-M.)

2 Unidad de Biología Celular y Molecular, Corporación para Investigaciones Biológicas (CIB), Universidad de Antioquia, Medellín 050010, Colombia

3 Departamento de Química, Facultad de Ciencias, Sede Bogotá, Universidad Nacional de Colombia, Av. Carrera 30 # 45-03, Bogotá 111321, Colombia; lcastellanosh@unal.edu.co

* Correspondence: jhonny.colorado@udea.edu.co; Tel.: +57-604-2198456

Abstract

Macroalgae are valuable natural sources for bioprospection and the development of raw materials applicable to the nutrition, health, and agriculture industries. To build a basis for the sustainable use of marine organisms from the Colombian Caribbean, a preliminary study was conducted focusing on known functional compounds in two genera of macroalgae, including the species *Acanthophora spicifera* (Rhodophyta), *Sargassum ramifolium*, and *Sargassum fluitans* (Ochrophyta). This study included the extraction and identification of polysaccharides using ultrafiltration, nuclear magnetic resonance (^{1}H-NMR), Fourier-transform infrared spectroscopy (FT-IR), and size exclusion chromatography (SEC); fatty acids by gas chromatographic (GC) profiling; and phenolic composition and antioxidant activity by complementary semi-quantitative methods (ABTS, DPPH, FRAP, and ORAC assays). Carrageenan-type polysaccharides were detected in *A. spicifera*, while alginate and fucoidan types were found in *S. ramifolium* and *S. fluitans*; palmitic acid was the predominant fatty acid in *A. spicifera* and *S. ramifolium*, but it was not detected in *S. fluitans*. *S. ramifolium* showed the highest ABTS, DPPH, and ORAC activities and phenolic compounds, while *S. fluitans* exhibited the highest FRAP activity. This study contributes to the chemical knowledge on Colombian macroalgae to establish potential applications in various fields, including biomedicine, cosmetics, functional foods, and nutraceutical ingredients.

Keywords: macroalgae; Colombia; fatty acids; polysaccharides; polyphenols; antioxidants

1. Introduction

Macroalgae are a valuable source of valuable compounds with critical industrial ap-plications, among which polysaccharides (PSs), fatty acids, and antioxidants have commercial recognition with applications in the food, pharmaceutical, and cosmetic industries [1,2] and a promising economic potential for coastal communities where these samples may be collected. The studies about raw material from macroalgae have focused on the use of high value products such as polyunsaturated fatty acids, phenols, and polysaccharides, mainly to be incorporated in foods and as drug delivery systems [3,4].

Alginates and carrageenan, due to their polysaccharide nature, are significant components of seaweed that constitute the cell wall [5]. Alginates have gel-forming properties that are very well appreciated for food, pharmaceutical, and cosmetic applications due to their rheological and suspending properties and their wound-healing effects [6–9]. Carrageenans are widely used as raw materials for food products such as gelling agents, emulsifiers, thickeners, or stabilizers [10,11]. Brown seaweed commonly present alginates, which are arranged in the linear backbone of blocks composed of β-D-mannuronic acid (M) and α-L-guluronic acid (G) residues, both linked by 1→4 glycosidic bonds [8]. Otherwise, red seaweeds are known for producing polysaccharides mainly composed of galactose, such as carrageenan, that are made by repeating disaccharide units conformed by 3-linked β-D-galactopyranose (G) and 4-linked α-D-galactopyranose (D) or 4-linked 3,6-anhydro-α-D-galactopyranose (DA); these units could be sulphated [12]. The sugar backbone of polysaccharides obtained from different macroalgae families can vary their expected molecular weight, their sulfation substitution and degree, and their biological activities [1].

Carbohydrates are not the only valuable compounds that can be obtained from algae, and although the content of lipids is not as high as in the case of polysaccharides, they represent an alternative source of polyunsaturated fatty acids, especially those belonging to long-chain omega-3 polyunsaturated fatty acids (*n*-3 PUFAs), which traditionally have been obtained from fish or fish oil and are essential in the human diet because of their functionality in cardiovascular and inflammatory diseases, brain development, cancer, anti-aging, and mental health [13,14]. Algae represent a sustainable and non-traditional alternative source of *n*-3 PUFAs since decades of overfishing have significantly declined stocks [14]. While red and brown algae are notable for their eicosapentaenoic acid (EPA) and arachidonic acid (AA) content, green seaweeds primarily contain oleic and palmitic acid [1].

Polyphenolic compounds are also present in macroalgae, such as flavonoids, phenolics acids, phenolic terpenoids, and phlorotannins, the latter being exclusive to brown algae [15,16]. They are essential for the growth and development of these organisms, and they are involved in protective functions since they are produced in response to stimuli that includes predator attacks, diseases, injures, and UV radiation [17–19]. Due to these properties, these substances are of interest for developing similar functions that may contribute to healing various diseases, showing a wide range of possible applications in the pharmaceutical and biomedical areas. Among their specific bioactivities, the antioxidant properties of algae are of interest to food industries to improve the nutritional value and sensory characteristics of several processed products such as cheese, yogurt, and desserts [1,20]. Additionally, their cosmetic applications have been investigated by incorporating phenolic compounds from algae, aiming to develop skincare and anti-aging products that leverage their protective effects against the loss of skin elasticity associated with aging [21]. Antioxidant activity is one of the most explored effects of phenolic compounds from macroalgae, but it is not an exclusive property of this type of substance. Other primary and secondary metabolites, such as polysaccharides, chlorophylls, and carotenoids exhibit these properties, which make them extremely valuable bioactive agents that can impact human health through the prevention of oxidative stress and the mitigation of prevalent modern diseases [18,21,22].

Considering the above, it is evident that research on marine algae has become a global trend. However, research remains insufficiently advanced within the Colombian national context to indicate that this area has been thoroughly explored. This may be explained by the fact that, despite having coastlines along both the Atlantic and Pacific Oceans, there is a lack of interest from the national scientific community, multiple coastal regions are challenging and expensive to access, and there are sociopolitical factors that impede access to different regions [23,24]. Additionally, marine macroalgae, as a source of bioactive substances, can be used as a renewable and sustainable natural resource. Nevertheless, several outcomes have demonstrated that the biomass produced by these organisms has a broad spectrum of substances, which varies according to the species and the environmental conditions [1]. Those differences could be evidenced in the explored region when compared with those previously reported in other countries and even continents since Colombia is a transcontinental country situated in the northwest of South America, bordered by the Caribbean Sea and the Pacific Ocean. Simultaneously, investigating these locally occurring organisms may yield novel compounds that have not yet been characterized [23,24].

A bibliographic review conducted through Scopus reveals that, of the 16,223 articles published globally on macroalgae and 32,676 on seaweed, just 23 and 48, respectively, have been produced in Colombia, where around 50% of the research has been focused on agriculture, biological, ecological, and Earth and planetary sciences. At the same time, those related to chemistry, biochemistry, and other fields of knowledge represent a percentage lower than 16%. *Acanthophora spicifera* is an edible red marine alga, widely distributed in subtropical and tropical seas [25], which has been documented as a rich source of carbohydrates, lipids, proteins, minerals, fatty acids, essential amino acids, and functional substances including flavonoids, phenolic compounds, and polysaccharides [26,27]. This species has been mainly studied in the United States and India, countries where environmental conditions differ significantly from those of Colombia, which could suggest that composition may be different among the specimens of this species that are collected in our country.

Regarding the algae of the genus *Sargassum*, growing in the tropical Atlantic Ocean and extending from the Gulf of Mexico to the Gulf of Guinea, they can make massive aggregations in the open ocean and on the coast, which in recent years has conducted negative environmental consequences and has led to the local communities exploring solutions to prevent its accumulation and subsequent decomposition [28,29]. *Sargassum fluitans* is found in the Caribbean's coastal waters as part of a surface-dwelling species inundating the Caribbean's shores [30]. Despite its overgrowth, this species acts as a biofilter that could reduce pollution and accumulate toxic metals in the marine environment [31]. In *S. fluitans*, fucoidan extracts have shown antifibrotic and anti-inflammatory effects [32], and organic extracts have shown antioxidant and antibacterial activities [33]. *Sargassum ramifolium* has been less documented, but there are some reports from Caribbean species, more specifically from Cuba and the Yucatán Peninsula [34,35], where they have shown antioxidant activity and the presence of phenolic compounds; however, a complete chemical characterization has not yet been carried out [36].

This research investigates Colombian macroalgae biodiversity, focusing on comparing these algae with those of the same species from different regions. Additionally, a characterization of its promissory substances could represent a strategy to be exploited by the locals since these species can be easily collected. In this way, the methodologies were designed to facilitate extraction in case these results could be transferred to the local communities to contribute to the biomass valorization of Colombian macroalgae as a resource for extracting products with high market potential. The relatively great cost-effectiveness supports this due to the large number of possible target products and the simple processes with reduced operational costs and environmental burdens.

2. Results and Discussion

Macroalgae represent an important source of valuable bioactive substances that are promissory for preventing and treating different human conditions. In this way, they are used to develop new food products, nutraceuticals, cosmetics, and other pharmaceutical products of interest. Among those, bioactive substances, minerals, vitamins, essential amino acids, proteins, enzymes, fatty acids, carotenoids, polyphenols, and carbohydrates have been described. These compounds offer excellent benefits that allow humans to use them directly as food or in the production of hydrocolloids, medicines, biofuel, paper, fertilizers, etc. Nowadays, they are considered prized raw materials due to their cultivation, which does not require fresh water, arable land, or fertilizers, and fast growth rates [4].

To build the basis for developing a sustainable use of Colombian biodiversity, a preliminary study of some primary and secondary metabolites in several macroalgae, including *Acanthophora spicifera* (Rhodophyta), *Sargassum ramifolium*, and *Sargassum fluitans* (Ochrophyta), was carried out. Algae samples were collected from El Rodadero (Santa Marta, Colombia), El Cabo de la Vela (La Guajira, Colombia), and Playita Jacobo (Providence, RI, USA), respectively.

2.1. Fatty Acids

The fatty acid composition of the seaweed species was explored (Table 1). The total fat content in all species was 0.59, 0.67, and 0.14 per 100 g for *A. spicifera*, *S. ramifolium*, and *S. fluitans*, respectively. The three species showed myristic acid (14:0), palmitoleic acid (16:1ω7), oleic acid (18:1ω9), and linoleic acid (18:2ω6). Other saturated and unsaturated fatty acids identified were linolenic acid (18:3ω3), behenic acid (22:0), and arachidonic acid (20:4ω6). While some polyunsaturated fatty acids (PUFAs) were present, they were not present in high percentage. Also, there was no evidence of important fatty acids such as EPA (eicosapentaenoic acid; 20:5ω3) and DHA (Docosahexaenoic acid; 22:6ω3). Oleic acid was the major fatty acid for *S. fluitans*, the main monounsaturated fatty acid (MUFA) in all species, and was reported as the main MUFA of *A. spicifera* [37]. Meanwhile, linoleic acid was the main polyunsaturated fatty acid (PUFA) in the three species.

Table 1. Fatty acid content in g/100 g DW of the studied Colombian macroalgae.

Fatty Acid	*Acanthophora spicifera*	*Sargassum ramifolium*	*Sargassum fluitans*
14:0	0.05	0.04	0.02
15:0	0.01	ND [1]	ND [1]
16:0	0.33	0.31	ND [1]
16:1ω7	0.02	0.04	0.01
18:0	ND [1]	0.01	ND [1]
18:1ω9	0.10	0.13	0.04
18:2ω6	0.02	0.03	0.02
18:3ω3	ND [1]	0.01	ND [1]
20:4ω6	ND [1]	0.03	0.01
22:0	ND [1]	0.01	ND [1]

[1] ND: not detected or <0.01 g/100 g DW.

As expected, the lipid content in seaweed is low. However, the percentage of different fatty acids was less than the reports; some of them were not even detected. Despite being stored in a controlled environment protected from light and heat, lipid oxidation occurred, which could serve as a basis to explore the rate of degradation during storage and drying processes, thereby helping to evaluate the quality and stability of organic compounds such as fatty acids and even phenolic compounds in the selected algae. Previous reports found lipid oxidation during storage to be low [38]. Although freeze drying yields the highest amount of compounds, oven drying is a better cost-effective alternative than freeze drying [39]. Therefore, freeze drying was not selected to process the samples. Some reports indicate that seaweed species are a balanced source of ω3 and ω6 PUFAs; like those studies, the Colombian analyzed seaweeds contain ω3, ω6 and ω3 and ω9. The algae contain linoleic acid (ω6), which, along with linolenic acid (ω3), is an essential fatty acid that must be obtained through diet, but linolenic acid was only present in *S. ramifolium*. In previous research, fatty acids like EPA (ω3), arachidonic acid (ω6), oleic acid, and palmitic acid have shown the highest percentage in total FAME analysis; in this case, eicosapentaenoic acid was not detected, and palmitic acid was the main component of the analyzed FAMEs, but it was not detected in *Sargassum* spp. Arachidonic acid was not detected in *A. spicifera*. Oleic acid is present in the three species, mainly in *A. spicifera* and *S. ramifolium* [37,40].

The fact that the studied algae contain some of the reported fatty acids could validate their use as a nutritional source since PUFAs and MUFAs are needed for normal growth and development, neuronal activity regulation, cellular function and signaling, obesity prevention, immune response, and hypertension regulation, among others [40–42]. However, it is mandatory to go beyond these results to explore other nutritional components like proteins, vitamins, amino acids, and minerals; these are the reason why they have been consumed as food in Asian countries since ancient times and might be presented to regional communities as a food source, as they are produced in large quantities during various seasons [43]. This study aimed to detect relevant concentrations of distinctive fatty acids commonly found in macroalgae, including the presence of specific long-chain polyunsaturated fatty acids (PUFAs), such as EPA, DHA, and arachidonic acid (ARA), which have recognized nutritional, biomedical, and industrial value. Even at low concentrations, the identification of fatty acids in macroalgae contributes valuable insights into their biochemical potential, ecological role, and commercial relevance.

2.2. Polysaccharides

From about 5 g of dry mass of each macroalgae, 17, 6.3, and 4.9% of total polysaccharides were obtained from *A. spicifera*, *S. ramifolium*, and *S. fluitans*, respectively. The dried extracts were subjected to FT-IR analysis. The spectra of the aqueous extract obtained from the three species present typical carbohydrate bands related to hydroxyl (3600–3050 cm^{-1}), methylidyne or methine (3050–2800 cm^{-1}), carbonyl groups (1700–1400 cm^{-1}), C-O/C-C (1200–800 cm^{-1}) bonds, and pyranoses or their derivatives (fingerprint region) [44].

The specific bands are different when comparing the spectrum of the extract of *A. spicifera* with those obtained from *Sargassum* spp.; the main difference is associated with the prominent band between 1220 and 1260 cm^{-1}, which can be related to sulfation [44–47].

In the infrared spectrum of the aqueous extract from *A. spicifera* (Figure 1a), a broad band at 3406 cm^{-1} was assigned to hydroxyl group O-H stretching vibrations. A similar band is also present in the spectra obtained from both *Sargassum* algae (Figure 1b,c) as well as a weak band around 2930 cm^{-1} that corresponds to the C-H stretching vibrations and two bands related to the asymmetric and symmetric stretching vibrations of carboxylate group O-C-O around 1600 and 1400 cm^{-1} [48–50].

Polysaccharides in the aqueous extract from *A. spicifera* showed signals commonly present for carbohydrates such as 1221, 1157, 1071, 934, and 891 cm^{-1} bands. The band at 1072 cm^{-1} is attributed to the main structure of galactan-type polysaccharides reported previously for red algae, which are producers of galactans like agarans and carrageenan (Figure 1a) [26,51,52]. Additionally, a band related to 3,6 sugar is observed at 931 cm^{-1}, and this is also consistent with the fact that 3,6-anhydrogalactose (3,6-AG) is a component of polysaccharides such as galactans [52,53].

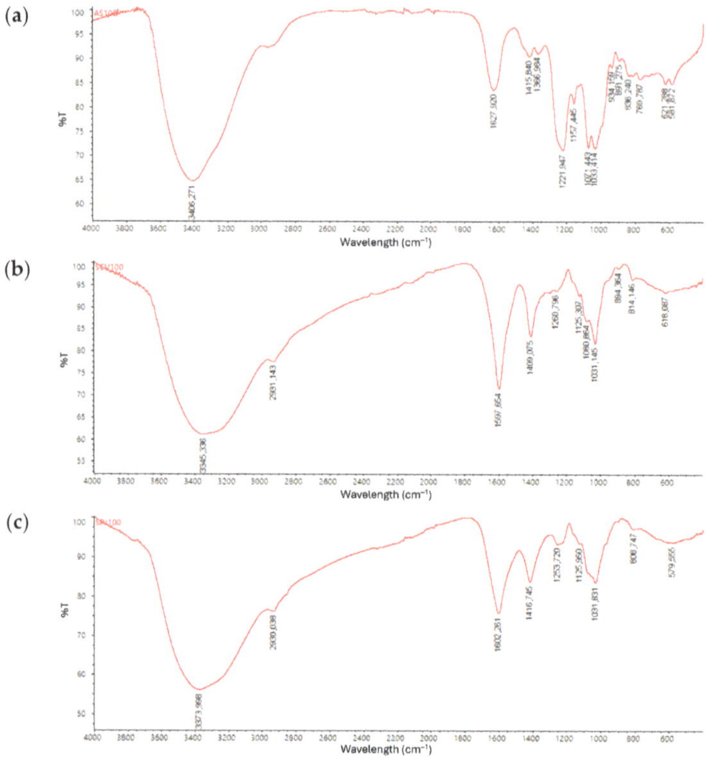

Figure 1. FT-IR spectra of polysaccharides in aqueous extracts from (**a**) *A. spicifera*, (**b**) *S. ramifolium*, and (**c**) *S. fluitans*.

Additionally, the bands found at 1249 and 891 cm^{-1} are related to a sulfated agar due to corresponding to the sulfated and agar groups, respectively. This is supported by the band at 836 cm^{-1} assigned to 2-O-sulfate of the D-galactose residues [26,44,47]. A similar band around 1260 cm^{-1} is associated with the asymmetric S=O stretching vibrations in the sulfuric acid group that appears in the spectra obtained from *Sargassum* spp. The band around 840 cm^{-1} is only present in the *S. fluitans* spectrum. These differences might suggest that the aqueous extraction from *A. spicifera* allowed it to obtain a polysaccharide with prevalent sulfation. A low intensity band at 1157.445 cm^{-1} in this spectrum can correspond to the C-OH deformation of secondary alcohol or to -SO_3 asymmetric stretching, as it has been previously reported for sulfated carbohydrates. The high-intensity band at 1033.414 cm^{-1} can be related to C-O deformation and vibration of the pyranose rings; this band is also present in *Sargassum* spp. extracts [48,54]. At 1366 cm^{-1}, a low-intensity band can also correspond to C-C-H and O-C-H deformations, which is not present in the spectrum of the other extracts [50].

At the fingerprint or so called anomeric region between 950 and 750 cm^{-1}, common bands discussed in carbohydrates such as alginate, fucoidan, carrageenan, and agaran are observed. In this way, bands around 814 and 808 cm^{-1} in polysaccharides obtained from *Sargassum* spp. have been associated with the presence of hexuronic acids such as mannuronic or guluronic acid residues, which can suggest that polysaccharides obtained from *Sargassum* spp. contain acid sugars, as reported in different characterization studies for this genus [44,48,50,54,55]. A band near 1125 cm^{-1} is present in the IR spectrum of the polysaccharides obtained from *S. fluitans* and *S. ramifolium* and it is also related to C-O stretching vibrations [48,54].

Based on the signals reported in various analyses of algal-derived polysaccharides, it is possible to identify the structural features of mixtures of polysaccharides using a single infrared spectrum, even exhibiting overlapping signals that are not necessarily associated with the same structural features. The bands 3374, 2930, 1602, 1417, 1254, 1032, and 809 cm^{-1} in the IR spectrum of the *S. fluitans* polysaccharide is consistent with the previously reported signals in a fucoidan extract from *S. fluitans* Borgesen, collected off the coast of Puerto Morelos, Mexico [32]. This analysis suggests that polysaccharides from these raw materials can be extracted through simple aqueous extraction with ultrafiltration steps.

Through chromatographic separation (Figure 2) by size exclusion chromatography, it was possible to observe that the extracts of *Sargassum* species showed a sharp peak while the extract of *A. spicifera* showed two broad peaks, suggesting the presence of heterodisperse polysaccharides, which could explain the number of signals in the infrared spectrum of this algae species.

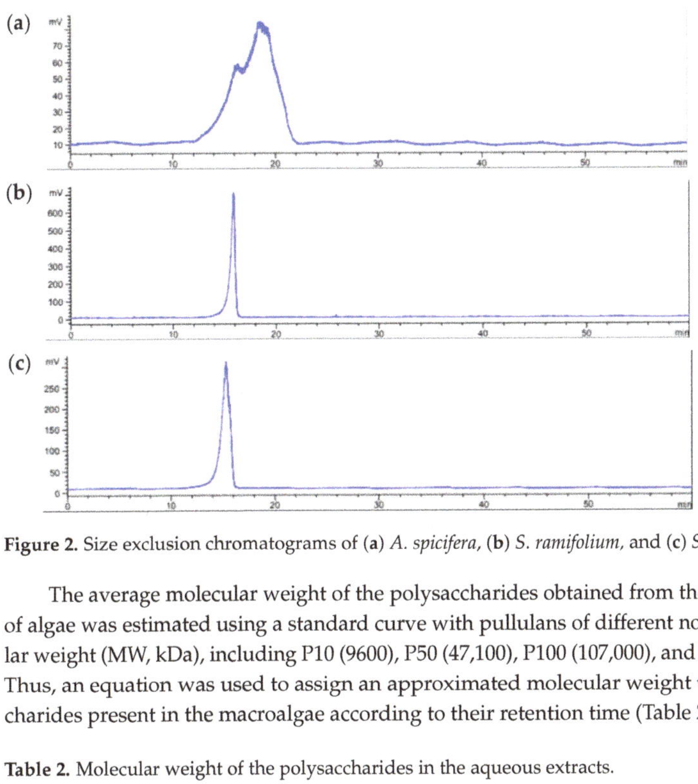

Figure 2. Size exclusion chromatograms of (**a**) *A. spicifera*, (**b**) *S. ramifolium*, and (**c**) *S. fluitans*.

The average molecular weight of the polysaccharides obtained from the three species of algae was estimated using a standard curve with pullulans of different nominal molecular weight (MW, kDa), including P10 (9600), P50 (47,100), P100 (107,000), and P200 (194,000). Thus, an equation was used to assign an approximated molecular weight to the polysaccharides present in the macroalgae according to their retention time (Table 2).

Table 2. Molecular weight of the polysaccharides in the aqueous extracts.

Sample	Rt	Log MW	Mp (kDa) *
A. spicifera	16.30–18.60	5.204	92–160
S. ramifolium	15.90	5.246	176
S. fluitans	15.70	5.267	185

* $y = -0.105x + 6.9155$ ($r^2 = 0.9934$).

The polysaccharides present in the aqueous extract of *A. spicifera* have a molecular weight between 92 and 160 kDa. *S. ramifolium* apparently possesses a single polysaccharide with a uniform distribution of weight near 176 kDa, similar to one of those found in *A. spicifera*, while the polysaccharide from *S. fluitans* presents the highest weight (185 kDa), larger than the molecular weight of the previously reported fucoidan of 60 kDa [32]. As it is known, the high molecular weight of polysaccharides from algae make them interesting to incorporate into different formulations, such as cosmetics and alimentary, mainly due to their capacity to be used as carriers or gelling agents, as well as actives with several pharmacological effects (antioxidant, anti-inflammatory, immunomodulator, antitumor) [56]. Other potential advantages of these carbohydrates is their biocompatibility and bioavailability, which allow them to be used in different matrices and applications [57–60].

Polysaccharides that are typically synthesized by seaweed possess a distinct chemical composition that may differ according to several factors, such as the species' life cycle, environmental conditions, and even the extraction techniques [61]. Comprehensive structural characterization of algal polysaccharides requires highly purified samples to allow for the accurate determination of their monosaccharide composition, substitution patterns, and sulfate content, among other features. Since direct interpretation by ^{1}H-NMR was not enough to encompass those multiple features, it was decided to compare the proton spectrum of the carbohydrates present in aqueous extracts with the obtained spectra from standard algae polysaccharides such as fucoidan, alginate, and carrageenan as well as with other polysaccharides previously reported in several studies. The ^{1}H-NMR spectra obtained for the extracts of the three algae show signals with chemical shifts in a spectral range from 6.0 to 3.0 ppm, which is expected for carbohydrates. In addition, some of them present typical signals from the chemical groups attached to the sugar rings around 1.0–2.0 ppm, which are commonly correlated with methyl protons located in different positions of the backbone.

Although the acquired spectra of the carbohydrate extract obtained from the red algae *A. spicifera* (Figure 3), did not enable homo- and heteronuclear correlation analyses, many observed chemical shifts were consistent with previously reported values for monomeric units found in various types of carrageenans and agarans, as noted in red seaweed studies [61]. It is possible to observe chemical shifts in the anomeric signals between 5.10 and 5.47 ppm like those that appear in the spectrum obtained for carrageenan, which can correspond to α-D-galactopyranose and its 3,6-anhydro-derivative. Other anomeric signals appear at around 4.4 and 5.0 ppm; however, they show expected overlapping. There are ^{1}H-NMR chemical shifts (ppm) consistent with those reported for the DA (4-linked 3,6-anhydro-α-D-galactopyranosyl) unit typical for carrageenans which includes H-1 5.11, H-2 4.15, H-3 4.55, and H-5 4.65 ppm. Furthermore, they are coincident with chemical shifts (H-1 5.49, H-2 3.60, H-3 3.95, H-4 4.22, H-5 4.18, H-6 3.95–3.82) related to L2M (4-linked 2-O-methyl-α-L-galactopyranosyl) units that can be present in agarans. The anomeric proton at 5.34 ppm and other observed signals have been reported for L (4-linked α-L-galactopyranosyl) monomers, the usual constituents of agarans [62,63]. Different from the carrageenan standard, an intense signal at 1.49 ppm suggests the presence of methyl groups along the main backbone [62]. This signal has been related to the 4,6-O- (1′-O-carboxyethylidene) pyruvate group present in an agar-type polysaccharide of high molecular weight previously obtained from *A. spicifera*, suggesting that the main polysaccharide of this extract possesses a characteristic structure of agaran. In addition, this polymer can be composed using small amounts of other monomers, such mannose, arabinose, or xylose, as substituents of its main galactose backbone [26,64,65].

Sargassum spp. are rich in diverse polysaccharides with physicochemical characteristics that identify them as phycocolloids, which include fucoidan, alginate, and laminarin. They are recognized for exhibiting neuroprotective, antitumor, antimicrobial, and antioxidant effects [66,67]. When the signals in the spectrum of the aqueous extract obtained from *S. ramifolium* were compared with those of the alginate standard (Figure 4), a proton spectrum with similar chemical shifts was observed, alluding to the presence of an alginate-type polysaccharide in the analyzed extract. Thus, the observed spectrum displayed signals corresponding to the anomeric protons of guluronic (G) and mannuronic (M) acid units, which have a chemical shift of around 5.1 ppm and 4.67 ppm, respectively. At the region between 4.67 and 4.76 ppm, the frequencies of the diads and triads of uronic acid blocks can be observed; for example, diads such as MM and MG and triads like MGM have been reported around 4.65, 4.68, and 4.70 ppm [68,69]. The region between 4.4 and 3.6 ppm displays multiplets corresponding to the H-2, H-3, and H-4 protons of the ring of both mannuronic and guluronic acid residues. Additionally, low intensity signals in this region can be attributed to minor amounts of hexoses, indicating the possible presence of other neutral sugars but in lower proportions [50,55,69].

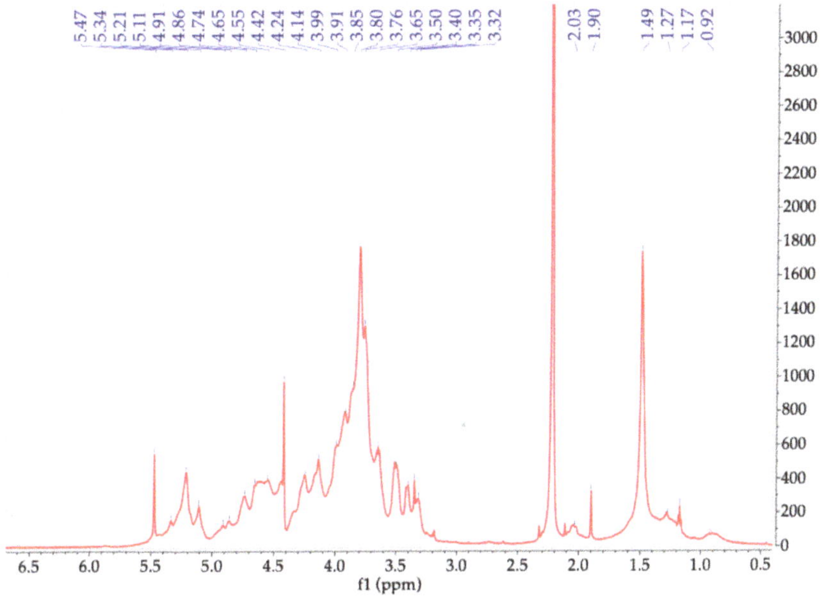

Figure 3. ^{1}H-NMR spectrum of aqueous extract of *A. spicifera;* recorded at 60 °C with acetone (2.22 ppm) as internal standard. Sample dissolved in deuterium oxide.

On the other hand, the ^{1}H-NMR spectrum of the algal extract obtained from *S. fluitans*, shown in Figure 5, displays the characteristic proton signals of fucose in the 1.0–1.6 ppm range, corresponding to the methyl groups (H-6) of this monosaccharide. The strong intensity of these signals suggests that fucose is a major component of the polymer backbone, supporting observations from comparisons between the algal spectrum and that of a fucoidan standard. This polysaccharide is claimed as the primary bioactive compound found in *Sargassum* species [66]. Additionally, the chemical shift in the signals in this range varies, pointing to alternating linkages or a different substitution pattern of fucose residues, including sulfate groups. The presence of signals within the ranges of 4.5–5.7 ppm has been attributed to the anomeric protons of fucoidan, where 4.35 ppm is reported to sulfate fucopyranose, and signals around 5.1 and 5.7 ppm could be assigned to α-L-fucopyranoside rings [55,70]. Finally, a chemical shift around 2.2 ppm can be observed as a signal associated with the methyl protons of O-acetyl groups, and signals of the ring region between 3.6 and 3.85 ppm can be related to other monomers like hexoses (galactose, mannose, glucose) and xylose [70,71].

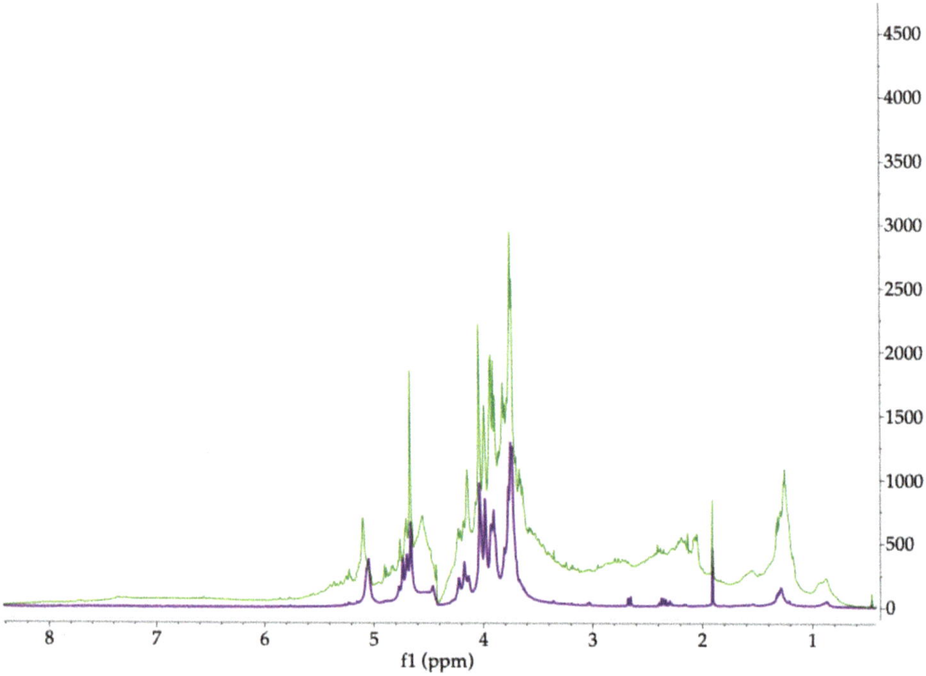

Figure 4. Comparison of ^{1}H-NMR spectra of commercial alginate (purple) and aqueous extract of *S. ramifolium* (green). Samples dissolved in deuterium oxide.

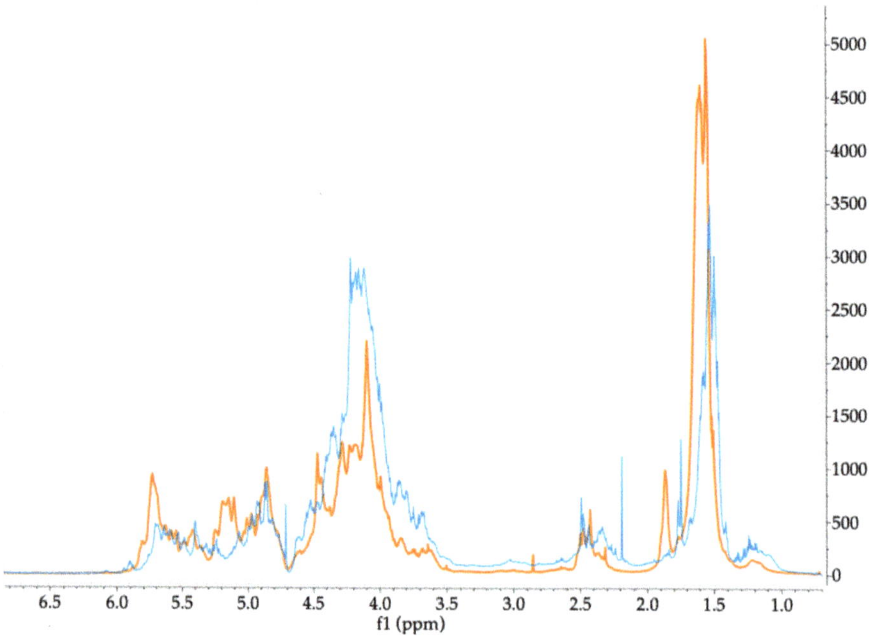

Figure 5. Comparison of ^{1}H-NMR spectra of commercial fucoidan (orange) and aqueous extract of *S. fluitans* (blue). Samples dissolved in deuterium oxide.

Following this carbohydrate analysis, it was possible to demonstrate through various techniques that the aqueous extracts from the different algae exhibited distinct compositions. This is consistent with the observations made in the acquired spectra, based on previously reported signals in the literature or through comparison with different standards.

2.3. Polyphenols and Antioxidant Activity

Different macroalgae are sessile organisms subjected to high UV radiation and temperatures, conditions that make them develop defense mechanisms such as antioxidants, which allow them to prevent, scavenge, and repair systems. This antioxidant capacity is an important tool against oxidative stress as an imbalance of free radicals and antioxidants in the body leads to cell damage related to many diseases [72]. Extensive exposure to stress, the sun, pollution, and toxins can cause the body to increase the level of free radicals, and several natural products rich in antioxidants could help to counteract their effect. Macroalgae have been shown to contain potent natural antioxidant compounds known as polyphenols, which act against oxidative damage and possess biological effects such as being anti-diabetic, anti-allergic, anti-inflammatory, anti-microbial, anti-viral, anti-photoaging, and anticancer [64,73].

In order to evaluate the phenolic content and its antioxidant effect, the extracts of the macroalgae were tested using Folin–Ciocalteu reagent to estimate the total phenolic compounds (TPCs) and by different assays, known as the 3-ethylbenzothiazoline-6-sulfonic acid (ABTS) assay, ferric reducing ability of plasma (FRAP) assay, 2,2-diphenyl1picrylhydrazyl (DPPH) radical scavenging capacity assay, and oxygen radical absorbance capacity (ORAC) assay, for the antioxidant effect [74]. The results of polyphenol and antioxidant activity are summarized in Table 3.

Table 3. Total polyphenol compounds and antioxidant activity via DPPH, ORAC, FRAP, and ABTS tests.

Alga	TPC	DPPH	ORAC	FRAP	ABTS
A. Spicifera	366.04 ± 6.76	39.17 ± 1.73	541.09 ± 21.89	49.19 ± 0.98	283.42 ± 5.67
S. ramifolium	936.67 ± 18.25	102.84 ± 3.34	3362.67 ± 99.85	113.24 ± 6.18	1830.69 ± 88.62
S. fluitans	449.43 ± 6.06	57.69 ± 2.42	1898.04 ± 65.70	128.74 ± 2.55	1237.45 ± 18.08

TPC values are expressed in milligrams of Gallic Acid Equivalent per 100 g of dried sample (mg GAE/100 g dw); FRAP in milligrams of Ascorbic Acid Equivalent per 100 g of dried sample (AAE/100 g dw); and ABTS, ORAC, and DPPH in milligrams of Trolox Equivalent per 100 g of dried sample (TE/100 g dw). Each value is presented as mean value (n = 3) ± standard deviation.

Total Phenolic Compounds and Antioxidant Potential

The red seaweed *A. spicifera* presents the lowest total phenolic content (366.08 mg GAE/100 g dw), followed by the brown seaweed *S. ramifolium* (450.30 mg GAE/100 g dw). The highest TPC was observed in the brown alga *S. fluitans* (936.79 mg GAE/100 g dw) (Table 3). Although the Folin Ciocalteau assay is commonly used to determine phenolic compounds content, it is known that other oxidizable groups interact with the reagent, so these results also suggest that some of the compounds present in the algae have a reduction capacity, which directly correlates with antioxidant activity [75]. Substances such as pigments (carotenoids), chlorophylls and derivates, and polysaccharides have been shown to interact with the Folin–Ciocalteu reagent, contributing to the positive result of this test. They also enhance radical scavenging potential when mixed with other antioxidant compounds [76,77]. Since TPC analysis was conducted using aqueous extracts, the presence of water-soluble compounds may have led to an overestimation of the phenolic content, and the actual concentration of phenolic compounds in each algal species could be lower. Previous studies have reported the TPC values for the same species. For instance, *S.*

ramifolium has shown TPC values ranging from 6.86 to 29.2 mg GAE/g dw [78], while *A. spicifera* exhibited values between 0.109 and 0.941 mg GAE/g dw [79]. In the case of *S. fluitans*, the presence of phenolic compounds and flavonoids has been confirmed; however, direct comparison with the current study is not possible due to differences in the sample preparation. Previous reports indicated TPC values of 62 mg GAE/g in acetone extract and 69 mg quercetin equivalents/g in ethanol extract [33]. The process should be validated to establish the reported impact of the storage time in declining the content of phenolic compounds and antioxidant activities in some *Sargassum* species [80].

The reducing capacity was evaluated by the FRAP method, which was also based on a SET reaction and possessed high sensitivity and precision [75]. A comparison between the TPC results and the subsequent data obtained by the FRAP assay revealed an inconsistent trend, wherein the sample with the highest reducing capacity did not exhibit a direct correlation with the concentration of phenolic compounds. Nevertheless, the red alga *A. spicifera* presented the lowest values in both tests.

Considering that the ABTS assay is not highly specific for phenolic compounds and may be influenced by the presence of other antioxidants, such as carotenoids, as well as vitamins E and C, it is advisable to verify the results using the FRAP method, which offers greater specificity for phenolics [75]. However, the ABTS values align with the TPC assay outcomes, where *S. ramifolium* has the highest scavenging activity toward this free radical. Another free radical to test scavenging capacity is DPPH; this sample also yielded results consistent with those of the TPC analysis, as evidenced in the previous assay.

A comparative analysis of the results obtained from the ABTS and FRAP assays provides insights into the approximate carotenoid content present in the studied extracts. The necessity of employing both methods becomes particularly evident in the case of the *S. fluitans* and *S. ramifolium* species. While the ABTS assay indicates a high antioxidant capacity in these samples, the FRAP assay reveals significantly lower antioxidant levels. This result suggests substantial amounts of non-phenolic antioxidant compounds, such as carotenoids, which are more effectively detected by the ABTS method. Consequently, these samples are likely rich in other antioxidant compounds that are not efficiently quantified by either method alone.

Through the oxygen radical absorbance capacity (ORAC) determination, the species *S. ramifolium* once again demonstrated the highest activity with a media of 3363.65 mg Trolox/100 g dw, indicating a strong peroxyl radical scavenging capacity. This high antioxidant activity is likely attributable to its levels of phenolic compounds, as previously observed in the TPC assay [81]. This ORAC value was followed by *S. fluitans* and *A. spicifera*, which also demonstrated considerable antioxidant activities, though to a lesser extent (1898.79 and 541.39 mg Trolox/100 g dw, respectively). Additionally, the outcomes observed in the ORAC assay closely matched the trends identified in the ABTS and DPPH assays, reinforcing the consistency of antioxidant profiles across different methods.

After conducting normality and homogeneity of variances tests, the findings from each of the assays were statistically analyzed using a one-way ANOVA test; the results are presented in Table 4.

Table 4. One-way ANOVA for TPC and antioxidant activity.

Statistical Measure	Test				
	TPC	**FRAP**	**ABTS**	**DPPH**	**ORAC**
F-value	482.57	351.23	668.87	482.57	1214.40
p-Value *	2.36×10^{-7}	6.07×10^{-7}	8.90×10^{-8}	2.36×10^{-7}	1.50×10^{-8}

* $p < 0.05$.

Given that the one-way ANOVA indicated statistically significant differences across all assays, a post hoc analysis was subsequently conducted using Tukey's Honest Significant Difference (HSD) test to identify pairwise differences between groups (Table 5).

Table 5. Multiple Comparison of Means—Tukey HSD.

Groups	Statistical Measure *	Test				
		TPC	FRAP	ABTS	DPPH	ORAC
A. spicifera –*S. fluitans*	Mean difference	83.37	79.56	954.08	18.52	1357.4
	p-Value	0.0003	0.0	0.0	0.0003	0.0
A. spicifera –*S. ramifolium*	Mean difference	570.71	64.15	1548.64	63.68	2822.26
	p-Value	0.0	0.0	0.0	0.0	0.0
A. spicifera –*S. fluitans*	Mean difference	487.34	−15.41	594.56	45.16	1464.86
	p-Value	0.0	0.0069	0.0	0.0	0.0

* $\alpha < 0.05$.

Post hoc analysis using Tukey's test revealed statistically significant differences between all the groups since comparisons yielded *p*-values below 0.05, confirming that the observed differences were unlikely to have occurred by chance. The most pronounced difference was observed between *A. spicifera* and *S. ramifolium*, with a mean difference of 2822.26 units, indicating a substantial increase in the measured ORAC assay in *S. ramifolium*. Additionally, a significant but more moderate difference was found in the FRAP test between *A. spicifera* and *S. fluitans*, with *A. spicifera* exhibiting a mean value that was 15.41 units lower than that of the other algae.

The seaweed *A. spicifera* has been described as a natural source of antibacterial, antitumoral, antiproliferative, procoagulant, and antioxidant substances such as phenolic compounds, flavonoids, and polysaccharides [26,64]. For instance, a flavonoid rich fraction were tested on rats, and an anti-diabetic action were observed, which is related to the anti-oxidative action of the flavonoids [82]. This algae also has bromophenols, tannins, and terpenoids that exhibit biological activities such as anticancer, anti-inflammatory, antiproliferative, antimicrobial, and antioxidant activities [83,84]. Additionally, it has been reported that sulphated polysaccharides from this species possess a reducing effect and scavenging activity against DPPH radicals, which strengthens the notion that carbohydrates, along with phenols, may contribute to enhancing the antioxidant effect [64,85]. Similarly, polysaccharides extracted from *Sargassum* macroalgae have also shown antioxidant effects. Fucoidan, for example, has shown activity both alone and in synergy with others against free radicals such as DPPH or in reducing the ferric ion in the FRAP assay. On the other hand, alginate is an antioxidant agent that has already been used as an active agent and as a carrier in different formulations [66]. Although there are not many reports related to the antioxidant effect of the studied *Sargassum* species, carotenoids such as β-carotene and canthaxanthin obtained from other species have been shown to be potential antioxidants [86]. At the same time, seaweed extracts containing sodium alginate and carrageenan increased the activity of some enzymes or cells that were the key indicators of antioxidant status [76]. However, it has been demonstrated that the antioxidant activity of fucoidan extracted from *Fucus vesiculosus* was exerted by the co-extracted phenolic compounds (e.g., phlorotannins) or terpenoids (e.g., fucoxanthins), which are truly responsible for the antioxidant effects rather than fucoidan itself [87]. Co-extraction of phenolic compounds with fatty acids and terpenoids is expected when using methanol to prepare the extracts for the DPPH, FRAP, and ABTS tests and, to a lesser extent, with oligo or polysaccharides (fucoidan or carrageenan) when water is employed as a solvent for TPC and ORAC tests. Accordingly, antioxidant effects involve compounds with different reactivities and solubilities extracted specifically from each sample being screened, requiring a more specific, structural, multifactorial, and quantitative approach.

All findings align with previously reported studies and reinforce the understanding that marine macroalgae are a valuable natural source of antioxidant agents, consistent with the existing scientific literature. Both brown and red algae have been shown to contain a variety of bioactive compounds with notable antioxidant properties. Specifically, the substantial mean difference observed between certain groups supports the presence of compounds different from polyphenols such as pigments, tocopherols, and other non-phenolics that display a marked antioxidant effect [28,51,88,89].

3. Materials and Methods

3.1. Sample Collection

The algae samples were collected in different regions of Colombia, including the La Guajira, Providencia, and Magdalena regions (Table 6). The *Sargassum ramifolium* sample was obtained from El Cabo de la Vela (12°12′22.20″ N, 72°9′21.96″ W), *Sargassum fluitans* from Playita Jacobo (12°35′36.69″ N, 81°42′28.44″ W), and *Acanthophora spicifera* from El Rodadero (11°7′46.73″ N, 74°13′48.79″ W). All the specimens were collected and supported with environmental permission granted by the Ministerio de Ambiente y Desarrollo Sostenible through contract 121 of 22 January 2016 (otro-sí N° 7), which regulates research permission of marine samples. The samples were collected by scuba diving conducted by biologists Monica Puyana Hegedus, Brigitte Gavio, and Felipe De La Roche Zogby. A sample of each species was identified and registered for preservation and comparison under the code in Table 6, in the collection of Instituto de Ciencias Naturales, Universidad Nacional de Colombia (Herbario JIWUKORI).

Table 6. Codification of the studied macroalgae.

Species	Group	Order	Family	Collection Date	Collection Site	Voucher Number
A. spicifera	Red macroalgae	Ceramiale	Rhodomelacea	28 February 2021	Santa Marta	JIW00005017
S. ramifolium	Brown macroalgae	Fucales	Sargassaceae	1 March 2021	Guajira	JIW00004940
S. fluitans		Fucales	Sargassaceae	1 February 2021	San Andrés	JIW00004945

From each sample, foreign material was removed by washing with seawater. Then, the macroalgae were left exposed to the sun and dried in an oven at 40 °C for 48 h. The dried algae were ground, and the resulting material was stored protected from light and heat.

3.2. Reagents

Alginic acid ref. A3249 was purchased from PanReac AppliChem (Saint Louis, MO, USA); carrageenan and fucoidan were obtained from Sigma (Saint Louis, MO, USA). With the exception of the ethanol used to wash the algae (96%, special purity, L&F, Medellin, Colombia), the solvents were of analytical grade (Merck, Darmstadt, Germany). The reagents used in the different assays were Folin–Ciocalteu reagent (analytical grade; Merck), sodium carbonate (>99%; Merck), potassium persulfate (>99%; Merck), 2,2′-azino-bis(3-ethylbenzothiazoline-6-sulfonic acid) diammonium salt (ABTS; >98%; Merck), and 2,2-diphenyl-1-picrylhydrazil (DPPH; >99%; Merck). For the antioxidant tests, gallic acid (>99%; Merck) and 6-hydroxy-2,5,7,8-tetramethylchroman-2-carboxylic acid ("Trolox"; >97%; Merck) were used as reference standards.

3.3. Fatty Acid Analysis

The dried and ground algae were analyzed by preparing methyl esters of fatty acids using BF_3 in methanol according to the AOAC Official Method 996.06 -Fat (Total, Saturated, and Unsaturated) in Foods: Hydrolytic Extraction Gas Chromatographic Method [90,91]. In total, 0.5 g of dry macroalgae sample was mixed with 2 mL of ethanol 96%, 100 mg of pyrogallic acid, and 2.0 mL of glyceril-triundecanoate (4.982 mg/mL) as internal standard, followed by the addition of 10 mL of hydrochloric acid (8.3 M) and heating at 70 °C for 40 min, in a tightly capped tub. The fatty acids were extracted with 10 mL ethanol, 25 mL ethyl ether, and methylated using 7% BF_3 in methanol at 100 °C (in a dry block) for 45 min. The phase containing fatty acid methyl esters (FAMEs) was dehydrated with Na_2SO_4 and anhydrous sodium sulfate and transferred to 1.5 mL vials for capillary gas chromatography coupled with mass spectrometry (GC-MS) in a Shimadzu (GCMS-TQ8050 NX) equipped with a ZB-FAME capillary column (30 m length × 0.25 mm i.d. × 0.2 μm). The oven temperature was held at 100 °C for 2 min, increased to 250 °C at a rate of 3 °C/min, and then held at 260 °C for 2 min. The injector and ion source temperatures were 250 °C and 260 °C, respectively. One microliter of each sample was injected with a split ratio of 50:1. The carrier gas was nitrogen at a constant flow rate of 0.71 mL/min. The areas and retention times of FAMEs in the samples and in the standard solution of mix FAMEs (Supelco 37 Component FAME Mix) were quantitatively measured against the $C_{11:0}$ internal standard (incorporated into each sample and standard vial) (See Supplementary Materials). Values are given as grams of fatty acid in 100 g of dry weight sample. Fatty acids below 0.01 g/100 g DW were regarded as not detected.

3.4. Carbohydrate Analysis

3.4.1. Aqueous Extract

Before polysaccharide extraction, the dried seaweeds were incubated overnight in an 80% ethanol solution at room temperature. The pretreated biomass was then filtered and rinsed with distilled water. Polysaccharides were subsequently extracted from 5 g of seaweed through four successive extraction cycles, each involving 100 mL of distilled water. Seaweeds of the *Sargassum* genus were submitted to heating (60 °C) and stirring (100 rpm) while the extract of *A. spicifera* was obtained by an ultrasound-assisted extraction using a PEX3 Sonifier (REUS, Contes, France) at 60 °C and 80 Hz. Finally, the aqueous extracts were diluted with water until a fluid suspension and ultrafiltered using a Sartorius Vivaflow 200 system with a 10 kDa molecular weight cutoff membrane followed by a 100 kDa membrane. Retained extracts in the 100 kDa membranes were freeze dried and then used for structural analysis.

3.4.2. FT-IR Analysis

Infrared spectroscopy was used to identify the presence of carbohydrates in the aqueous extract obtained from *S. ramifolium*, *S. fluitans*, and *A. spicifera*. FT-IR spectra of lyophilized extracts were acquired with a Nicolet™ Summit™ 912A1139, with an attenuated total reflectance (ATR) accessory; measurements were performed at 20 °C in a range from 4000 to 400 cm^{-1}, with a resolution of 4 cm^{-1} and 16 scans.

3.4.3. Size Exclusion Chromatographic Analysis

Chromatography was performed using an Agilent 1100 HPLC (Waldbronn, Germany) system equipped with a UV detector set at 280 nm, followed by an evaporative light scattering detector (ELSD; Varian 380-LC, Shropshire, UK). A Superose 12 10/300 GL (GE Healthcare, Uppsala, Sweden) column (11 μm, 300 mm × 10 mm) was used for separation, and elution was carried out with water at a flow rate of 0.5 mL/min for 60 min.

A pullulan standard kit (Standard P-82, Shodex, Kawasaki, Japan) with various molecular weights was used to estimate the average molecular weight of the polysaccharides in the aqueous extracts.

3.4.4. ^{1}H-NMR Analysis

The proton NMR spectra of the extracts were recorded on a 600 MHz Bruker Avance III (Ettlingen, Germany) by dissolving 10 mg of extract with 0.75 mL of D_2O (99.9%) and transferring it to an NMR tube. Spectra were acquired at 60 °C, a spectral width of 3000 Hz, 64 scans, and a 90° pulse; acquisition mode = 2 s, recovery = 5 s (for a complete return after a 90° pulse). Acetone was used as internal reference for the extract from *A. spicifera* because the standard was not available for comparing chemical shifts.

3.5. Total Phenolic Compounds and Antioxidant Potential Assays

3.5.1. Total Phenolic Compounds (TPC)

TPCs were determined using the Folin–Ciocalteau method of the AOAC 2017.13 [92]. The sample of each alga was prepared by mixing 1.0 g of algae with 100.0 mL of water. An aliquot of 50 µL from the sample solution was mixed with 100 µL of Folin–Ciocalteau reagent, 300 µL of 20% sodium carbonate solution, and 15 mL of deionized water. The resulting mixture was incubated in the darkness at 25 °C for two hours, and its absorbance at 765 nm was measured in a spectrofluorophotometer (Synergy H1, Biotek®, Winooski, VT, USA). Methanol was used as a negative control. The total phenolic content in each algae extract was determined using a standard curve of gallic acid (40–200 mg/L), and results were expressed as milligrams of gallic acid equivalents (GAE) per 100 g of dried sample.

3.5.2. Antioxidant Assays

ABTS Assay

The ABTS assay was conducted by mixing 10 µL of a sample solution (500 mg of dry sample in 10 mL of methanol) with 190 µL of a 3.5 mM solution of ABTS. The absorbance of this mixture was acquired at 732 nm after being incubated at room temperature in darkness for 30 min. The ABTS radical-scavenging activity was estimated through the Trolox Equivalent Antioxidant Capacity (TEAC) value [93].

DPPH Assay

The DPPH test was performed by mixing 10 µL of a sample solution (500 mg of dry sample in 10 mL of methanol) with 190 µL of a 200 ppm solution of the 2,2-diphenyl-1-picrylhydrazyl (DPPH) radical. This mixture was incubated at room temperature in the dark for 30 min, and absorbance was acquired at 517 nm. Scavenging activity was estimated through the Trolox Equivalent Antioxidant Capacity (TEAC) value [94].

FRAP Assay

The FRAP assay was conducted by incubating 10 µL of a sample solution (500 mg of dry sample in 10 mL of methanol) with 180 µL of FRAP solution that contains acetate buffer, TPTZ, and $FeCl_3$. After 60 min of incubation at room temperature in darkness, the absorbance was acquired at 593 nm; ascorbic acid was used as the standard [95].

ORAC Assay

The ORAC assay was performed according to the AOAC 2012.23 Method (Official Methods of Analysis, 21st Edition, 2019 [96]). Previously, the sample was pretreated by dissolving 500 mg of dry material in 20 mL of solvent, using both hydrophilic (acetone–water) and lipophilic media (acetone). The test involved mixing 25 µL of the sample solution with 150 µL of fluorescein sodium salt, followed by incubation at 37 °C for 30 min in darkness. After this initial incubation, 25 μL of 2,2′-azobis(2-amidino-propane) dihydrochloride (AAPH) solution was added, and fluorescence was recorded for 60 min at an excitation wavelength of 485 ± 20 nm and an emission wavelength of 530 ± 25 nm. Standard solutions of Trolox were used to calculate the Oxygen Radical Absorbance Capacity (ORAC) values of the algae [81].

3.6. Statistical Data Analysis

The results of antioxidant tests and polyphenol quantification were statistically analyzed using Python software 3.10.10. Each antioxidant activity assay was performed three times from the same extract in order to determine their reproducibility. Statistical analyses were achieved with the Python software. First, normality and equal variances tests were carried out to assess if data had a normal distribution and if the variance of the groups was similar. Subsequently, a one-way ANOVA was used to test differences in chemical parameters and activity between species. When the model was significant ($p < 0.05$), Tukey's HSD test was used as post hoc.

4. Conclusions

Macroalgae represent valuable natural resources for bioprospecting and sustainable development, owing to their high biomass yield and potential as raw materials for industries such as nutrition, medicine, agriculture, and cosmetics. Despite the numerous studies on macroalgae, those found in Colombia remain largely unexplored as a source of functional ingredients. This study contributes to unlocking the potential of these and other seaweeds for the development of aquaculture enterprises, thereby supporting local communities in benefiting from these resources by promoting bioeconomic diversification in Colombia and other tropical countries through the sustainable use of marine biodiversity.

As a result, functional components such as fatty acids, polysaccharides, and antioxidants were detected in the three macroalgae. More specifically, although all of them showed similar results, the content of mono and polyunsaturated fatty acids was potentially higher in *Sargassum* algae than in the algae of the genus *Acanthophora*. Furthermore, regarding the partial state of purification of the polysaccharides analyzed, the lack of monosaccharide composition, linkage, sulfate patterns, and a deeper structural analysis, the spectroscopic chemical analyses by NMR, FT-IR, and SEC were useful to identify structural features consistent with carrageenan, alginate, and fucoidan in the aqueous extracts of *A. spicifera*, *S. ramifolium*, and *S. fluitans*, respectively. These findings indicate that the algae may have diverse application potentials since these polymers have shown a diverse group of biological effects and uses. This difference has been observed in the total polyphenol composition of the algae and their antioxidant potentials. Among them, the alga *S. ramifolium* showed the most favorable antioxidant profile, followed by *S. fluitans*, and *A. spicifera*.

While the results suggest potential applications in several fields, including the biomedicine, cosmetics, functional foods, and nutraceutical industry, the effect of seasonal variation on the composition of polysaccharides, fatty acids, and antioxidant compounds needs to be thoroughly analyzed. This is essential to ensure the continuous valorization of different species and to support further research into the chemical composition of seaweeds, the standardization of methodologies for biomass transformation to add value, and the confirmation of the functionality of both known and novel compounds.

Supplementary Materials: The following supporting information can be downloaded at: https://www.mdpi.com/article/10.3390/molecules30163333/s1, Table S1: Calculation formulas used for fatty acids detected; Table S2: Conversion factors for conversion of FAMEs to their corresponding fatty acids detected in macroalgae; Table S3: Experimental data of fatty acid methyl esters from macroalgae samples.

Author Contributions: Conceptualization, J.C.-R., A.M.-M., and D.C.R.-E.; methodology, Y.R.-M., J.D.M., and J.C.-R.; resources, A.M.-M., D.M.M.-F., L.C., and J.C.-R.; writing—original draft preparation, A.M.-M., J.C.-R., and D.C.R.-E.; writing—review and editing, A.M.-M., D.C.R.-E., and J.C.-R.; supervision, A.M.-M., D.M.M.-F., and L.C.; project administration, L.C., D.M.M.-F., A.M.-M., and J.C.-R.; funding acquisition, A.M.-M., D.M.M.-F., J.C.-R., and L.C. All authors have read and agreed to the published version of the manuscript.

Funding: This research was funded by the Ministry of Science; this work has received financial support from the Ministry of Science, Technology and Innovation of Colombia (Minciencias) with resources from the "Fondo Nacional Autónomo de Financiación del Patrimonio Para la Ciencia, la Tecnología y la Innovación: Francisco José de Caldas", the Jorge Tadeo Lozano University Foundation, the National University of Colombia, and the University of Antioquia, within the framework of the contingent recovery financing contract 80740-739-2020 concluded between Fiduciaria la Previsora S.A.—Fiduprevisora S.A. acting as spokesperson and administrator of the national financing fund for science, technology and innovation, Francisco José de Caldas Fund, and the National University of Colombia—Bogota Headquarters.

Institutional Review Board Statement: Not applicable.

Informed Consent Statement: Not applicable.

Data Availability Statement: The original data presented in the study is included in the article; further information can be requested directly from the corresponding author.

Acknowledgments: The authors acknowledge all the authors for their contributions to the research, data curation, and writing—reviewing and editing. Heartfelt thanks for the funding from Ministry of Science, Technology and Innovation of Colombia (Minciencias), Universidad Nacional de Colombia (UNAL), and Universidad de Antioquia (UdeA); Brigitte Gavio from UNAL and Vanessa Urrea Victoria from Pontificia Universidad Javeriana for assistance in taxonomical identification; the Max Planck Tandem Group in Nanobioengineering (UdeA) for recording FT-IR spectra; Elkin Galeano Jaramillo, from UdeA, for recording ^{1}H-NMR spectra; Maria Carmen Dominguez Gomez from Aoxlab S.A.S. for assistance in recording GC-MS analysis; and Freimar Segura, Biopolimer Group—UdeA for assistance in ultrafiltration processes.

Conflicts of Interest: The authors declare no conflicts of interest.

Abbreviations

The following abbreviations are used in this manuscript:

TPC	Total phenolic compounds
ORAC	Oxygen Radical Absorbance Capacity
FRAP	Ferric-reducing antioxidant power
TEAC	Trolox equivalent antioxidant capacity
ABTS	2,2-azino-bis-3-ethylbenzothiazoline-6-sulphonic acid
GAE	Gallic acid equivalent
NMR	Nuclear magnetic resonance
HPLC	High performance liquid chromatography
FT-IR	Fourier-transform infrared spectroscopy
FAME	Fatty acid methyl ester

References

1. Biris-Dorhoi, E.-S.; Michiu, D.; Pop, C.R.; Rotar, A.M.; Tofana, M.; Pop, O.L.; Socaci, S.A.; Farcas, A.C. Macroalgae—A Sustainable Source of Chemical Compounds with Biological Activities. *Nutrients* **2020**, *12*, 3085. [CrossRef]
2. Arias, A.; Feijoo, G.; Moreira, M.T. Macroalgae Biorefineries as a Sustainable Resource in the Extraction of Value-Added Compounds. *Algal Res.* **2023**, *69*, 102954. [CrossRef]
3. Hentati, F.; Tounsi, L.; Djomdi, D.; Pierre, G.; Delattre, C.; Ursu, A.V.; Fendri, I.; Abdelkafi, S.; Michaud, P. Bioactive Polysaccharides from Seaweeds. *Molecules* **2020**, *25*, 3152. [CrossRef]

4. Pal, A.; Kamthania, M.C.; Kumar, A. Bioactive Compounds and Properties of Seaweeds—A Review. *Open Access Libr. J.* **2014**, *1*, 1–17. [CrossRef]
5. Lomartire, S.; Gonçalves, A.M.M. Algal Phycocolloids: Bioactivities and Pharmaceutical Applications. *Mar. Drugs* **2023**, *21*, 384. [CrossRef]
6. Bi, D.; Yang, X.; Yao, L.; Hu, Z.; Li, H.; Xu, X.; Lu, J. Potential Food and Nutraceutical Applications of Alginate: A Review. *Mar. Drugs* **2022**, *20*, 564. [CrossRef]
7. Pournaki, S.K.; Aleman, R.S.; Hasani-Azhdari, M.; Marcia, J.; Yadav, A.; Moncada, M. Current Review: Alginate in the Food Applications. *J* **2024**, *7*, 281–301. [CrossRef]
8. Abka-khajouei, R.; Tounsi, L.; Shahabi, N.; Patel, A.K.; Abdelkafi, S.; Michaud, P. Structures, Properties and Applications of Alginates. *Mar. Drugs* **2022**, *20*, 364. [CrossRef] [PubMed]
9. Tomić, S.L.; Babić Radić, M.M.; Vuković, J.S.; Filipović, V.V.; Nikodinovic-Runic, J.; Vukomanović, M. Alginate-Based Hydrogels and Scaffolds for Biomedical Applications. *Mar. Drugs* **2023**, *21*, 177. [CrossRef] [PubMed]
10. Pacheco-Quito, E.-M.; Ruiz-Caro, R.; Veiga, M.-D. Carrageenan: Drug Delivery Systems and Other Biomedical Applications. *Mar. Drugs* **2020**, *18*, 583. [CrossRef] [PubMed]
11. Kokkuvayil Ramadas, B.; Rhim, J.-W.; Roy, S. Recent Progress of Carrageenan-Based Composite Films in Active and Intelligent Food Packaging Applications. *Polymers* **2024**, *16*, 1001. [CrossRef]
12. Hilliou, L. Structure–Elastic Properties Relationships in Gelling Carrageenans. *Polymers* **2021**, *13*, 4120. [CrossRef]
13. Sohrabipour, J.; Rabiei, R.; Pirian, K. Fatty Acids Composition of Marine Macroalgae (Review). *J. Phycol. Res.* **2019**, *3*, 348–374. [CrossRef]
14. Pereira, H.; Barreira, L.; Figueiredo, F.; Custódio, L.; Vizetto-Duarte, C.; Polo, C.; Rešek, E.; Engelen, A.; Varela, J. Polyunsaturated Fatty Acids of Marine Macroalgae: Potential for Nutritional and Pharmaceutical Applications. *Mar. Drugs* **2012**, *10*, 1920–1935. [CrossRef] [PubMed]
15. Zhang, J.; Xing, L.; Meng, W.; Zhang, X.; Li, J.; Dong, P. Molecular Weight Distribution and Structure Analysis of Phlorotannins in Sanhai Kelp (*Saccharina Japonica*) and Evaluation of Their Antioxidant Activities. *Food Chem.* **2025**, *469*, 142569. [CrossRef] [PubMed]
16. Shrestha, S.; Zhang, W.; Smid, S.D. Phlorotannins: A Review on Biosynthesis, Chemistry and Bioactivity. *Food Biosci.* **2021**, *39*, 100832. [CrossRef]
17. Aina, O.; Bakare, O.O.; Daniel, A.I.; Gokul, A.; Beukes, D.R.; Fadaka, A.O.; Keyster, M.; Klein, A. Seaweed-Derived Phenolic Compounds in Growth Promotion and Stress Alleviation in Plants. *Life* **2022**, *12*, 1548. [CrossRef]
18. Cotas, J.; Leandro, A.; Monteiro, P.; Pacheco, D.; Figueirinha, A.; Gonçalves, A.M.M.; da Silva, G.J.; Pereira, L. Seaweed Phenolics: From Extraction to Applications. *Mar. Drugs* **2020**, *18*, 384. [CrossRef]
19. Jimenez-Lopez, C.; Pereira, A.G.; Lourenço-Lopes, C.; Garcia-Oliveira, P.; Cassani, L.; Fraga-Corral, M.; Prieto, M.A.; Simal-Gandara, J. Main Bioactive Phenolic Compounds in Marine Algae and Their Mechanisms of Action Supporting Potential Health Benefits. *Food Chem.* **2021**, *341*, 128262. [CrossRef]
20. Eom, S.-H.; Kim, Y.-M.; Kim, S.-K. Antimicrobial Effect of Phlorotannins from Marine Brown Algae. *Food Chem. Toxicol.* **2012**, *50*, 3251–3255. [CrossRef]
21. Liu, M.; Hansen, P.E.; Lin, X. Bromophenols in Marine Algae and Their Bioactivities. *Mar. Drugs* **2011**, *9*, 1273–1292. [CrossRef]
22. Thomas, N.V.; Kim, S.-K. Potential Pharmacological Applications of Polyphenolic Derivatives from Marine Brown Algae. *Environ. Toxicol. Pharmacol.* **2011**, *32*, 325–335. [CrossRef] [PubMed]
23. Campos, N.H. (Ed.) Gavio Brigitte Historia de La Ficología En Colombia. In *Colombia Bioazul: Dos Mares un País; Territorios por Explorar*; Universidad Nacional de Colombia. (Sede Caribe): Saint Andrew, Colombia; Instituto de Estudios en Ciencias del Mar (CECIMAR): Santa Marta, Colombia, 2023; pp. 239–253, ISBN 978-958-505-136-2.
24. Quintana-Manotas, H.L.; Hernández-Contreras, D.A.; Gavio, B.; Quintana-Manotas, H.L.; Hernández-Contreras, D.A.; Gavio, B. Updated List and New Records of Macroalgae from the Gulf of Morrosquillo, Colombian Caribbean. *Acta Botánica Mex.* **2024**, *131*, 1–23. [CrossRef]
25. Kilar, J.A.; McLachlan, J. Ecological Studies of the Alga, *Acanthophora Spicifera* (Vahl) Børg. (Ceramiales: Rhodophyta): Vegetative Fragmentation. *J. Exp. Mar. Biol. Ecol.* **1986**, *104*, 1–21. [CrossRef]
26. Pereira Júnior, L.C.; Nascimento, F.G.; Oliveira, S.R.B.D.; Lima, G.C.; Chagas, F.D.S.; Sombra, V.G.; Feitosa, J.P.A.; Soriano, E.M.; Souza, M.H.L.P.; Zocolo, G.J.; et al. Protective Effect against Gastric Mucosa Injury of a Sulfated Agaran from *Acanthophora spicifera*. *Carbohydr. Polym.* **2021**, *261*, 117829. [CrossRef]
27. Guillén, P.O.; Motti, P.; Mangelinckx, S.; De Clerck, O.; Bossier, P.; Van Den Hende, S. Valorization of the Chemical Diversity of the Tropical Red Seaweeds Acanthophora and Kappaphycus and Their Applications in Aquaculture: A Review. *Front. Mar. Sci.* **2022**, *9*, 957290. [CrossRef]

28. Fagundo-Mollineda, A.; Robledo, D.; Vásquez-Elizondo, R.M.; Freile-Pelegrín, Y. Antioxidant Activities in Holopelagic *Sargassum* Species from the Mexican Caribbean: Temporal Changes and Intra-Thallus Variation. *Algal Res.* **2023**, *76*, 103289. [CrossRef]
29. Debue, M.; Guinaldo, T.; Jouanno, J.; Chami, M.; Barbier, S.; Berline, L.; Chevalier, C.; Daniel, P.; Daniel, W.; Descloitres, J.; et al. Understanding the *Sargassum* Phenomenon in the Tropical Atlantic Ocean: From Satellite Monitoring to Stranding Forecast. *Mar. Pollut. Bull.* **2025**, *216*, 117923. [CrossRef]
30. Davis, D.; Simister, R.; Campbell, S.; Marston, M.; Bose, S.; McQueen-Mason, S.J.; Gomez, L.D.; Gallimore, W.A.; Tonon, T. Biomass Composition of the Golden Tide Pelagic Seaweeds *Sargassum fluitans* and *S. natans* (Morphotypes I and VIII) to Inform Valorisation Pathways. *Sci. Total Environ.* **2021**, *762*, 143134. [CrossRef]
31. Ortega-Flores, P.A.; Serviere-Zaragoza, E.; De Anda-Montañez, J.A.; Freile-Pelegrín, Y.; Robledo, D.; Méndez-Rodríguez, L.C. Trace Elements in Pelagic *Sargassum* Species in the Mexican Caribbean: Identification of Key Variables Affecting Arsenic Accumulation in *S. fluitans*. *Sci. Total Environ.* **2022**, *806*, 150657. [CrossRef]
32. Chale-Dzul, J.; Pérez-Cabeza de Vaca, R.; Quintal-Novelo, C.; Olivera-Castillo, L.; Moo-Puc, R. Hepatoprotective Effect of a Fucoidan Extract from *Sargassum Fluitans* Borgesen against CCl4-Induced Toxicity in Rats. *Int. J. Biol. Macromol.* **2020**, *145*, 500–509. [CrossRef]
33. Emu, S.A.; Dulal, M.A.; Kali, T.D.; Chadni, M.S.; Rasul, M.G.; Mondal, M.N.; Ahsan, M.E.; Khan, M.; Shah, A.K.M.A. Effects of Extracting Solvents on Phytochemical, Antioxidant, and Antibacterial Activity of Some Seaweeds from the Bay of Bengal Offshore Island. *Food Humanit.* **2023**, *1*, 1157–1166. [CrossRef]
34. Robledo, D.; Vázquez-Delfín, E.; Freile-Pelegrín, Y.; Vásquez-Elizondo, R.M.; Qui-Minet, Z.N.; Salazar-Garibay, A. Challenges and Opportunities in Relation to Sargassum Events Along the Caribbean Sea. *Front. Mar. Sci.* **2021**, *8*, 699664. [CrossRef]
35. Pech-Puch, D.; Pérez-Povedano, M.; Lenis-Rojas, O.A.; Rodríguez, J.; Jiménez, C. Marine Natural Products from the Yucatan Peninsula. *Mar. Drugs* **2020**, *18*, 59. [CrossRef]
36. Zubia, M.; Robledo, D.; Freile-Pelegrin, Y. Antioxidant Activities in Tropical Marine Macroalgae from the Yucatan Peninsula, Mexico. *J. Appl. Phycol.* **2007**, *19*, 449–458. [CrossRef]
37. D'Armas, H.; Jaramillo-Jaramillo, C.; D'Armas, M.; Ordaz-González, G.J. Fatty acid profile, total phenolic content and antioxidant capacity of seaweeds in Salinas Bay, Ecuador. *Rev. De Biol. Mar. Y Oceanogr.* **2023**, *58*, 128–136. [CrossRef]
38. Wazir, H.; Chay, S.Y.; Zarei, M.; Hussin, F.S.; Mustapha, N.A.; Wan Ibadullah, W.Z.; Saari, N. Effects of Storage Time and Temperature on Lipid Oxidation and Protein Co-Oxidation of Low-Moisture Shredded Meat Products. *Antioxidants* **2019**, *8*, 486. [CrossRef]
39. Dhakal, S.; Pandey, D.; van der Heide, M.E.; Nørgaard, J.V.; Vrhovsek, U.; Khanal, P. Effect of Different Drying Methods on the Nutritional Composition and Phenolic Compounds of the Brown Macroalga, Fucus Vesiculosus (Fucales, Phaeophyceae). *J. Appl. Phycol.* **2024**, *36*, 3649–3663. [CrossRef]
40. Matos, J.; Cardoso, C.; Serralheiro, M.L.; Bandarra, N.M.; Afonso, C. Seaweed Bioactives Potential as Nutraceuticals and Functional Ingredients: A Review. *J. Food Compos. Anal.* **2024**, *133*, 106453. [CrossRef]
41. Calderon, D.; Juarez, H.; Osnaya, N.; Ortiz, M.; Trujillo, F.; Valenzuela, A.; Labra, N.; Santamaria, D.; Barragan, G. Oleic Acid Reduces Oxidative Stress in Rat Brain Induced by Some Anticancer Drugs. *Chem.-Biol. Interact.* **2024**, *398*, 111086. [CrossRef]
42. Burns, J.L.; Nakamura, M.T.; Ma, D.W.L. Differentiating the Biological Effects of Linoleic Acid from Arachidonic Acid in Health and Disease. *Prostaglandins Leukot. Essent. Fat. Acids* **2018**, *135*, 1–4. [CrossRef]
43. Quitral, V.; Morales, C.; Sepúlveda, M.; Schwartz, M. Propiedades Nutritivas y Saludables de Algas Marinas y Su Potencialidad Como Ingrediente Funcional. *Rev. Chil. De Nutr.* **2012**, *39*, 196–202. [CrossRef]
44. Vandanjon, L.; Burlot, A.-S.; Zamanileha, E.F.; Douzenel, P.; Ravelonandro, P.H.; Bourgougnon, N.; Bedoux, G. The Use of FTIR Spectroscopy as a Tool for the Seasonal Variation Analysis and for the Quality Control of Polysaccharides from Seaweeds. *Mar. Drugs* **2023**, *21*, 482. [CrossRef] [PubMed]
45. Tipson, R.S. *Infrared Spectroscopy of Carbohydrates: A Review of the Literature*; National Bureau of standards: Washington, DC, USA, 1968.
46. Wiercigroch, E.; Szafraniec, E.; Czamara, K.; Pacia, M.Z.; Majzner, K.; Kochan, K.; Kaczor, A.; Baranska, M.; Malek, K. Raman and Infrared Spectroscopy of Carbohydrates: A Review. *Spectrochim. Acta Part A Mol. Biomol. Spectrosc.* **2017**, *185*, 317–335. [CrossRef] [PubMed]
47. Yao, Z.; Xu, L.; Wang, B.; Ye, T.; Li, Y.; Wu, H. Optimization of Preparation Conditions, Molecular Structure Analysis and Antitumor Activity of Sulfated Sodium Alginate Oligosaccharides. *Eur. Polym. J.* **2023**, *201*, 112571. [CrossRef]
48. Leal, D.; Matsuhiro, B.; Rossi, M.; Caruso, F. FT-IR Spectra of Alginic Acid Block Fractions in Three Species of Brown Seaweeds. *Carbohydr. Res.* **2008**, *343*, 308–316. [CrossRef] [PubMed]
49. Pereira, R.; Tojeira, A.; Vaz, D.C.; Mendes, A.; Bártolo, P. Preparation and Characterization of Films Based on Alginate and Aloe Vera. *Int. J. Polym. Anal. Charact.* **2011**, *16*, 449–464. [CrossRef]

50. Marcin, N.; Thesnor, V.; Duvauchelle, V.; Ponce-Mora, A.; Gimeno-Mallench, L.; Narayanin-Richenapin, S.; Brelle, L.; Bejarano, E.; Yacou, C.; Sylvestre, M.; et al. Characterization of Alginates of Sargassum from the Archipelago of Guadeloupe. *Separations* **2024**, *11*, 226. [CrossRef]
51. Ganesan, A.R.; Shanmugam, M.; Palaniappan, S.; Rajauria, G. Development of Edible Film from Acanthophora Spicifera: Structural, Rheological and Functional Properties. *Food Biosci.* **2018**, *23*, 121–128. [CrossRef]
52. Schnoller, V.C.G.; Hernández-Carmona, G.; Hernández-Garibay, E.; López-Vivas, J.M.; Muñoz-Ochoa, M. Chemical Characterization of the Soluble Polysaccharides of the Red Alga Acanthophora Spicifera from La Paz Bay, Baja California Sur, México. *Cienc. Mar.* **2020**, *46*, 165–176. [CrossRef]
53. Temjensangba, I.; Konark, T.; Reshmitha, R.; Krishnap, A. Evaluation of the Proximate Composition and Antioxidant Capacity of Some Seaweeds from the Konkan Coast of India. *Algal Res.* **2024**, *83*, 103730. [CrossRef]
54. Singh, J.; Vishavnath; Sharma, V.; Singh, B. Development of Agar-Alginate Marine Polysaccharides-Based Hydrogels for Agricultural Applications to Reduce Environmental Hazards. *Int. J. Biol. Macromol.* **2025**, *295*, 139659. [CrossRef]
55. Premarathna, A.D.; Ahmed, T.A.E.; Sooaar, A.; Rjabovs, V.; Critchley, A.T.; Hincke, M.T.; Tuvikene, R. Extraction and Functional Characterization of Fucoidans and Alginates from Ecklonia Maxima: A Focus on Skin, Immune, and Intestinal Health. *Food Hydrocoll.* **2025**, *159*, 110668. [CrossRef]
56. Yu, Y.; Shen, M.; Song, Q.; Xie, J. Biological Activities and Pharmaceutical Applications of Polysaccharide from Natural Resources: A Review. *Carbohydr. Polym.* **2018**, *183*, 91–101. [CrossRef] [PubMed]
57. Dong, Q.; Wu, D.; Li, M.; Dong, W. Polysaccharides, as Biological Macromolecule-Based Scaffolding Biomaterials in Cornea Tissue Engineering: A Review. *Tissue Cell* **2022**, *76*, 101782. [CrossRef]
58. Williams, D.F. Chapter 36—Hydrogels in Regenerative Medicine. In *Principles of Regenerative Medicine*, 3rd ed.; Atala, A., Lanza, R., Mikos, A.G., Nerem, R., Eds.; Academic Press: Boston, UK, 2019; pp. 627–650, ISBN 978-0-12-809880-6.
59. Raza, Z.A.; Munim, S.A.; Ayub, A. Recent Developments in Polysaccharide-Based Electrospun Nanofibers for Environmental Applications. *Carbohydr. Res.* **2021**, *510*, 108443. [CrossRef] [PubMed]
60. Cui, R.; Zhu, F. Ultrasound Modified Polysaccharides: A Review of Structure, Physicochemical Properties, Biological Activities and Food Applications. *Trends Food Sci. Technol.* **2021**, *107*, 491–508. [CrossRef]
61. Ramadan, N.E.; Youssef, F.R.; Alshishtawy, A.A.K.; Elshikh, F.M.; Newir, O.; Abdelazeem, S.H.; Ma'ruf, N.K.; Shouman, H.; Ali, S.S.; El-Sheekh, M.M. Marine Algal Polysaccharides for Drug Delivery Applications: A Review. *Int. J. Biol. Macromol.* **2025**, *295*, 139551. [CrossRef]
62. Rodríguez Sánchez, R.A.; Matulewicz, M.C.; Ciancia, M. NMR Spectroscopy for Structural Elucidation of Sulfated Polysaccharides from Red Seaweeds. *Int. J. Biol. Macromol.* **2022**, *199*, 386–400. [CrossRef]
63. Knutsen, S.H.; Myslabodski, D.E.; Larsen, B.; Usov, A.I. A Modified System of Nomenclature for Red Algal Galactans. *Bot. Mar.* **1994**, *37*, 163–170. [CrossRef]
64. Anand, J.; Sathuvan, M.; Babu, G.V.; Sakthivel, M.; Palani, P.; Nagaraj, S. Bioactive Potential and Composition Analysis of Sulfated Polysaccharide from *Acanthophora spicifera* (Vahl) Borgeson. *Int. J. Biol. Macromol.* **2018**, *111*, 1238–1244. [CrossRef]
65. Duarte, M.E.R.; Cauduro, J.P.; Noseda, D.G.; Noseda, M.D.; Gonçalves, A.G.; Pujol, C.A.; Damonte, E.B.; Cerezo, A.S. The Structure of the Agaran Sulfate from *Acanthophora spicifera* (Rhodomelaceae, Ceramiales) and Its Antiviral Activity. Relation between Structure and Antiviral Activity in Agarans. *Carbohydr. Res.* **2004**, *339*, 335–347. [CrossRef] [PubMed]
66. Flores-Contreras, E.A.; Araújo, R.G.; Rodríguez-Aguayo, A.A.; Guzmán-Román, M.; García-Venegas, J.C.; Nájera-Martínez, E.F.; Sosa-Hernández, J.E.; Iqbal, H.M.N.; Melchor-Martínez, E.M.; Parra-Saldivar, R. Polysaccharides from the Sargassum and Brown Algae Genus: Extraction, Purification, and Their Potential Therapeutic Applications. *Plants* **2023**, *12*, 2445. [CrossRef]
67. Muthu, S.; Altemimi, A.B.; Lakshmikanthan, M.; Krishnan, K.; ALKaisy, Q.H.; Awlqadr, F.H.; Hesarinejad, M.A. Phycocolloids from *Sargassum Microcystum*: Immunomodulatory and Antioxidant Activities of Alginic Acid and Fucoidan. *Food Hydrocoll. Health* **2025**, *7*, 100209. [CrossRef]
68. Faidi, A.; Becheikh, M.E.H.; Lassoued, M.A.; stumbé, J.F.; Safta, F.; Sfar, S. Isolation of Sodium Alginate-like Polysaccharide from *Padina Pavonica*: Optimization, Characterization and Antioxidant Properties. *J. Mol. Struct.* **2025**, *1321*, 139737. [CrossRef]
69. El-Sheekh, M.; Kassem, W.M.A.; Alwaleed, E.A.; Saber, H. Optimization and Characterization of Brown Seaweed Alginate for Antioxidant, Anticancer, Antimicrobial, and Antiviral Properties. *Int. J. Biol. Macromol.* **2024**, *278*, 134715. [CrossRef]
70. Roy, D.; Sobuj, M.K.A.; Islam, M.S.; Haque, M.M.; Islam, M.A.; Islam, M.M.; Ali, M.Z.; Rafiquzzaman, S.M. Compositional, Structural, and Functional Characterization of Fucoidan Extracted from *Sargassum polycystum* Collected from Saint Martin's Island, Bangladesh. *Algal Res.* **2024**, *80*, 103542. [CrossRef]
71. Mabate, B.; Daub, C.D.; Malgas, S.; Pletschke, B.I. Characterisation of *Sargassum elegans* Fucoidans Extracted Using Different Technologies: Linking Their Structure to α-Glucosidase Inhibition. *Algal Res.* **2025**, *85*, 103885. [CrossRef]
72. Urrea-Victoria, V.; Furlan, C.M.; dos Santos, D.Y.A.C.; Chow, F. Antioxidant Potential of Two Brazilian Seaweeds in Response to Temperature: *Pyropia spiralis* (Red Alga) and *Sargassum stenophyllum* (Brown Alga). *J. Exp. Mar. Biol. Ecol.* **2022**, *549*, 151706. [CrossRef]

73. Santos, J.M.; Jesus, B.C.; Ribeiro, H.; Martins, A.; Marto, J.; Fitas, M.; Pinto, P.; Alves, C.; Silva, J.; Pedrosa, R.; et al. Extraction of Macroalgae Phenolic Compounds for Cosmetic Application Using Eutectic Solvents. *Algal Res.* **2024**, *79*, 103438. [CrossRef]
74. Pradas-Baena, I.; Moreno-Rojas, J.M.; Luque de Castro, M.D. Chapter 1—Effect of Processing on Active Compounds in Fresh-Cut Vegetables. In *Processing and Impact on Active Components in Food*; Preedy, V., Ed.; Academic Press: San Diego, CA, USA, 2015; pp. 3–10, ISBN 978-0-12-404699-3.
75. Rumpf, J.; Burger, R.; Schulze, M. Statistical Evaluation of DPPH, ABTS, FRAP, and Folin-Ciocalteu Assays to Assess the Antioxidant Capacity of Lignins. *Int. J. Biol. Macromol.* **2023**, *233*, 123470. [CrossRef]
76. Siddik, M.A.B.; Francis, P.; Rohani, M.F.; Azam, M.S.; Mock, T.S.; Francis, D.S. Seaweed and Seaweed-Based Functional Metabolites as Potential Modulators of Growth, Immune and Antioxidant Responses, and Gut Microbiota in Fish. *Antioxidants* **2023**, *12*, 2066. [CrossRef]
77. Oluwagunwa, O.A.; Alashi, A.M.; Riedl, K.; Aluko, R.E. Effect of Chlorophyll Content on the Multifunctional Properties of *Telfairia Occidentalis* Aqueous Leaf Polyphenolic Concentrate. *S. Afr. J. Bot.* **2024**, *174*, 85–95. [CrossRef]
78. Tamayo-Rincón, V.M.; Colorado-Ríos, J.; Alvarez-Bustamante, D.J.; Urrea-Victoria, V.; Márquez-Fernández, D.M.; Salamanca, C.H.; Dall'Acqua, S.; Castellanos-Hernandez, L.; Martínez-Martínez, A. Sustainable Extraction of Prospective Cosmetic Ingredients from Colombian Marine Macroalgae Using Natural Deep Eutectic Solvents. *Mar. Drugs* **2025**, *23*, 239. [CrossRef]
79. Valdez N, A.; Choez, I.; Van Der Hende, S.; Ruìz, O.; Manzano, P. Condiciones óptimas de extracción de compuestos antioxidante del alga roja Acanthophora spicifera. *Rev. Bionatura* **2023**, *8*, 1–8. [CrossRef]
80. Cuong, D.X.; Boi, V.N.; Van, T.T.T.; Hau, L.N. Effect of Storage Time on Phlorotannin Content and Antioxidant Activity of Six Sargassum Species from Nhatrang Bay, Vietnam. *J. Appl. Phycol.* **2016**, *28*, 567–572. [CrossRef]
81. Prior, R.L.; Hoang, H.; Gu, L.; Wu, X.; Bacchiocca, M.; Howard, L.; Hampsch-Woodill, M.; Huang, D.; Ou, B.; Jacob, R. Assays for Hydrophilic and Lipophilic Antioxidant Capacity (Oxygen Radical Absorbance Capacity (ORACFL)) of Plasma and Other Biological and Food Samples. *J. Agric. Food Chem.* **2003**, *51*, 3273–3279. [CrossRef]
82. Vuppalapati, L.; Velayudam, R.; Nazeer Ahamed, K.F.H.; Cherukuri, S.; Kesavan, B.R. The Protective Effect of Dietary Flavonoid Fraction from *Acanthophora Spicifera* on Streptozotocin Induced Oxidative Stress in Diabetic Rats. *Food Sci. Hum. Wellness* **2016**, *5*, 57–64. [CrossRef]
83. Sivakumar, S.; Sadaiyandi, V.; Swaminathan, S.; Ramalingam, R. Biocompatibility, Anti-Hemolytic, and Antibacterial Assessments of Electrospun PCL/Collagen Composite Nanofibers Loaded with *Acanthophora spicifera* Extracts Mediated Copper Oxide Nanoparticles. *Biocatal. Agric. Biotechnol.* **2024**, *55*, 102983. [CrossRef]
84. Sali, V.K.; Malarvizhi, R.; Manikandamathavan, V.M.; Vasanthi, H.R. Isolation and Evaluation of Phytoconstituents from Red Alga *Acanthophora spicifera* as Potential Apoptotic Agents towards A549 and HeLa Cancer Cells Lines. *Algal Res.* **2018**, *32*, 172–181. [CrossRef]
85. Liu, Z.; Sun, X. A Critical Review of the Abilities, Determinants, and Possible Molecular Mechanisms of Seaweed Polysaccharides Antioxidants. *Int. J. Mol. Sci.* **2020**, *21*, 7774. [CrossRef]
86. Santos, A.K.F. de S.; da Fonseca, D.V.; Salgado, P.R.R.; Muniz, V.M.; de Arruda Torres, P.; Lira, N.S.; da Silva Dias, C.; de Morais Pordeus, L.C.; Barbosa-Filho, J.M.; de Almeida, R.N. Antinociceptive Activity of *Sargassum polyceratium* and the Isolation of Its Chemical Components. *Rev. Bras. Farmacogn.* **2015**, *25*, 683–689. [CrossRef]
87. Lahrsen, E.; Liewert, I.; Alban, S. Gradual Degradation of Fucoidan from *Fucus Vesiculosus* and Its Effect on Structure, Antioxidant and Antiproliferative Activities. *Carbohydr. Polym.* **2018**, *192*, 208–216. [CrossRef]
88. Ruiz-Medina, M.A.; Sansón, M.; González-Rodríguez, Á.M. Changes in Antioxidant Activity of Fresh Marine Macroalgae from the Canary Islands during Air-Drying Process. *Algal Res.* **2022**, *66*, 102798. [CrossRef]
89. Esim, N.; Dawar, P.; Arslan, N.P.; Orak, T.; Doymus, M.; Azad, F.; Ortucu, S.; Albayrak, S.; Taskin, M. Natural Metabolites with Antioxidant Activity from Micro-and Macro-Algae. *Food Biosci.* **2024**, *62*, 105089. [CrossRef]
90. DeVries, J.W.; Kjos, L.; Groff, L.; Bob, M.; Kristi, C.; Patel, H.; Payne, M.; Leichtweis, H.; Shay, M.; Newcomer, L. Studies in Improvement of Official Method 996.06. *J. AOAC Int.* **1999**, *82*, 1146–1155. [CrossRef]
91. House, S.D. Determination of Total, Saturated, and Monounsaturated Fats In Foodstuffs by Hydrolytic Extraction and Gas Chromatographic Quantitation: Collaborative Study. *J. AOAC Int.* **1997**, *80*, 555–563. [CrossRef] [PubMed]
92. Kupina, S.; Fields, C.; Roman, M.C.; Brunelle, S.L. Determination of Total Phenolic Content Using the Folin-C Assay: Single-Laboratory Validation, First Action 2017.13. *J. AOAC Int.* **2018**, *101*, 1466–1472. [CrossRef] [PubMed]
93. Arnao, M.B.; Cano, A.; Acosta, M. The Hydrophilic and Lipophilic Contribution to Total Antioxidant Activity. *Food Chem.* **2001**, *73*, 239–244. [CrossRef]
94. Plank, D.W.; Szpylka, J.; Sapirstein, H.; Woollard, D.; Zapf, C.M.; Lee, V.; Chen, C.-Y.O.; Liu, R.H.; Tsao, R.; Düsterloh, A.; et al. Determination of Antioxidant Activity in Foods and Beverages by Reaction with 2,2′-Diphenyl-1-Picrylhydrazyl (DPPH): Collaborative Study First Action 2012.04. *J. AOAC Int.* **2012**, *95*, 1562–1569. [CrossRef]

95. Benzie, I.F.F.; Strain, J.J. The Ferric Reducing Ability of Plasma (FRAP) as a Measure of "Antioxidant Power": The FRAP Assay. *Anal. Biochem.* **1996**, *239*, 70–76. [CrossRef] [PubMed]
96. *AOAC 2012.23*; Total Antioxidant Activity Oxygen Radical Absorbance Capacity (ORAC) Using Fluorescein as the Fluorescence Probe. AOAC Official Methods of Analysis, Online, Ed.; Association of Official Analytical Chemists: Washington, DC, USA, 2019.

molecules

MDPI

Article

Bio-Compounds, Antioxidant Activity, and Phenolic Content of Broccoli After Impregnation with Beetroot Juice

Magdalena Kręcisz [1,*], Joanna Kolniak-Ostek [2], Bogdan Stępień [1] and Maciej Combrzyński [3]

[1] Institute of Agricultural Engineering, Wrocław University of Environmental and Life Sciences, Chełmońskiego Street 37a, 51-630 Wrocław, Poland; bogdan.stepien@upwr.edu.pl
[2] Department of Fruit, Vegetable and Grain Technology, Wroclaw University of Environmental and Life Sciences, Chełmońskiego Street 37/41, 51-630 Wrocław, Poland; joanna.kolniak-ostek@upwr.edu.pl
[3] Department of Food Process Engineering, University of Life Sciences in Lublin, Głęboka 31, 20-612 Lublin, Poland; maciej.combrzynski@up.lublin.pl
* Correspondence: magdalena.krecisz@upwr.edu.pl

Abstract: The study presented in this paper examined the effects of vacuum impregnation (VI) with beetroot juice and drying medium temperature on selected properties of broccoli. Broccoli florets were dried using the convection-drying method (CD) at a constant drying factor speed (1 m/s) at temperatures of 50 and 70 °C. The bioactive compound content, antioxidant capacity, and polyphenol content of the broccoli before and after vacuum impregnation were determined. The Page and logistic models showed good compliance with the experimental data obtained for all of the tested versions of the materials. In addition, the water activity, density, and color were examined. The use of the vacuum impregnation process resulted in an increase in the drying time, the determination of six betalains characteristic of beetroots, an increase in the polyphenol content, and an increase in the antioxidant activity (FRAP). The material after VI was characterized by a darker color, a red color, and an increased density. Increasing the drying factor temperature resulted in a shorter drying time and a higher antioxidant activity value and content of polyphenols. These findings provide valuable insights into the relationship between VI, the drying temperature, and the broccoli tissue's characteristics, offering guidance for optimizing processing conditions and the production of innovative dried materials that can be added to dishes or serve as a healthy snack.

Keywords: broccoli; beetroot; bioactive compounds; antioxidant activity; phenols; kinetics; vacuum impregnation; drying

1. Introduction

Broccoli (*Brassica oleracea* L. var *italica)* is one of the most widely grown vegetables in the world. It originates from the Mediterranean region and belongs to the cabbage family [1]. Since 2019, a doubling in broccoli production has been observed compared with the latter part of the 19th century. The largest producers of broccoli are India, the USA, Spain, and Italy. Broccoli is rich in bioactive compounds such as tocopherols, which are the most abundant in the Brassicaceae family. In addition, many glucosinolates have been identified in broccoli, which have been shown to prevent chronic diseases. Broccoli also contains carotenoids, such as lutein, β-carotene, neoxanthin, and violaxanthin [2]; minerals (zinc, selenium, iron, magnesium, potassium, calcium, and phosphorus); and ascorbic acid. The compounds listed above are probably responsible for reducing the risk of cancer and cardiovascular disease [3,4].

 https://doi.org/10.3390/molecules30102143

Due to its high betalain content, beetroot is among the top ten vegetables with the highest antioxidant properties. In addition, beetroot contains bioactive compounds, thanks to which its consumption has a positive effect on the human body [5].

Under normal temperature and humidity conditions (i.e., 25 °C and 50%), the quality of vegetables deteriorates rapidly. Fresh vegetables should be stored at temperatures below ambient temperature, i.e., around 15 °C. Otherwise, they must be packaged and frozen to enhance their storage stability [3]. Drying is an important step in the food industry that makes it possible to extend the shelf life of fruits and vegetables [6,7]. This is mainly due to the reduction in the water content in the product, which limits the growth of microbiological contaminants and prevents the occurrence of unwanted chemical reactions. Drying allows the preservation of nutrients, such as bioactive compounds (catechins, phenolic compounds, and isoflavones), protein, fiber, sugars, vitamins, and minerals [8–10]. An important advantage of dried materials is that they are easier and cheaper to transport due to their reduced volume and weight [11]. Other authors have shown that, of the various drying methods studied, samples obtained by the convection method have the highest-rated physicochemical properties, including bioactive ones, and thus, this method is optimal for drying quince [11] and coriander [12]. In the food industry, taking energy efficiency into account, more than 85% of all industrial thermal dryers are convectional [9]. Convective drying (CD) is still the most popular drying technique implemented in food-processing technologies due to the simplicity of the equipment, the financial efficiency of the method, and the preservation of bioactive compounds. Therefore, due to the numerous advantages of convective drying, it is crucial to use this technique to examine the content of bioactive components and optimize the drying process, especially since the modification of the plant material matrix affects the drying process [11–13].

The regular consumption of vegetables and fruits, which are a component of a balanced diet, has a positive effect on health, as proven by numerous studies [14]. In addition, increased consumer awareness and the extended promotion of a healthy lifestyle and nutrition have resulted in the significant growth of the functional food market and the search for effective methods of food enrichment. Vacuum impregnation (VI) is one of the methods that can be used before the drying process to enrich food, and it is also one of the non-destructive methods that allow the formation of a functional food with specific ingredients, such as probiotics, minerals, and vitamins, in order to improve its thermal, sensory, and bioactive properties [15,16]. This is possible thanks to the porous structure of vegetables and fruits. In the intercellular spaces of the materials, gas exchange with an aqueous solution takes place [17–19]. This occurs because the pressure in the cylinder is lowered, causing the pores to expand and the native gases to be displaced. The next stage of vacuum impregnation is called relaxation and is associated with the filling of the pores with the impregnating solution and their shrinkage [19]. VI is considered a valuable process that allows for the development of high-quality food products with desirable characteristics [18]. Pre-treatment can minimize unfavorable changes occurring in the tissue during drying and, as a result, obtain dried material of an appropriate quality [12]. VI with calcium ions can improve texture [20]. Other researchers have reported an increased firmness of honeydew melons after vacuum impregnation with calcium [21]. The use of grape juice resulted in an increase in bioactive compounds in apple tissue [22]. The type of impregnation solution has an impact on the qualitative and metabolic parameters of apples [17]. Vacuum impregnation has also been used to change the properties of beef. Researchers have observed that the use of onion juice reduces lipid oxidation and increases the taste rating of beef [23]. VI has also been used to enrich broad bean flour with iron. The results of these studies also confirmed the positive effect of vacuum impregnation [24]. In turn, De Olivier et al. [25] compared the impact of two pre-treatments on melon processing: soaking and vacuum impregnation. Beetroot juice was used in fruit and vegetable matrices and had a positive effect on the parameters studied [16,26]. The VI value largely depends on the structure of the fruit and vegetable tissue [15,27]. Popular impregnating solutions include calcium, iron, sucrose, probiotics, and sodium chloride. Currently, in addition to estimating the effect of VI on the physical properties of materials, the focus is on the bioactive properties of polyphenol content and antioxidant activity, which is why vegetable and fruit juices with high nutritional properties are used in the vacuum impregnation process, such as onion juice, kale juice, red beet juice, grape juice, or aloe vera gel [15,17,20,23,24,28]. Their research showed that the use of VI was a more effective method of maintaining the viability of probiotics. Vacuum impregnation as a pre-treatment method can be used to create new, innovative, and functional food. Current trends in the consumption of health-promoting foods indicate a greater demand in this sector. Therefore, it is necessary to use vacuum impregnation using beetroot juice with high bioactive properties to produce innovative dried products.

There is still a lack of comprehensive reports in the literature on the impact of convective drying and vacuum impregnation with beetroot juice on bioactive properties, antioxidant activity, polyphenols, drying kinetics, and selected physical properties, i.e., water activity, color, and density.

This review presents a comprehensive and innovative study of the latest trends in the creation of functional foods based on broccoli with beetroot juice. The aim of this study was to examine the effect of beet juice vacuum impregnation (VI) and drying agent temperature on selected bioactive and physical properties of fresh and dried broccoli and their potential industry applications in functional foods, emphasizing the novelty of the bioactive compounds in broccoli. The suitability of the vacuum impregnation process was evaluated through the analysis of the following parameters: bioactive compounds, antioxidant activity, polyphenols, drying kinetics, water activity, density, and color.

2. Results and Discussion

2.1. *Bioactive Compounds of Broccoli Extracts*

Table 1 shows the list of 30 phenolic compounds, eight glucosinolates, and six betalains identified in broccoli samples. Among the phenolic compounds, hydroxycinnamic acids, kaempferol, and quercetin derivatives were the dominant groups. After hydrolysis to aglycons of specific phenolic compounds, Fernandez-Leon et al. [29] investigated the bioactive components in fresh broccoli heads of the cultivars 'Monaco' and 'Parthenon,' finding a higher concentration of quercetin derivatives than kaempferol. According to Vallejo et al. [30], the predominant flavonoids in broccoli inflorescence samples after alkaline hydrolysis are complex acylated tri- or tetra-glycosides of kaempferol and quercetin. In the broccoli samples used in this study, 10 kaempferol glycosides and four quercetin derivatives were tentatively identified. Additionally, the analysis showed the presence of 15 derivatives of phenolic acids—mostly caffeic and sinapic acid derivatives.

Table 1. Bioactive compounds of broccoli (B) and broccoli impregnated in beetroot juice (BB) dried by convective drying at 50 °C (CD50) and 70 °C.

Rt (min)	$[M-H]^-$ (m/z) [a]	MS/MS Fragments (m/z) [a]	Compound	B	B CD50	B CD70	BB	BB CD50	BB CD70
2.56	341.0826	179.0250/161.0179	Caffeoyl hexoside	16.02 ± 0.25 ^{e}	0.25 ± 0.04 ^{b}	0.40 ± 0.12 ^{c}	4.60 ± 0.62 ^{d}	0.19 ± 0.05 ^{a}	0.19 ± 0.06 ^{a}
3.28	353.0844	191.0560/179.0348	Caffeoylquinic acid	87.02 ± 2.15 ^{f}	38.34 ± 1.15 ^{e}	33.39 ± 1.18 ^{d}	23.89 ± 1.26 ^{c}	13.57 ± 0.74 ^{a}	15.91 ± 0.84 ^{b}
3.35	353.0811	179.0290	Caffeoylquinic acid	0.49 ± 0.04 ^{b}	0.29 ± 0.11 ^{a}	0.66 ± 0.09 ^{c}	7.26 ± 0.35 ^{e}	0.94 ± 0.04 ^{d}	0.92 ± 0.14 ^{d}
3.40	447.0410	357.0850	Orientin [b]	0.80 ± 0.02 ^{c}	0.56 ± 0.54 ^{b}	0.28 ± 0.03 ^{a}	7.01 ± 0.24 ^{d}	0.20 ± 0.26 ^{a}	0.19 ± 0.03 ^{a}
3.85	609.1469	447.0531/285.0361	Kaempferol diglucoside	239.69 ± 4.13 ^{e}	4.85 ± 0.16 ^{a}	5.17 ± 0.12 ^{b}	41.04 ± 1.32 ^{d}	8.28 ± 0.86 ^{c}	4.61 ± 0.24 ^{a}
4.03	337.0337	191.0497/163.0337	Coumaroyl-quinic acid	1.94 ± 0.06 ^{c}	1.18 ± 0.04 ^{b}	1.27 ± 0.15 ^{b}	9.61 ± 0.36 ^{d}	0.79 ± 0.26 ^{a}	0.89 ± 0.36 ^{a}
4.20	353.0904	191.0596/	Caffeoylquinic acid [b]	21.95 ± 1.18	1.25 ± 0.14	1.95 ± 0.08	16.35 ± 1.65	1.78 ± 0.42	1.44 ± 0.05
4.22	1111.3350	949.2182/301.0816	Quercetin-3-caffeoyltriglucoside-7-glucoside	2.69 ± 0.08 ^{c}	1.11 ± 0.06 ^{b}	0.27 ± 0.06 ^{a}	5.50 ± 0.54 ^{d}	0.41 ± 0.32 ^{a}	5.41 ± 0.23 ^{d}
4.48	1095.0083	933.4816/787.2160	Kempferol-3-caffeoyltriglucoside-7-glucoside	6.31 ± 0.04 ^{c}	12.09 ± 0.45 ^{d}	11.24 ± 0.12 ^{d}	1.33 ± 0.26 ^{a}	5.69 ± 0.16 ^{b}	13.77 ± 0.54 ^{e}
4.83	1139.2931	977.2447/285.0431	Kempferol-3-sinapoylsophorotrioside-7-glucosided	2.03 ± 0.19 ^{a}	2.28 ± 0.08 ^{a}	2.64 ± 0.20 ^{b}	3.84 ± 0.36 ^{c}	4.39 ± 0.54 ^{d}	3.00 ± 0.64 ^{c}
4.94	385.1083	205.0451/189.0714	Sinapoyl hexose	56.49 ± 2.53 ^{g}	7.63 ± 0.34 ^{d}	4.10 ± 0.26 ^{b}	10.60 ± 0.64 ^{f}	5.99 ± 0.12 ^{c}	1.21 ± 0.08 ^{a}
5.80	609.1398	447.0898/285.0439	Kaempferol diglucoside	68.74 ± 2.64 ^{d}	11.12 ± 0.04 ^{a}	10.04 ± 0.42 ^{a}	31.68 ± 0.64 ^{c}	11.14 ± 0.24 ^{a}	18.58 ± 01.24 ^{b}
6.51	341.0989			12.58 ± 1.24 ^{b}	18.13 ± 1.06 ^{c}	12.20 ± 0.65 ^{b}	31.01 ± 0.68	10.38 ± 0.46 ^{a}	18.10 ± 0.67 ^{c}
6.53	301.0023	723.1643/429.1104	Quercetin [b]	11.52 ± 1.36 ^{a}	38.35 ± 1.74 ^{c}	19.17 ± 0.34 ^{b}	60.20 ± 1.12 ^{d}	17.53 ± 0.84 ^{b}	25.00 ± 1.29 ^{b}
6.91	359.1560	197.0451/179.1125/161.0216	Rosmarinic acid [b]	1.62 ± 0.02 ^{b}	2.32 ± 0.06 ^{c}	2.23 ± 0.08 ^{c}	0.90 ± 0.04 ^{a}	2.78 ± 0.22 ^{d}	4.23 ± 0.46 ^{e}
7.15	947.2666	785.2501/293.0054	Kempferol-3-feruloyldiglucoside-7-glucoside	47.88 ± 2.54 ^{e}	8.61 ± 0.13 ^{c}	6.97 ± 0.64 ^{b}	111.59 ± 2.65 ^{f}	5.28 ± 0.46 ^{a}	23.65 ± 0.58 ^{d}
7.35	1095.2855	787.1799/285.1093	Kempferol-3-caffeoyltriglucoside-7-glucoside	5.90 ± 0.42 ^{a}	24.87 ± 0.54 ^{e}	15.52 ± 0.16 ^{b}	17.72 ± 1.12 ^{c}	22.98 ± 0.98 ^{d}	17.24 ± 1.16 ^{c}
7.58	577.1445	285.0321	Kempferol-3,7-*O*-di-rhamnopyranoside	15.28 ±0.65 ^{f}	5.26 ± 0.32 ^{d}	1.06 ± 0.08 ^{a}	10.56 ± 1.24 ^{e}	1.81 ± 0.21 ^{c}	1.42 ± 0.28 ^{b}
8.12	919.3005	723.1643/429.1104/301.0721	Quercetin derivative	10.12 ± 0.24 ^{c}	1.62 ± 0.14 ^{a}	1.90 ± 0.16 ^{b}	9.28 ± 1.16 ^{c}	2.13 ± 0.08 ^{b}	2.02 ± 0.62 ^{b}
8.31	753.2167	523.1585/223.0616/205.0515	1,2-Disinapoyl-gentobioside	5.40 ± 0.16 ^{a}	70.13 ± 2.25 ^{d}	74.18 ± 2.14 ^{d}	23.12 ± 1.54 ^{b}	90.89 ± 2.54 ^{e}	48.47 ± 2.12 ^{c}
8.60	723.2103	499.1444/175.0398	1-sinapoyl-2-feruloyl-gentibiose	21.13 ± 1.31 ^{b}	93.64 ± 7.32 ^{d}	104.85 ± 3.16 ^{e}	3.94 ± 0.62 ^{a}	122.49 ± 3.25 ^{f}	73.89 ± 1.98 ^{c}
8.81	1139.2924	977.4442/285.1507	Kempferol-3-sinapoylsophorotrioside-7-glucoside	3.90 ± 0.24 ^{a}	20.55 ± 1.02 ^{e}	19.85 ± 1.08 ^{d}	14.22 ± 0.52 ^{c}	11.99 ± 1.12 ^{b}	10.20 ± 0.52 ^{b}
8.93	693.2132	499.1516/259.5630	1,2-diferuoyl-diglucoside	1.19 ± 0.14 ^{c}	0.93 ± 0.24 ^{c}	0.80 ± 0.08 ^{b}	9.29 ± 0.32 ^{d}	0.39 ± 0.36 ^{a}	0.87 ± 0.26 ^{b}
9.21	959.2661	735.3117/511.1374	Trisinapoyl-gentionbiose	2.72 ± 0.04 ^{a}	62.78 ± 2.47 ^{c}	62.23 ± 1.74 ^{c}	85.71 ± 3.52	60.22 ± 0.76 ^{b}	52.04 ± 1.14 ^{d}
9.49	929.2539	723.2125	Feruloyl-disinapoyl-gentionbiose	1.99 ± 0.27 ^{a}	18.96 ± 1.12 ^{e}	16.63 ± 1.54 ^{d}	5.85 ± 0.24 ^{b}	22.22 ± 0.24 ^{f}	11.90 ± 0.76 ^{c}
9.81	1109.3099	947.0086/285.0297	Kempferol-3-feruloylsophorotrioside	5.32 ± 0.67 ^{b}	10.00 ± 0.64 ^{c}	9.86 ± 0.68 ^{c}	2.61 ± 0.12 ^{a}	9.77 ± 0.56 ^{c}	6.86 ± 1.08 ^{a}
10.07	929.2347	705.1979	Feruloyl-disinapoyl-gentionbiose	1.11 ± 0.17 ^{b}	1.61 ± 0.18 ^{b}	2.06 ± 0.16 ^{c}	1.66 ± 0.32 ^{b}	1.16 ± 0.06 ^{b}	0.52 ± 0.36 ^{a}
10.56	489.2639		Kaempferol 3-*O*-(6″-acetyl-hexoside)	9.01 ± 0.63 ^{f}	2.11 ± 0.14 ^{b}	1.66 ± 0.24 ^{a}	6.90 ± 0.68 ^{e}	4.28 ± 0.23 ^{d}	3.62 ± 0.09 ^{c}
10.73	959.2738	735.1979/511.2109	Trisinapoyl-gentionbiose	446.37 ± 0.42 ^{e}	3.69 ± 0.08 ^{b}	2.37 ± 0.35 ^{a}	15.50 ± 0.54 ^{d}	5.13 ± 0.42 ^{c}	3.28 ± 0.11 ^{b}
10.85	625.4776	/463.2062/301.0021	Quercetin-3,4′-*O*-di-beta-glucoside	0.81 ± 0.06 ^{a}	2.43 ± 0.12 ^{b}	2.86 ± 0.42 ^{b}	166.88 ± 4.54 ^{c}	2.21 ± 0.09 ^{b}	2.44 ± 0.25 ^{b}
			Total [mg/100g]	**1107.87 ± 33.79**	**466.92 ± 16.54**	**427.82 ± 13.12**	**739.64 ± 24.98**	**446.95 ± 11.86**	**371.85 ± 9.46**

Abbreviations: Rt—retention time; $[M-H]^-$ (m/z)—masses of identified compounds; MS/MS fragments (m/z)—masses of identified fragments. Values (mean of three replications) ± standard deviation followed by different letters (a–f) are different ($p \leq 0.05$) according to Duncan's test. B—broccoli; B CD50 and B CD70—broccoli dried by convective drying at 50 and 70 °C, respectively; BB—broccoli after impregnation with beetroot juice; and BB CD50 and BB CD70—broccoli after impregnation with beetroot juice and dried by convective drying at 50 and 70 °C, respectively. [a] Experimental data. [b] Identification confirmed by commercial standards.

Glucosinolates were identified in all tested samples (Table 2). We identified compounds typical for broccoli, whose presence in broccoli has been confirmed by other studies [31,32]. The compound at *m/z* 195 and the resulting product ions at *m/z* 177 and 129 were tentatively identified as gluconic acid [33]. The compound at *m/z* 436 and product ions at *m/z* 372 and 178 were identified as glucoraphanin [33], while the compound with the $[M-H]^-$ ion at *m/z* 447 and product ions at *m/z* 259 and 134 was identified as glucobrassicin [33]. The compound at *m/z* 447 and resulting product ions at *m/z* 254 and 139 were identified as indolymethyl glucosinolate [33], while the compound at *m/z* 422 and product ions at *m/z* 358 and 259 were tentatively identified as glucoiberin [34]. Three compounds had the same $[M-H]^-$ ions, but due to the different fragmentation patterns, they were identified as neoglucobrassicin (product ions at *m/z* 284 and 154) and two isomers of methoxyglucobrassicin (product ions at *m/z* 235).

Table 2. Glucosinolates identified in broccoli (B) and broccoli impregnated in beetroot juice (BB) dried by convective drying at 50 °C (CD50) and 70 °C.

Rt (min)	$[M-H]^-$ (*m/z*)	MS/MS Fragments (*m/z*)	Compound
2.60	341.0860		Vulgaxanthin II
2.63	356.0997		Cyclodopa glucoside
2.93	385.1063		N-Formylcyclodopa glucoside
5.29	551.1737	389.1350	Betanin
9.15	535.1428		Mono-decarboxy betanin

Abbreviations: Rt—retention time; $[M-H]^-$ (*m/z*)—masses of identified compounds; MS/MS fragments (*m/z*)—masses of identified fragments.

In samples with the addition of beetroot juice, we identified six betalains, characteristic for beetroots (Table 3): 2,17-bidecarboxy-betanidin/isobetanidin ($[M-H]^-$ ion at *m/z* 463 and resulting product ion at 301), vulgaxanthin ($[M-H]^-$ ion at *m/z* 341), cyclodopa glucoside ($[M-H]^-$ ion at *m/z* 356), N-formylcyclodopa glucoside ($[M-H]^-$ ion at *m/z* 385), betanin ($[M-H]^-$ ion at *m/z* 551 and resulting product ion at 389), and mono-decarboxy betanin ($[M-H]^-$ ion at *m/z* 535) [5,35].

Table 3. Betalains identified in broccoli (B) and broccoli impregnated in beetroot juice (BB) dried by convective drying at 50 °C (CD50) and 70 °C.

Rt (min)	$[M-H]^-$ (*m/z*)	MS/MS Fragments (*m/z*)	Compound
0.90	195.0461	177.0476/129.0088	Gluconic acid
1.87	436.0401	372.0553/178.0165	Glucoraphanin
3.19	447.0482	259.0295/134.0551	Glucobrassicin
3.76	447.0535	254.1377/139.0027	Indolymethyl glucosinolate
4.66	422.0568	358.1490/259.0676	Glucoiberin
4.97	477.0605	284.0360/154.0144	Neoglucobrassicin
6.16	477.0588	235.9673	Methoxyglucobrassicin 1
6.32	477.0568	235.9234	Methoxyglucobrassicin 2

Abbreviations: Rt—retention time; $[M-H]^-$ (*m/z*)—masses of identified compounds; MS/MS fragments (*m/z*)—masses of identified fragments.

The process of vacuum impregnation is influenced by a variety of factors, which can be categorized into internal and external factors. Among variables of internal origin, features characteristic of impregnated tissue are distinguished, like its size, porosity, mechanical properties, and shape of capillaries. In turn, key external factors determining the impregnation rate encompass parameters such as the vacuum level applied, the concentration and composition of the impregnating solution, the proportion of the solution to the product, the temperature, the intensity of mixing, the vacuum process duration, and the moment of the restoration of atmospheric pressure [28,36].

The use of vacuum impregnation technology not only allowed the introduction of new compounds characteristic of beet, but also a significant increase in other compounds also present in fresh broccoli. The largest change was noted for quercetin-3,4′-O-di-beta-glucoside; the use of VI allowed the tested compound to be increased by 20,464%. Significant changes in the content of bioactive compounds after the vacuum impregnation process were also noted for trisinapoyl-gentionbiose (3,056%), caffeoylquinic acid (1 381%), 1,2-diferuoyl-diglucoside (738%), orientin (723%), coumaroyl-quinic acid (396%), 1,2-disinapoyl-gentobioside (328%), kempferol-3-sinapoylsophorotrioside-7-glucoside (265%), caffeoyl hexoside (235%), kempferol-3-caffeoyltriglucoside-7-glucoside (200%), and feruloyl-disinapoyl-gentionbiose (194%). However, in these studies, the total content of bioactive compounds decreased after the vacuum impregnation process. This indicates the characteristics of the vacuum impregnation process and the mass transfer between the vegetable tissue and the impregnation solution [36]. The vacuum impregnation process can increase the nutritional value of products, but at the same time, changes in the structure can lead to the degradation of some bioactive compounds due to contact with oxygen or enzymes [36]. Studies by other authors have shown that appropriate VI parameters (i.e., time and pressure) can increase the content of phenols and flavonoids in apples. However, excessive process intensity can cause losses of these compounds [37].

2.2. Total Phenolic Content (TPC) and Antioxidant Capacity (AC)

The results for antioxidant activity and fresh polyphenols (B), after vacuum impregnation with beetroot juice (BB) and dried broccoli florets at 50 °C (CD50) and 70 °C (CD70), are shown in Table 4.

Table 4. Antioxidant capacity (μMol Trolox/100 g of dry matter) and total phenolic content of broccoli (B) and broccoli impregnated in beetroot juice (BB) dried by convective drying at 50 °C (CD50) and 70 °C.

Method	ABTS	DPPH	FRAP	TPC
B	58.98 ± 2.28 ^{f}	88.60 ± 3.13 ^{e}	41.60 ± 2.22 ^{e}	9.82 ± 0.58 ^{d}
B CD50	19.07 ± 0.24 ^{b}	21.78 ± 0.72 ^{b}	15.50 ± 1.08 ^{b}	2.96 ± 0.38 ^{a}
B CD70	29.55 ± 0.74 ^{d}	22.39 ± 0.38 ^{b}	22.92 ± 1.73 ^{d}	4.81 ± 0.46 ^{c}
BB	44.79 ± 2.42 ^{e}	66.03 ± 2.62 ^{d}	47.79 ± 3.12 ^{f}	13.06 ± 0.97 ^{e}
BB CD50	16.97 ± 0.76 ^{a}	16.57 ± 0.56 ^{a}	13.20 ± 0.62 ^{a}	2.63 ± 0.14 ^{a}
BB CD70	24.07 ± 1.56 ^{c}	24.34 ± 1.98 ^{c}	19.72 ± 1.04 ^{c}	3.50 ± 0.32 ^{b}

Values (mean of three replications) ± standard deviation followed by different letters (a–f) are different ($p \leq 0.05$) according to Duncan's test. Abbreviations: ABTS—2,2′-azino-bis(3-ethylbenzothiazoline-6-sulfonic acid); DPPH—2,2-diphenyl-1-(2,4,6-trinitrophenyl)hydrazyl; FRAP—ferric reducing antioxidant power assay; B—broccoli; B CD50 and B CD70—broccoli dried by convective drying at 50 and 70 °C, respectively; BB—broccoli after impregnation with beetroot juice; BB CD50 and BB CD70—broccoli after impregnation with beetroot juice and dried by convective drying at 50 and 70 °C, respectively.

Antioxidant capacity (AC) was tested using the ABTS, DPPH, and FRAP methods. The highest AC value for ABTS and DPPH was recorded for fresh broccoli (88.60 μMol/g), and the lowest was recorded for broccoli with VI after drying at 50 °C (16.57 μMol/g). Other authors, studying the effect of VI with the use of apple and pear juice on the properties of chokeberry, observed a decrease in antioxidant activity. In addition, the authors observed that with the increase in pressure during the vacuum impregnation process, the AC value decreases [38]. The impregnation process is influenced by many agents, such as material structure, vacuum pressure, VI time, impregnating solution, and solution particle size [28]. In the case of the FRAP method, the highest value was recorded for broccoli after the vacuum impregnation process (47.79 μMol/g), and the lowest was recorded for broccoli without VI after drying at 50 °C (13.20 μMol/g). The samples dried after VI had a lower AC than the samples dried without pre-treatment. Matys. et al., who studied the effect of pre-treatment with pulsed electric fields in their studies, obtained observations consistent with those presented in this study [13]. Other studies show that in the case of drying sweet potatoes, a higher AC value was recorded when a vacuum impregnation process was used with onion juice and kale [39] and for celery after the VI of onion juice, kale, and celery leaves [40]. A higher antioxidant activity value, tested by ABTS, DPPH, and FRAP methods in broccoli dried by convection at 70 °C, was observed by 54.96, 2.80, and 73.64% for broccoli without VI and by 41.84, 46.89, and 27.23% for broccoli after VI compared to broccoli dried at a lower temperature. Higher AC values with increasing drying process temperatures were observed by other researchers for spray-dried broccoli stem and broccoli florets powders [3].

The used VI process resulted in the highest polyphenol value (13.06 μMol/g). In the case of broccoli not subjected to the drying process, the TPC value was 32.99% higher in broccoli after VI (BB) than for broccoli without pre-treatment. In the study, it was observed that the temperature of the drying medium influenced the increase in polyphenol value by 62.5% in the case of untreated broccoli and by 33.08% for broccoli after impregnation with beetroot juice. An increase in TPC with increasing temperature from 50 to 70 °C during convective drying was observed in other studies in which celery and celery after VI were dried using onion juice, kale, and celery [40]. Saavedra-Leos et al. [3] observed that the TPC value increased with increasing temperature from 170 to 220 °C when spray-drying broccoli stems and florets [3]. Similar observations were made by Sarabandi et al. [41] when spray-drying eggplant peel extracts enclosed in gum arabic and maltodextrin. The authors explained that the increase in TPC at higher temperatures may be due to the faster formation of a protective film around the materials studied. As a result, more polyphenols are enclosed in the microstructure of the materials [41]. In addition, a greater loss of polyphenols was observed in the material dried after VI by 11.15% after CD50 and by 27.23% after CD70. These losses may be related to the partial loosening of the broccoli tissue. This loosening can lead to the leakage of the tested solutions and the activation of reaction substrates and/or oxidizing enzymes (flavonoids and phenols) from the vegetable materials [13,42]. Other studies indicate an increase in TPC value for sweet potatoes impregnated with onion juice and kale [39]. Many researchers report that the changes in the phenolic compound values can be influenced by agents such as the type of raw material, process temperature, pre-treatment time, and the type of osmotic compound [14,43,44].

2.3. *Vacuum Impregnation*

The weight gain (WG), Brix degrees (°Bx), and dry mass (DM) are shown in Table 5. In this study, in which broccoli juice was used, the weight gain of the broccoli was 14.88% at 10.3 °Bx, compared to the broccoli before vacuum impregnation. This indicates the porous structure of the tested material. Other authors, studying the effect of the vacuum impregnation process with the use of an isotonic solution (13–14 °Bx) on the properties of apples, observed a WG of 20.1–23.4% [17].

Table 5. Weight gain (WG), Brix degrees (°Bx), and dry mass (DM).

Material	WG (%)	°Bx	DM (%)
B	-	-	12.87 ± 0.57
BB	14.88 ± 0.43	10.3 ± 0.2	11.95 ± 0.43

B—broccoli; BB—broccoli after impregnation with beetroot juice.

2.4. Moisture Ratio Curves and Water Content Curves

The changes in moisture ratio (MR) and moisture content (MC) of broccoli samples without pre-treatment (B) and after vacuum impregnation (BB) dried using the CD method at 50 and 70 °C are shown in Figures 1 and 2, respectively. The figures show that different drying temperatures and the use of vacuum impregnation (VI) had a significant impact on the change in moisture content and drying time in all samples tested. The moisture content of broccoli florets decreases with increasing temperature, and thus the drying time decreases. The time required to reach the equilibrium moisture content of the broccoli was 150 (B CD70), 170 (BB CD70), 290 (B CD50), and 350 (BB CD50) minutes. The required drying time for CD 70 was 48.28% shorter for broccoli without pre-treatment and 51.43% shorter for broccoli after the VI process compared to convective drying at 50 °C. These studies confirm that increasing the temperature of the drying medium improves the diffusion and evaporation of moisture, thus shortening the drying time. These results are in line with previous studies on broccoli stems [45], carrots [46], coriander [12], celery [40,47], and green bananas [6].

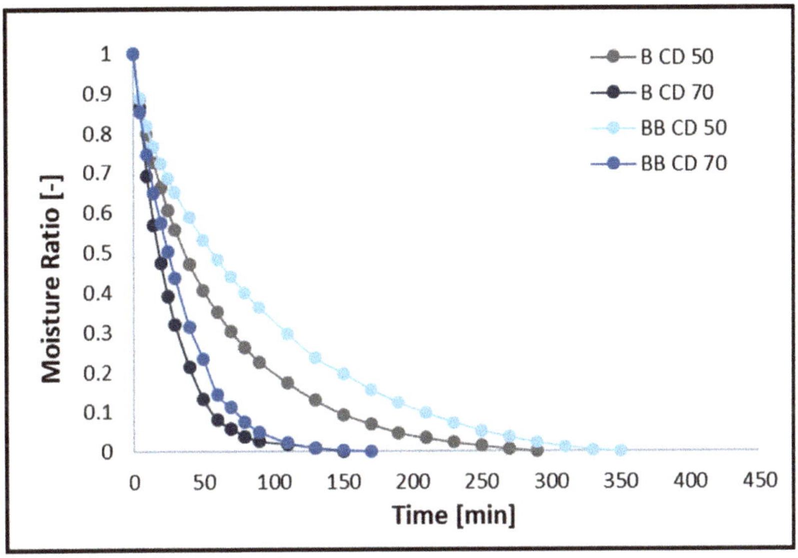

Figure 1. Drying kinetics for convective drying at 50 °C (CD50) and 70 °C (CD70). B—broccoli without VI; BB—broccoli after VI.

The use of the vacuum impregnation process, using beet juice as an impregnating solution, resulted in an increase in drying time. In broccoli samples dried at 50 °C (CD50) with VI, the drying time increased by 20.69%, and in samples dried at 70 °C (CD70), it increased by 20%. In the material after the vacuum impregnation process, an increase in water content of 13.33% was observed, which probably contributes to the prolonged drying time of broccoli (BB). In addition, the weight gain in the VI samples was 14.88%, which may also contribute to the prolonged drying time.

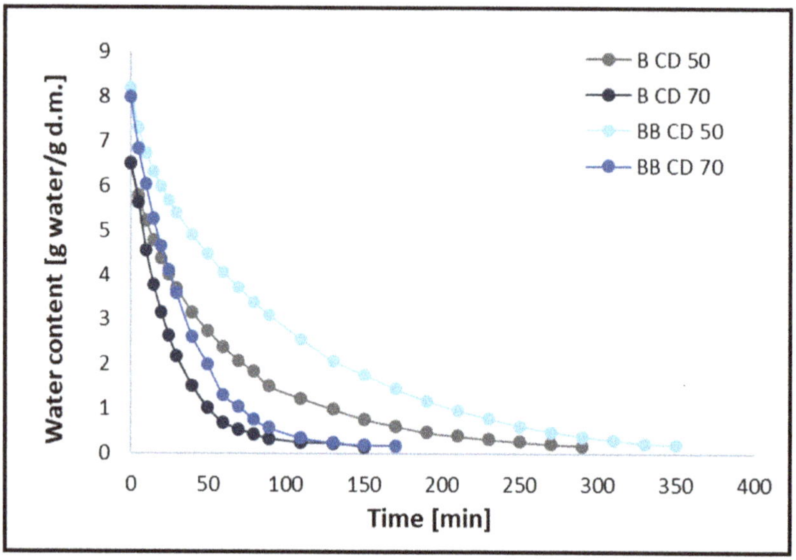

Figure 2. Water content during convective drying at 50 °C (CD50) and 70 °C (CD70). B—broccoli without VI; BB—broccoli after VI.

2.5. Modeling of Broccoli Drying Process

The model parameters and statistical parameters describing the kinetics of the broccoli drying process are presented in Table 6. For convective drying at 50 and 70 °C, all five models provided an excellent fit to the experimental data with an R^2 value above 0.99. Of these, the logistic model proved to be the best model for convective drying at 70 °C, taking into account the highest R^2 values (0.9995 and 0.9992) and the lowest RSME values (0.0072 and 0.0093), V_e (2.1 and 2.9), and χ^2 (0.0001). Interestingly, in the case of convective drying at 50 °C, the Page model achieved the best fit in terms of high R^2 values (0.9995 and 0.9961) and the lowest RSME values (0.0075 and 0.0203). The best fit of the logistic model was demonstrated by researchers drying celery [47]. Other researchers have shown the best fit of Page's model when drying quince [11], and this model is also commonly used in other studies on drying coriander [12].

Table 6. Parameter values a, b, k, R^2, RMSE, χ^2, and V_e of the function describe the drying kinetics for courgette samples dried by convection at different temperatures.

Drying Method	Material	Model Parameters			Statistical Parameters				Drying Time [min]
		k	a	b	RMSE	V_e [%]	R^2	χ^2	
				Logistical Model					
CD50	B	0.0167	1962.7203	1870.3274	0.0165	5.1	0.9972	0.0003	290
	BB	0.0110	1589.9455	1488.6300	0.0990	5.6	0.9959	0.0004	350
CD70	B	0.0388	2.4187	3.3763	0.0072	2.1	0.9995	0.0001	150
	BB	0.0359	2.1818	3.1279	0.0093	2.9	0.9992	0.0001	170
				Logarithmic Model					
CD50	B	0.0163	0.9270	0.0041	0.0113	3.8	0.9983	0.0001	290
	BB	0.0110	0.9320	0.0000	0.0989	5.6	0.9959	0.0004	350
CD70	B	0.0330	1.0199	0.0000	0.0134	4.6	0.9982	0.0002	150
	BB	0.0300	1.0149	0.0000	0.0153	5.5	0.9976	0.0003	170
				Henderdon and Pabis Model					
CD50	B	0.0167	0.9525	-	0.01652	5.1	0.9972	0.0003	290
	BB	0.0110	0.9322	-	0.0199	5.6	0.9959	0.0004	350
CD70	B	0.0326	1.0097	-	0.0135	4.0	0.9986	0.0002	150
	BB	0.0297	1.0078	-	0.0150	4.8	0.9982	0.0003	170

Table 6. *Cont.*

Drying Method	Material	Model Parameters				Statistical Parameters			Drying Time [min]
		k	a	b	RMSE	V_e [%]	R^2	χ^2	
				Newton Model					
CD50	B	0.0179	-	-	0.0235	7.2	0.9972	0.0006	290
	BB	0.0121	-	-	0.0331	9.3	0.9941	0.0012	350
CD70	B	0.0322	-	-	0.0139	4.2	0.9988	0.0002	150
	BB	0.0294	-	-	0.0153	4.8	0.9984	0.0003	170
				Page Model					
CD50	B	0.0297	0.8734	-	0.0075	2.3	0.9995	0.0001	290
	BB	0.0224	0.8620	-	0.0203	5.7	0.9961	0.0004	350
CD70	B	0.0276	1.0338	-	0.0071	2.2	0.9995	0.0001	150
	BB	0.0236	1.0624	-	0.0119	3.8	0.9987	0.0002	170

B—broccoli; BB—broccoli after impregnation with beetroot juice; CD50—dried by convective drying at 50 °C; and CD70—dried by convective drying at 70 °C.

2.6. Dry Matter (DM), Water Activity (AW), and Density (ρb)

The water activity (AW) for all tested material versions is shown in Table 7. As expected, the highest values of the tested parameter were recorded for fresh broccoli (0.987) and broccoli after the vacuum impregnation process (0.984). This is consistent with previous studies [26]. Anaya-Esparza et al., while studying the effect of vacuum impregnation on the properties of apples, observed an increase in water activity in apples after VI [37]. The use of the drying process allowed for a reduction in the AW by 64.01–52.45%, depending on the drying process temperature and the pre-treatment used. Lower water activity values were recorded for broccoli without VI: 0.469 (B CD50) and 0.436 (B CD70). Increasing the drying factor temperature resulted in a 18.49% reduction in water activity for fresh broccoli without VI and a 18.72% reduction for broccoli after VI. This is in line with our previous studies on broccoli [26], courgette [26,48], and celery [40].

Table 7. Water activity (AW) and density (ρb).

Method	Water Activity [-]	Density [kg/m^3]
B	0.987 ± 0.007 ^{e}	240.94 ± 5.05 ^{d}
B CD50	0.469 ± 0.008 ^{c}	111.34 ± 4.00 ^{b}
B CD70	0.436 ± 0.001 ^{a}	84.16 ± 1.73 ^{a}
BB	0.382 ± 0.008 ^{e}	288.90 ± 5.98 ^{d}
BB CD50	0.354 ± 0.010 ^{d}	116.16 ± 2.95 ^{b}
BB CD70	0.459 ± 0.005 ^{b}	93.75 ± 2.87 ^{c}

Values (mean of three replications) ± standard deviation followed by different letters (a–e) are different ($p \leq 0.05$) according to Duncan's test. B—broccoli; B CD50 and B CD70—broccoli dried by convective drying at 50 and 70 °C, respectively; BB—broccoli after impregnation with beetroot juice; and BB CD50 and BB CD70—broccoli after impregnation with beetroot juice and dried by convective drying at 50 and 70 °C, respectively.

The density for fresh broccoli was 240.94 kg/m^3, and that for broccoli after the vacuum impregnation process was 288.90 kg/m^3. As can be seen from the data presented in Table 5, broccoli after VI before and after drying are characterized by a higher density. These results are consistent with previous studies by the authors of the publication, which concerned celery impregnated with beetroot juice [47] and courgette impregnated with tomato juice [49]. The use of a higher drying factor temperature resulted in a lower density of the tested material. A decrease in the density of the tested material with increasing temperature was observed in previous studies when drying celery [47] and courgette [49].

2.7. Color

In the study presented in this paper, the color parameters (L*, a*, b*) of fresh broccoli, after the vacuum impregnation process, and dried broccoli were determined. Then, the saturation, browning, and color difference in relation to fresh material without VI were calculated, and the results are presented in Table 8.

Table 8. Color parameters of raw and dried broccoli: L*—lightness; a* for (+) redness/(−) greenness and b* for (+) yellowing; BI—browning index; C*—saturation; and ΔE—total color of vegetables.

Color Parameters	B	B CD50	B CD70	BB	BB CD50	BB CD70
L	32.54 ± 1.09 [e]	18.35 ± 0.59 [c]	15.75 ± 0.91 [b]	23.86 ± 0.56 [d]	16.74 ± 0.40 [b]	14.62 ± 1.02 [a]
A	−5.12 ± 0.61 [a]	−1.90 ± 0.16 [b]	−0.66 ± 1.12 [b]	1.35 ± 0.04 [c]	2.85 ± 0.53 [d]	3.40 ± 0.26 [e]
B	6.04 ± 0.76 [c]	10.24 ± 0.38 [e]	7.95 ± 0.33 [d]	1.36 ± 0.11 [a]	7.45 ± 0.55 [d]	5.56 ± 0.71 [b]
C*	5.60 ± 0.78 [b]	10.15 ± 0.38 [e]	7.91 ± 0.34 [d]	1.79 ± 0.08 [a]	7.64 ± 0.54 [d]	5.86 ± 0.68 [b]
BI	1.99 ± 2.09 [a]	62.31 ± 3.2 [c]	61.85 ± 10.59 [c]	12.03 ± 0.69 [b]	80.45 ± 6.17 [e]	77.62 ± 9.87 [d]
ΔE	-	15.15 [b]	17.48 [c]	11.80 [a]	17.75 [c]	19.85 [d]

Values (mean of three replications) ± standard deviations followed by different letters (a–e) are different ($p \leq 0.05$) according to Duncan's test. B—broccoli; B CD50 and B CD70—broccoli dried by convective drying at 50 and 70 °C, respectively; BB—broccoli after impregnation with beetroot juice; and BB CD50 and BB CD70—broccoli after impregnation with beetroot juice and dried by convective drying at 50 and 70 °C, respectively.

The vacuum impregnation process reduced the lightness (L*) and the b* value, which indicates a yellow tint. In addition, the a* value was higher and took on positive values, indicating a red tint. These results are in line with expectations because beet juice, which has an intense dark color, was used in the vacuum impregnation process. These results are consistent with studies that examined courgette and broccoli [39], celery [38], and apples [37].

The use of a higher drying factor temperature resulted in a decrease in the L* and b* parameters and an increase in the a* parameter. The higher a* values can be explained by the active enzymatic and non-enzymatic browning (Maillard reaction) during drying, which led to a red-brown color of the samples both with and without VI [50–52]. On the other hand, the darker color of broccoli may be caused by the high temperature of the process [53]. Szychowski et al. [11], when drying quince, also observed the darkest color in samples dried at 70 °C [11].

The smallest change in color was observed for broccoli after VI without drying. The application of the drying process in broccoli after VI resulted in an increase in ΔE of 50.42% at CD50 and an increase of 68.22% at CD70. As predicted, a higher ΔE value was observed in the material after the vacuum impregnation process. This is consistent with the darker color of the samples (L*). In other studies, which examined the effect of tomato juice on the properties of courgette [49], kale and onion juice on the properties of courgette [48], and beet juice on the properties of celery [47], a similar relationship was observed. In addition, the greater color difference is due to the use of a strongly colored juice as an impregnation solution. The change in color difference is also confirmed by the browning index (BI). Higher values of the index were recorded in the material after the vacuum impregnation process. However, the highest change in this index was recorded in the samples after the drying process. The color saturation (C*) was recorded for BB and was the highest for B CD50. A decrease in the value of the tested parameter was observed in the material after VI. The drying process caused an increase in saturation, but as the temperature of the drying agent increased, the saturation value decreased.

2.8. Pearson Correlation of Drying Kinetics and Selected Broccoli Quality Attributes

As shown in Figure 3, Pearson's correlation was used to examine the association between selected broccoli properties. The data showed a significant ($p < 0.05$) positive correlation between vacuum impregnation and the material with or without drying (r = 0.88), water activity (r = 0.88), and bulk density (r = 0.88). The results also showed a significant positive correlation of the material with or without drying with water activity (r = 1), color difference (r = 0.68), and bulk density (r = 1) and a negative correlation with FRAP (r = −0.53) and DPPH (r = −0.50). The data obtained indicate that the material with or without drying had a greater impact on BC, FRAP, and ABTS than the drying methods. Both variables had a similar effect on water activity, color difference, bulk density, and total phenolic content. Moreover, a significant positive correlation was observed between water activity and bulk density (r = 1) and color difference (r = 0.68). Water activity negatively correlates with FRAP (r = −0.53) and ABTS (r = −0.50). The results also showed a positive correlation of ABTS with TPC and BC (r = 0.46) and a negative correlation with DPPH (r = −0.49). DPPH significantly negatively correlates with bioactive compounds (r = −0.93). The negative correlation between the content of bioactive compounds and the DPPH value is beneficial because it indicates the high ability of these compounds to neutralize free radicals, which indicates their strong antioxidant properties. Such action may contribute to protecting the body from oxidative stress and related diseases.

-1 -0.80 -0.60 -0.40 -0.20 0 0.20 0.40 0.60 0.80 1

	VI	M	AW	L*	E	p	ABTS	DPPH	FRAP	TPC	BC
VI	1.00										
M	0.88	1.00									
AW	0.88	1.00	1.00								
L*	0.07	-0.35	-0.35	1.00							
E	0.47	0.68	0.68	-0.67	1.00						
p	0.88	1.00	1.00	-0.35	0.68	1.00					
ABTS	0.00	0.21	0.21	-0.09	0.32	0.21	1.00				
DPPH	-0.10	-0.50	-0.50	0.79	-0.76	-0.50	-0.49	1.00			
FRAP	-0.36	-0.53	-0.53	0.53	-0.53	-0.53	-0.03	0.17	1.00		
TPC	0.39	0.33	0.33	0.14	0.26	0.33	0.46	0.16	-0.64	1.00	
BC	-0.06	0.33	0.33	-0.73	0.62	0.33	0.46	-0.97	0.03	-0.34	1.00

Figure 3. Correlation matrix for selected broccoli parameters. VI: vacuum impregnation; M: material with or without drying; AW: water activity; L*: lightness; E: color difference; p: bulk density; ABTS, DPPH, FRAP: antioxidant capacity; TPC: total phenolic content; and BC: bioactive compounds.

2.9. Principal Component Analysis (PCA)

Approximately 96.95% of the variance in the sample data was explained by the first two principal components PC1 (65.59%) and PC2 (31.36%). PC1 correlated negatively with DPPH, ABTS, FRAP, L*, BC, AW, p, TPC, quercetin-3,4′-O-di-beta-glucoside, 1,2-diferuoyl-diglucoside, and caffeoylquinic acid and positively with ΔE and trisinapoyl-gentionbiose. PC2 correlated negatively with BC, DPPH, ABTS, L*, TPC, and AW and positively with FRAP, p, TPC, quercetin-3,4′-*O*-di-beta-glucoside, trisinapoyl-gentionbiose, 1,2-diferuoyl-diglucoside, caffeoylquinic acid, and ΔE (Figure 4).

The PCA diagram (Figure 5) reveals that the first component (PC1) describes the results of broccoli after the drying process by 65.59%. In the figure, positive PC1 values describe the results obtained for broccoli after the drying process. Negative PC1 values describe fresh broccoli, i.e., not subjected to the convective drying process. The second main component (PC2) refers to the pre-treatment used, which was vacuum impregnation, at 31.36%. In the figure, positive PC2 values describe fresh broccoli after vacuum impregnation. Negative PC2 values describe the results of fresh broccoli and broccoli after convective drying. In addition, three groups were observed which indicated significant differences. The first group included fresh broccoli, the second group included broccoli after vacuum impregnation, and the third group included samples of broccoli after convective drying.

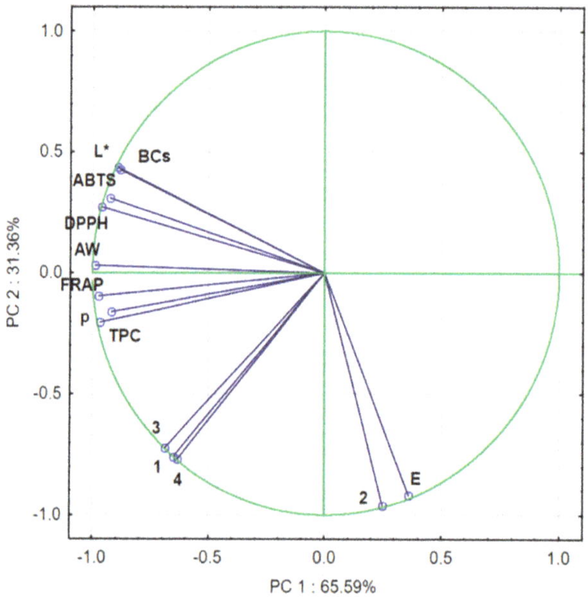

Figure 4. PCA of dried broccoli. AW: water activity; L*: lightness; E: color difference; p: bulk density; ABTS, DPPH, and FRAP: antioxidant capacity; TPC: total phenolic content; BCs: bioactive compounds; 1—quercetin-3,4′-*O*-di-beta-glucoside; 2—trisinapoyl-gentionbiose; 3—1,2-diferuoyl-diglucoside; and 4—caffeoylquinic acid.

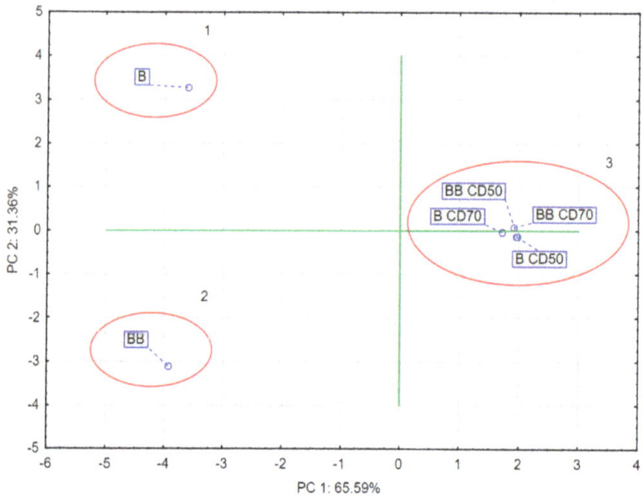

Figure 5. PCA of dried broccoli.

3. Materials and Methods

3.1. Plants

This study was conducted using broccoli purchased at a local vegetable market. The vegetables were stored in a refrigerator at 4 ± 1 °C (Samsung Electronics, Wronki, Poland). Before processing, the broccoli was washed, dried, and cut into evenly sized florets (1.5 cm in diameter and 2 cm in height).

3.2. Impregnation Solution

In the conducted research, organic, cold-pressed red beet juice was used as an impregnation solution (Haus Rabenhorst, Unkel, Germany). The average values per 100 mL were as follows: energy: 155 kJ (37 kcal), fat: <0.5, carbohydrate: 8.0 g, fiber: <0.5 g, protein: <0.5 g, and salt: 0.13 g.

3.3. Pre-Treatment Before Drying Process

A vacuum impregnation (VI) process was used as the pre-treatment. VI was carried out according to the procedure described in our previous publication [26]. For each pre-treatment, three independent vacuum impregnations were performed. Weight gain (WG) was calculated according to the method by Tappi et al. (2022) [17]:

$$WG = 100 \cdot \frac{m - m_0}{m_0} \quad (1)$$

where

m—mass of the impregnated sample;
m_0—initial mass.

After the vacuum impregnation process, the samples (Table 9) were analyzed for selected bioactive properties and physical properties, and the remaining samples were subjected to a drying process.

Table 9. Material codes for raw and dried broccoli.

Code	Material	Type of Drying
B	Broccoli	-
B CD50	Broccoli	Convective drying at 50 °C
B CD70	Broccoli	Convective drying at 70 °C
BB	Broccoli after impregnation with beetroot juice	-
BB CD50	Broccoli after impregnation with beetroot juice	Convective drying at 50 °C
BB CD70	Broccoli after impregnation with beetroot juice	Convective drying at 70 °C

3.4. Convective Drying (CD)

The convective drying process was carried out at two set temperatures, 50 °C (CD50) and 70 °C (CD70), and an air flow of 1 $m \cdot s^{-1}$. Broccoli weights of 80 g were placed in six baskets, and the entire process was carried out in a drought in a dryer designed and built at the Institute of Agricultural Engineering (Wrocław, Poland) [54].

3.5. Bioactive Compounds, Antioxidant Capacity, and Phenols

3.5.1. Extraction Procedure

The dried samples were ground in a laboratory mill (IKA 11A, Staufen, Germany) and then sent for extraction. An amount of 0.5 g of powder samples was extracted with 2 mL of 80% methanol acidified with 1% HCl (*v*/*v*) for 24 h under refrigeration. The samples were subjected twice to sonication (300 W, 40 kHz; Sonic 6D, Polsonic, Warsaw, Poland) for 20 min with periodic shaking. The slurry was centrifuged at 19,000× *g* for 10 min. The supernatant was then filtered over a hydrophilic PTFE 0.20 µm membrane (Millex SamplicityTM filter, Merck, Darmstadt, Germany) and used for analysis.

3.5.2. Identification of Bioactive Compounds by UPLC-PDA–MS Method

The bioactive compounds in the broccoli samples were identified using an ACQUITY Ultra-Performance LC system (Waters Corporation, Milford, MA, USA) equipped with a photodiode array detector with a binary solvent manager and a mass detector G2 Q-

TOF micro-mass spectrometer (Waters, Manchester, UK) equipped with an electrospray ionization (ESI) source operating in negative mode. Individual compound separations were performed at 30 °C using a UPLC BEH C18 column (1.7 µm, 2.1 mm, 100 mm, Waters Corporation, Milford, MA, USA). The samples (10 µL) were injected, and the elution took 15 min using the linear gradients and isocratic flow rates described previously by Kolniak-Ostek and Oszmiański [55]. Full-scan, data-dependent MS scanning from *m/z* 100 to 2500 was used for the analysis. The retention duration and precise molecular masses were used to characterize the individual components. Before and after fragmentation, each chemical was optimized to its predicted molecular mass in the negative mode. The retention periods and spectra were compared to genuine standards.

3.5.3. Antioxidant Capacity (AC) and Total Phenolic Content (TPC)

In these studies, three methods of antioxidant capacity were used: DPPH [56], ABTS [57], and FRAP [58]. AC was determined using a Synergy H1 plate reader (BioTek, Winooski, VT, USA). Various concentrations of Trolox were used to prepare standard curves. All data obtained are expressed as Trolox equivalents per 100 g of broccoli dry matter (mMol Tx/100 g DM).

TPC was determined by using a modified method previously presented by Gao et al. [59]. In this study, we used 5 µL of methanolic broccoli extract, 10 µL of Folin–Ciocalteu reagent, 100 µL of H_2O, and 50 µL of 10% sodium carbonate, and then everything was mixed and shaken for 30 s. Total phenolic content was read after 1 h. The measurements were recorded at 765 nm on a Synergy H1 (BioTek, Winooski, VT, USA) and saved as mg of gallic acid per 1 g of broccoli dry matter (DM).

3.6. *Mathematical Modeling*

The moisture ratio (MR) was determined using the following equation [60]:

$$MR = \frac{M_t - M_e}{M_0 - M_e} \tag{2}$$

where M_t, M_e, and M_0, denote the moisture content achieved after the drying time, the equilibrium moisture content, and the initial moisture content, respectively.

Table 10 presents five popular mathematical models that were used in this study. A comparison of these models provided an opportunity to select the best model that describes convective drying.

Table 10. Mathematical models.

Number	Model Name	Equation
1	Page Model [61]	$MR = \exp(-k \cdot \tau^a)$
2	Henderdon and Pabis Model [62]	$MR = a \cdot \exp(-k\tau)$
3	Newton Model [63]	$MR = \exp(-k\tau)$
4	Logarithmic Model [53]	$MR = a \cdot \exp(-k\tau) + b \cdot \exp(-k_{ja} \cdot \tau)$
5	Logistic Model [64]	$MR = \frac{b}{(1 + a \cdot \exp(k \cdot \tau))}$

k—drying coefficient [min^{-1}]; a and b—coefficients of the equations; n—exponent; τ—time [min]; and MR—moisture ratio.

3.7. Physical Properties

3.7.1. Dry Weight

The dry weight of broccoli was determined using the vacuum dryer (Memmert, VO101, Schwabach, Germany) at 70 °C for 24 h under reduced pressure (5 kPa). The result was recorded as the average of three repetitions.

3.7.2. Water Activity

Water activity was measured at constant temperature (25 °C) using AquaLab 4TE ± 0.003 (AquaLab, Warsaw, Poland). Four measurements were taken and the final result was the average.

3.7.3. Bulk Density

The bulk density measurement was carried out using a measuring cylinder into which the tested material was poured, ensuring its even distribution without excessive compaction [65]. To increase the reliability of the results, the measurement was repeated six times. The bulk density was calculated based on the obtained results using the following formula:

$$\rho_b = \frac{w_s}{V} \quad (3)$$

where ρ_b, w_s, and V denote the bulk density [kg·m^{-3}], the weight of the samples [kg], and the volume [m^3], respectively.

3.7.4. Color

In order to examine the influence of the vacuum impregnation process, using beet juice as an impregnation solution and the temperature of the drying agent, three parameters were measured: L*, a*, and b*. The color of the broccoli was measured using a Minolta Chroma Meter CR-200 (Minolta Corp., Osaka, Japan). The color meter was calibrated against a standard white calibration plate. The values L*, a*, and b* were the average of 10 readings. The lightness coordinate L* measures the whiteness of the color and ranges from white at 100 to black at zero. The chromaticity coordinate a* determines the redness when the values are positive and the greenness when the values are negative. The third color coordinate b* measures the shade of yellow when the values are positive and the color blue when the values are negative. In addition, the following are calculated based on the three chromaticity coordinates: chroma (C*), browning index (BI), and color difference (ΔE) [47].

3.8. Statistical Analysis

Statistical analyses were performed using Statistica version 13.1 (StatSoft, Tulsa, OK, USA). A one-way analysis of variance (ANOVA) was used to assess differences between mean values, supplemented with Duncan's test as a post hoc method. Differences were considered statistically significant at the significance level of $p < 0.05$. Additionally, principal component analysis (PCA) was performed to determine the relationships between physicochemical properties of broccoli and the drying method and vacuum impregnation process.

4. Conclusions

In this study, a vacuum impregnation process using beetroot juice and different hot-air drying temperatures (50 and 70 °C) was demonstrated to influence both the physical properties and bioactive compounds, antioxidant capacity, and polyphenol content of broccoli.

The best fit of the models to the experimental data was obtained using the modified Page model and a logistic model. In general, the process that gave good results and is the recommended drying method was CD at 70 °C; it showed higher values of bioactive compounds, antioxidant capacity, and polyphenols. The drying time required for CD 70 was 48.28% shorter for broccoli without pre-treatment and 51.43% shorter for broccoli after the VI process compared to convective drying at 50 °C.

The use of the vacuum impregnation process resulted in a 20.69% increase in drying time for broccoli samples dried at 50 °C (CD50) with VI and a 20% increase for samples dried at 70 °C (CD70). In the samples after VI, a higher polyphenol content and antioxidant capacity measured by the FRAP method were recorded. Additionally, bioactive compounds characteristic of beetroot were identified. In addition, the use of VI increased the density of the tested materials. The use of VI lowered the brightness value, which is related to the drying process and the type of impregnating solution used, and a higher red value was recorded.

In conclusion, the findings of this study provide crucial insights for industrial applications, suggesting that the vacuum impregnation process using beetroot juice may change the physical and chemical properties of broccoli. This research can provide inspiration for the development of innovative, healthy, and functional vegetable snacks. The vacuum impregnation process and the type of impregnation solution used significantly affect the properties of the vegetables studied. In addition, drying temperature is a core parameter for broccoli processing, which affects its properties and processing time. Future research may focus on the use of equally bioactive impregnation solutions and the application of additional drying methods such as microwave drying or vacuum drying. Therefore, the findings in this study serve as a platform for future research on the production of dried vegetables and the high-value and innovative usage of broccoli.

5. Patents

Patent Poland, no. 421913. Vacuum impregnating machine and method for initial processing of material. Wrocław University of Environmental and Life Sciences, Wrocław, PL. Authors: Bogdan Stępień, Radosław Maślankowski, Leszek Rydzak, and Marta Pasławska.

Author Contributions: Conceptualization, M.K.; Data Curation, M.K.; Formal Analysis, M.K.; Funding Acquisition, M.K.; Investigation, M.K. and J.L-O.; Methodology, M.K. and J.K.-O.; Project Administration, M.K.; Resources, M.K.; Software, M.K. and M.C.; Supervision, M.K.; Validation, M.K.; Visualization, M.K. and M.C.; Writing—Original Draft Preparation, M.K. and J.K.-O.; Writing—Review and Editing, M.K., J.L-O. and B.S. All authors have read and agreed to the published version of the manuscript.

Funding: The APC is financed by Wrocław University of Environmental and Life Sciences.

Institutional Review Board Statement: Not applicable.

Informed Consent Statement: Not applicable.

Data Availability Statement: Data are contained within the article.

Conflicts of Interest: The authors declare no conflicts of interest.

References

1. Manríquez-Zúñiga, A.N.; de la Torre, A.R.; Valdés-Santiago, L.; Hernández-Bustos, D.A.; Cuéllar-Sojo, S.; Hernández-Rayas, A.; Perez-Vega, S.; Molina-Guerrero, C.E. Broccoli Leaves (*Brassica oleracea* var. *italica*) as a Source of Bioactive Compounds and Chemical Building Blocks: Optimal Extraction Using Dynamic Maceration and Life Cycle Assessment. *Sustainability* **2023**, *15*, 16616. [CrossRef]
2. Fanesi, B.; Ismaiel, L.; Nartea, A.; Orhotohwo, O.L.; Kuhalskaya, A.; Pacetti, D.; Lucci, P.; Falcone, P.M. Bioactives and Technological Quality of Functional Biscuits Containing Flour and Liquid Extracts from Broccoli By-Products. *Antioxidants* **2023**, *12*, 2115. [CrossRef]
3. Saavedra-Leos, M.Z.; Leyva-Porras, C.; Toxqui-Terán, A.; Espinosa-Solis, V. Physicochemical Properties and Antioxidant Activity of Spray-Dry Broccoli (*Brassica oleracea var Italica*) Stalk and Floret Juice Powders. *Molecules* **2021**, *26*, 1973. [CrossRef]

4. Czarnowska-Kujawska, M.; Draszanowska, A.; Chróst, M.; Starowicz, M. Effect of Sous-Vide Processing Time on Chemical and Sensory Properties of Broccoli, Green Beans and Beetroots. *Appl. Sci.* **2023**, *13*, 4086. [CrossRef]
5. Sawicki, T.; Bączek, N.; Wiczkowski, W. Betalain profile, content and antioxidant capacity of red beetroot dependent on the genotype and root part. *J. Funct. Foods* **2016**, *27*, 249–261. [CrossRef]
6. Sujinda, N.; Saengsuwan, T.; Chaichana, N. A study on drying characteristics, color, and vitamin C preservation of green banana slices using a vacuum heat pump system. *Agric. Eng.* **2024**, *28*, 176–184. [CrossRef]
7. Malkina, V.; Kiurchev, S.; Hutsol, T.; Verkholantseva, V.; Kiurcheva, L.; Miroshnichenko, M.; Biliuk, M.; Pidlisnyj, V.; Gurgulu, H.; Kowalczyk, Z. Optimization of parameters of a vibroconveyor system for infrared drying of soy. *Agric. Eng.* **2022**, *26*, 157–166. [CrossRef]
8. Gavahian, M.; Nayi, P.; Masztalerz, K.; Szumny, A.; Figiel, A. Cold plasma as an emerging energy-saving pretreatment to enhance food drying: Recent advances, mechanisms involved, and considerations for industrial applications. *Trends Food Sci. Technol.* **2024**, *143*, 104210. [CrossRef]
9. Menon, A.; Stojceska, V.; Tassou, S.A. A systematic review on the recent advances of the energy efficiency improvements in non-conventional food drying technologies. *Trends Food Sci. Technol.* **2020**, *100*, 67–76. [CrossRef]
10. Kroehnke, J.; Szadzińska, J.; Radziejewska-Kubzdela, E.; Biegańska-Marecik, R.; Musielak, G.; Mierzwa, D. Osmotic dehydration and convective drying of kiwifruit (*Actinidia deliciosa*)—The influence of ultrasound on process kinetics and product quality. *Ultrason. Sonochemistry* **2021**, *71*, 105377. [CrossRef]
11. Szychowski, P.J.; Lech, K.; Sendra-Nadal, E.; Hernández, F.; Figiel, A.; Wojdyło, A.; Carbonell-Barrachina, A.A. Kinetics, biocompounds, antioxidant activity, and sensory attributes of quinces as affected by drying method. *Food Chem.* **2018**, *255*, 157–164. [CrossRef]
12. Łyczko, J.; Masztalerz, K.; Lipan, L.; Iwiński, H.; Lech, K.; Carbonell-Barrachina, Á.A.; Szumny, A. *Coriandrum sativum* L.—Effect of Multiple Drying Techniques on Volatile and Sensory Profile. *Foods* **2021**, *10*, 403. [CrossRef]
13. Matys, A.; Nowacka, M.; Witrowa-Rajchert, D.; Wiktor, A. Chemical and Thermal Characteristics of PEF-Pretreated Strawberries Dried by Various Methods. *Molecules* **2024**, *29*, 3924. [CrossRef]
14. Mieszczakowska-Frąc, M.; Dyki, B.; Konopacka, D. Effects of Ultrasound on Polyphenol Retention in Apples After the Application of Predrying Treatments in Liquid Medium. *Food Bioprocess Technol.* **2016**, *9*, 543–552. [CrossRef]
15. Panayampadan, A.S.; Alam, M.S.; Aslam, R.; Kaur, J. Vacuum Impregnation Process and Its Potential in Modifying Sensory, Physicochemical and Nutritive Characteristics of Food Products. *Food Eng. Rev.* **2022**, *14*, 229–256. [CrossRef]
16. Aguirre-García, M.; Hernández-Carranza, P.; Cortés-Zavaleta, O.; Ruiz-Espinosa, H.; Ochoa-Velasco, C.E.; Ruiz-López, I.I. Mass transfer analysis of bioactive compounds in apple wedges impregnated with beetroot juice: A 3D modelling approach. *J. Food Eng.* **2020**, *282*, 110003. [CrossRef]
17. Tappi, S.; Velickova, E.; Mannozzi, C.; Tylewicz, U.; Laghi, L.; Rocculi, P. Multi-Analytical Approach to Study Fresh-Cut Apples Vacuum Impregnated with Different Solutions. *Foods* **2022**, *11*, 488. [CrossRef]
18. Nuñez, H.; Jaques, A.; Belmonte, K.; Elitin, J.; Valdenegro, M.; Ramírez, C.; Córdova, A. Development of an Apple Snack Enriched with Probiotic Lacticaseibacillus rhamnosus: Evaluation of the Refractance Window Drying Process on Cell Viability. *Foods* **2024**, *13*, 1756. [CrossRef]
19. Trusińska, M.; Drudi, F.; Rybak, K.; Tylewicz, U.; Nowacka, M. Effect of the Pulsed Electric Field Treatment on Physical, Chemical and Structural Changes of Vacuum Impregnated Apple Tissue in Aloe Vera Juices. *Foods* **2023**, *12*, 3957. [CrossRef]
20. Assis, F.R.; Rodrigues, L.G.G.; Tribuzi, G.; de Souza, P.G.; Carciofi, B.A.M.; Laurindo, J.B. Fortified apple (*Malus* spp., var. Fuji) snacks by vacuum impregnation of calcium lactate and convective drying. *LWT* **2019**, *113*, 108298. [CrossRef]
21. Chong, J.X.; Lai, S.; Yang, H. Chitosan combined with calcium chloride impacts fresh-cut honeydew melon by stabilising nanostructures of sodium-carbonate-soluble pectin. *Food Control* **2015**, *53*, 195–205. [CrossRef]
22. González-Pérez, J.E.; Jiménez-González, O.; Ramírez-Corona, N.; Guerrero-Beltrán, J.A.; López-Malo, A. Vacuum Impregnation on Apples with Grape Juice Concentrate: Effects of Pressure, Processing Time, and Juice Concentration. *Innov. Food Sci. Emerg. Technol.* **2022**, *77*, 102981. [CrossRef]
23. Demir, H.; Çelik, S.; Sezer, Y.Ç. Effect of ultrasonication and vacuum impregnation pretreatments on the quality of beef marinated in onion juice a natural meat tenderizer. *Food Sci. Technol. Int.* **2021**, *28*, 340–352. [CrossRef]
24. Arnal, M.; Gallego, M.; Mora, L.; Talens, P. Vacuum impregnation as a sustainable technology to obtain iron-fortified broad bean (*Vicia faba*) flours. *Food Funct.* **2023**, *14*, 5429–5441. [CrossRef]
25. de Oliveira, P.M.; Ramos, A.M.; Martins, E.M.F.; Vieira, É.N.R.; de Souza Soares, A.; de Noronha, M.C. Comparison of vacuum impregnation and soaking techniques for addition of the probiotic Lactobacillus acidophilus to minimally processed melon. *Int. J. Food Sci. Technol.* **2017**, *52*, 2547–2554. [CrossRef]
26. Kręcisz, M.; Stępień, B.; Łyczko, J.; Kamiński, P. The Influence of the Vacuum Impregnation, Beetroot Juice, and Various Drying Methods on Selected Properties of Courgette and Broccoli Snacks. *Foods* **2023**, *12*, 4294. [CrossRef]

27. Alzamora, S.M.; Salvatori, D.; Tapia, M.S.; López-Malo, A.; Welti-Chanes, J.; Fito, P. Novel functional foods from vegetable matrices impregnated with biologically active compounds. *J. Food Eng.* **2005**, *67*, 205–214. [CrossRef]
28. Vinod, B.R.; Asrey, R.; Sethi, S.; Menaka, M.; Meena, N.K.; Shivaswamy, G. Recent advances in vacuum impregnation of fruits and vegetables processing: A concise review. *Heliyon* **2024**, *10*, e28023. [CrossRef]
29. Fernandez-Leon, M.F.; Fernandez-Leon, A.M.; Lozano, M.; Ayuso, M.C.; Gonzalez-Gómez, D. Identification, quantification and comparison of the principal bioactive compounds and external quality parameters of two broccoli cultivars. *J. Funct. Foods* **2012**, *4*, 465–473. [CrossRef]
30. Vallejo, F.; Gil-Izquierdo, A.; Perez-Vicente, A.; García-Viguera, C. In vitro gastrointestinal digestion study of broccoli inflorescence phenolic compounds, glucosinolates, and vitamin C. *J. Agric. Food Chem.* **2024**, *52*, 135–138. [CrossRef]
31. Li, S.; Lin, J.; Wei, J.; Zhou, L.; Wang, P.; Qu, S. Sinigrin Impedes the Breast Cancer Cell Growth through the Inhibition of PI3K/AKT/MTOR Phosphorylation-Mediated Cell Cycle Arrest. *J. Environ. Pathol. Toxicol. Oncol.* **2022**, *41*, 33–43. [CrossRef]
32. Li, Y.; Zhang, T. Targeting cancer stem cells with sulforaphane, a dietary component from broccoli and broccoli sprouts. *Future Oncol.* **2013**, *9*, 1097–1103. [CrossRef]
33. Gudino, I.; Martin, A.; Casquete, R.; Prieto, M.H.; Ayuso, M.C.; Córdoba, M.G. Evaluation of broccoli (*Brassica oleracea* var. italica) crop by-products as sources of bioactive compounds. *Sci. Hortic.* **2022**, *304*, 111284. [CrossRef]
34. Sallas-Millan, J.A.; Aznar, A.; Conesa, E.; Conesa-Bueno, A.; Aguayo, E. Functional food obtained from fermentation of broccoli by-products (stalk): Metagenomics profile and glucosinolate and phenolic compounds characterization by LC-ESI-QqQ-MS/MS. *LWT-Food Sci. Technol.* **2022**, *169*, 113915. [CrossRef]
35. Kujala, T.S.; Vienola, M.S.; Klika, K.D.; Loponen, J.M.; Pihjala, K. Betalain and phenolic compositions of four beetroot (*Beta vulgaris*) cultivars. *Eur. Food Res. Technol.* **2002**, *214*, 505–510. [CrossRef]
36. Radziejewska-Kubzdela, E.; Biegańska-Marecik, R.; Kidoń, M. Zastosowanie impregnacji próżniowej do modyfikacji właściwości fizykochemicznych, sensorycznych i odżywczych produktów pochodzenia roślinnego—Przegląd. *Int. J. Mol. Sci.* **2014**, *15*, 16577. [CrossRef]
37. Anaya-Esparza, L.M.; Rodríguez-Lafitte, E.; Villagrán, Z.; Aurora-Vigo, E.F.; Ruvalcaba-Gómez, J.M.; Símpalo-López, W.B.; Martínez-Esquivias, F.; Sarango-Córdova, C.H. Optimization of Vacuum Impregnation with Aqueous Extract from Hibiscus sabdariffa Calyces in Apple Slices by Response Surface Methodology: Effect on Soluble Phenols, Flavonoids, Antioxidant Activity, and Physicochemical Parameters. *Appl. Sci.* **2024**, *14*, 10850. [CrossRef]
38. Nawirska-Olszańska, A.; Pasławska, M.; Stępień, B.; Oziembłowski, M.; Sala, K.; Smorowska, A. Effect of Vacuum Impregnation with Apple-Pear Juice on Content of Bioactive Compounds and Antioxidant Activity of Dried Chokeberry Fruit. *Foods* **2020**, *9*, 108. [CrossRef]
39. Kręcisz, M.; Kolniak-Ostek, J.; Stępień, B.; Łyczko, J.; Pasławska, M.; Musiałowska, J. Influence of Drying Methods and Vacuum Impregnation on Selected Quality Factors of Dried Sweet Potato. *Agriculture* **2021**, *11*, 858. [CrossRef]
40. Kręcisz, M.; Kolniak-Ostek, J.; Łyczko, J.; Stępień, B. Evaluation of bioactive compounds, volatile compounds, drying process kinetics and selected physical properties of vacuum impregnation celery dried by different methods. *Food Chem.* **2023**, *413*, 135490. [CrossRef]
41. Sarabandi, K.; Jafari, S.M.; Mahoonak, A.S.; Mohammadi, A. Application of gum Arabic and maltodextrin for encapsulation of eggplant peel extract as a natural antioxidant and color source. *Int. J. Biol. Macromol.* **2019**, *140*, 59–68. [CrossRef] [PubMed]
42. Radziejewska-Kubzdela, E.; Szadzińska, J.; Biegańska-Marecik, R.; Spiżewski, T.; Mierzwa, D. Effect of ultrasound on mass transfer during vacuum impregnation and selected quality parameters of products: A case study of carrots. *Ultrason. Sonochemistry* **2023**, *99*, 106592. [CrossRef] [PubMed]
43. Yusoff, I.M.; Mat Taher, Z.; Rahmat, Z.; Chua, L.S. A review of ultrasound-assisted extraction for plant bioactive compounds: Phenolics, flavonoids, thymols, saponins and proteins. *Food Res. Int.* **2022**, *157*, 111268. [CrossRef]
44. Rahaman, A.; Zeng, X.A.; Kumari, A.; Rafiq, M.; Siddeeg, A.; Manzoor, M.F.; Baloch, Z.; Ahmed, Z. Influence of ultrasound-assisted osmotic dehydration on texture, bioactive compounds and metabolites analysis of plum. *Ultrason. Sonochemistry* **2019**, *58*, 104643. [CrossRef]
45. Md Salim, N.S.; Gariépy, Y.; Raghavan, V. Suszenie gorącym powietrzem i suszenie gorącym powietrzem wspomagane mikrofalami plastrów łodyg brokułów (*Brassica oleracea* L. var. *Italica). J. Food Process Preserv.* **2016**, *41*, e12905. [CrossRef]
46. Zielinska, M.; Markowski, M. Air drying characteristics and moisture diffusivity of carrots. *Chem. Eng. Process. Process Intensif.* **2010**, *49*, 212–218. [CrossRef]
47. Kręcisz, M.; Klemens, M.; Latański, A.; Stępień, B. The Use of Beetroot Juice as an Impregnating Solution to Change Volatile Compounds, Physical Properties and Influence the Kinetics of the Celery Drying Process. *Molecules* **2024**, *29*, 4050. [CrossRef] [PubMed]
48. Kręcisz, M.; Stępień, B.; Pasławska, M.; Popłoński, J.; Dulak, K. Physicochemical and Quality Properties of Dried Courgette Slices: Impact of Vacuum Impregnation and Drying Methods. *Molecules* **2021**, *26*, 4597. [CrossRef]

49. Kręcisz, M.; Stępień, B.; Pikor, K. Effect of Tomato Juice and Different Drying Methods on Selected Properties of Courgette. *Appl. Sci.* **2024**, *14*, 7105. [CrossRef]
50. Liu, K.; Hao, Y.; Chen, Y.; Gao, Q. Effects of dry heat treatment on the structure and physicochemical properties of waxy potato starch. *Int. J. Biol. Macromol.* **2019**, *132*, 1044–1050. [CrossRef]
51. Xu, H.; Wu, M.; Zhang, X.; Wang, B.; Wang, S.; Zheng, Z.; Li, D.; Wang, F. Application of blanching pretreatment in herbaceous peony (*Paeonia lactiflora* Pall.) flower processing: Improved drying efficiency, enriched volatile profile and increased phytochemical content. *Ind. Crops Prod.* **2022**, *188*, 115663. [CrossRef]
52. Mowafy, S.; Guo, J.; Lei, D.; Liu, Y. Application of novel blanching and drying technologies improves the potato drying kinetics and maintains its physicochemical attributes and flour functional properties. *Innov. Food Sci. Emerg. Technol.* **2024**, *94*, 103648. [CrossRef]
53. Arslan, D.; Musa Özcan, M.M.; Mengeş, H.O. Evaluation of drying methods with respect to drying parameters, some nutritional and colour characteristics of peppermint (*Mentha* x *piperita* L.). *Energy Convers. Manag.* **2010**, *51*, 2769–2775. [CrossRef]
54. Jałoszyński, K.; Szarycz, M.; Jarosz, B. The Effect of Convective and Microwave-Vacuum Drying on the Preservation of Aromatic Compounds in Parsley (PL). *Agric. Eng.* **2006**, *12*, 209–215.
55. Kolniak-Ostek, J.; Oszmianski, J. Characterization of phenolic compounds in different anatomical pear (*Pyrus communis* L.) parts by ultra-performance liquid chromatography photodiode detector-quadrupole/time of flight-mass spectrometry (UPLC-PDA-Q/TOF-MS). *Int. J. Mass Spectrom.* **2015**, *392*, 154–163. [CrossRef]
56. Yen, G.-C.; Chen, H.-Y. Antioxidant Activity of Various Tea Extracts in Relation to Their Antimutagenicity. *J. Agric. Food Chem.* **1995**, *43*, 27–32. [CrossRef]
57. Re, R.; Pellegrini, N.; Proteggente, A.; Pannala, A.; Yang, M.; Rice-Evans, C. Antioxidant activity applying an improved ABTS radical cation decolorization assay. *Free Radic. Biol. Med.* **1999**, *26*, 1231–1237. [CrossRef]
58. Benzie, I.F.F.; Strain, J.J. The ferric reducing ability of plasma (FRAP) as a measure of "antioxidant power": The FRAP assay. *Anal. Biochem.* **1996**, *239*, 70–76. [CrossRef]
59. Gao, X.; Ohlander, M.; Jeppsson, N.; Björk, L.; Trajkovski, V. Changes in antioxidant effects and their relationship to phytonutrients in fruits of Sea Buckthorn (*Hippophae rhamnoides* L.) during maturation. *J. Agric. Food Chem.* **2000**, *48*, 1485–1490. [CrossRef]
60. Kaushal, P.; Sharma, H.K. Osmo-convective dehydration kinetics of jackfruit (*Artocarpus heterophyllus*). *J. Saudi Soc. Agric. Sci.* **2016**, *15*, 118–126. [CrossRef]
61. Sarimeseli, A. Microwave drying characteristics of coriander (*Coriandrum sativum* L.) leaves. *Energy Convers. Manag.* **2011**, *52*, 1449–1453. [CrossRef]
62. Henderson, S.M.; Pabis, S. Grain Drying Theory II: Temperature Effect on Drying Coefficient. *J. Agric. Eng. Res.* **1961**, *6*, 169–174.
63. Demir, V.; Gunhan, T.; Yagcioglu, A.K.; Degrmencioglu, A. Mathematical modeling and the determination of some quality parameters of air-dried bay leaves. *Biosyst. Eng.* **2004**, *88*, 325–335. [CrossRef]
64. Soysal, Y.; Öztekin, S.; Eren, Ö. Microwave drying of parsley: Modeling, kinetics, and energy aspects. *Biosyst. Eng.* **2006**, *93*, 403–413. [CrossRef]
65. *ASAE S269.3*; Wafers, Pellet, and Crumbles—Definitions and Methods for Determining Density, Durability and Moisture Content. ASAE Standard: Washington, DC, USA, 1989.

molecules

MDPI

Article

In Vitro Multi-Bioactive Potential of Enzymatic Hydrolysis of a Non-Toxic *Jatropha curcas* Cake Protein Isolate

Olloqui Enrique Javier [1,*], González-Rodríguez Maurilio Alejandro [2], Contreras-López Elizabeth [2], Pérez-Flores Jesús Guadalupe [2], Pérez-Escalante Emmanuel [2,3], Moreno-Seceña Juan Carlos [4,*] and Martínez-Carrera Daniel [1,*]

1 Centro de Biotecnología de Hongos Comestibles, Funcionales y Medicinales (CB-HCFM), Colegio de Postgraduados, Campus Puebla, Boulevard Forjadores de Puebla no. 205, Puebla 72760, Mexico
2 Área Académica de Química, Instituto de Ciencias Básicas e Ingeniería, Universidad Autónoma del Estado de Hidalgo, Carretera Pachuca-Tulancingo km 4.5, Mineral de la Reforma, Hidalgo 42185, Mexico
3 Departamento de Biotecnología, División de Ciencias Biológicas y de la Salud, Universidad Autónoma Metropolitana, Campus Iztapalapa, Avenida San Rafael Atlixco 186, Mexico City 09340, Mexico
4 Colegio de Postgraduados, Campus Montecillo, Carretera Mexico-Texcoco km 36.5, Texcoco 56264, Mexico
* Correspondence: olloqui.jose@colpos.mx (O.E.J.); moreno.juancarlos@colpos.mx (M.-S.J.C.); dcarrera@colpos.mx (M.-C.D.)

Abstract: The *Jatropha curcas* cake, a protein-rich by-product of biofuel production, was the subject of our study. We identified and quantified the ACE inhibitory, antioxidant, and antidiabetic activities of bioactive peptides from a *Jatropha curcas* L. var Sevangel protein isolate. The protein isolate (20.44% recovered dry matter, 38.75% protein content, and 34.98% protein yield) was subjected to two enzyme systems for hydrolysis: alcalase (PEJA) and flavourzyme (PEJF), recording every 2 h until 8 h had passed. The highest proteolytic capacity in PEJA was reached at 2 h (4041.38 ± 50.89), while in PEJF, it was reached at 6 h (3435.16 ± 59.31). Gel electrophoresis of the PEJA and PEJF samples showed bands corresponding to peptides smaller than 10 kDa in both systems studied. The highest values for the antioxidant capacity (DPPH) were obtained at 4 h for PEJA (56.17 ± 1.14), while they were obtained at 6 h for PEJF (26.64 ± 0.52). The highest values for the antihypertensive capacity were recorded at 6 h (86.46 ± 1.85) in PEJF. The highest antidiabetic capacity obtained for PEJA and PEJF was observed at 6 h, 68.86 ± 8.27 and 52.75 ± 2.23, respectively. This is the first report of their antidiabetic activity. Notably, alcalase hydrolysate outperformed flavourzyme hydrolysate and the cereals reported in other studies, confirming its better multi-bioactivity.

Keywords: *Jatropha curcas*; bioactive peptides; antioxidant; antihypertensive; antidiabetic; alcalase; flavourzyme

1. Introduction

Global use of green technologies is necessary for a sustainable future. Biofuels are an alternative to meet the demand to overcome the detrimental dependence on fossil fuels [1]. One primary biofuel source is *Jatropha curcas*, widely cultivated worldwide due to its adaptability to different climatic conditions [2]. *Jatropha curcas* cake is obtained after the extraction of its oil for use as biofuel. This waste product of refining can play a crucial role in food and nutrition [3].

The main limiting factor for the consumption of *Jatropha curcas* is the presence of toxic phorbol esters. However, non-toxic genotypes have been reported to have the potential to be used in animal diets or for human consumption [3]. From a nutritional point of view, there are reports on the chemical composition of *Jatropha curcas*, which stands out for its high crude protein content and as a source of essential amino acids. These characteristics make it a source for obtaining bioactive peptides (BPs) reported to have antimicrobial, antidiabetic, antihypertensive, hypocholesterolemic, immunomodulatory, and other properties. Bioactive peptides are generally obtained by bacterial or enzymatic hydrolysis [4]. Enzymatic hydrolysis is a simple process that presents good regioselectivity and stereoselectivity, a higher reaction speed to cleave proteins, and enzymes that are easy to inactivate. The most popular commercial enzymes are alcalase® (USA, MA), protamex® (USA, MA), and flavourzyme® (USA, MA) [5]. This is in contrast to microbial fermentation, which is susceptible to low reproducibility with unexpected deviations in hydrolysis and inconsistency in the production of bioactive peptides industrially [5].

Marrufo-Estrada et al. [6] reported the generation of BPs from a protein isolate of *Jatropha curcas* L. (toxic genotype) by enzymatic hydrolysis of alcalase and pepsin–pancreatin, finding low-molecular-weight peptides with ACE inhibitory, antithrombotic and antioxidant activities.

The objectives of this work are to identify and quantify the ACE inhibitory, antioxidant, and antidiabetic activities of a protein isolate from *Jatropha curcas* L. var. Sevangel (no-toxic), which was hydrolyzed with alcalase and flavourzyme.

2. Results and Discussion

2.1. Protein Extraction

Jatropha curcas cake is mainly composed of glutelins and globulins [7]. Glutelins are soluble in acid and base solutions, while globulins are soluble in saline solutions. These factors are determinants of the solubility of the protein and, therefore, its yield [8]. The protein extract of *Jatropha* cake showed 20.44 ± 2.46% dry matter recovered, 38.75 ± 2.10% protein content, and 34.98 ± 1.92% protein yield. Specifically, the dry matter recovered, protein content, and protein yield in this work were equivalent to those Ahluwalia et al. [9] reported. *Jatropha* seed cake from Delhi, India, obtained values of 17.10% dry matter, 41.98% protein content, and 38.66% protein yield, suggesting a difference in agroecological conditions, a determinant of these parameters.

2.2. Proteolytic Capacity

2.2.1. Analysis of Free Amino Groups

As shown in Table 1, the amino groups increased as the hydrolysis times increased. An increase was observed in the PEJA system at 2 h, reaching 4041.38 ± 50.89 ppm with no statistical difference with subsequent measurements ($p \geq 0.05$). Therefore, under these conditions, the PEJA system obtained a higher degree of hydrolysis in a relatively short time. On the other hand, an increase was observed as time passed in the PEJF system up to 6 h, obtaining 3435.16 ± 59.31 ppm with no statistical difference with 8 h ($p \geq 0.05$). The concentration of free amino groups depends on the enzyme used in each proteolytic system. In the case of *Jatropha curcas* L. var. Sevangel cake, the primary amino acids present were tyrosine, glutamine, histidine, and proline [3], hydrophobic amino acids where alcalase can cleave the peptide bonds of the carboxylic termini, obtaining an increase in the degree of hydrolysis compared to the PEJF system [10]. On the other hand, flavourzyme possesses activity in relation to neutral proteases, alkaline protease, leucine aminopeptidase, dipeptidyl peptidase, and amylase, taking on the role of hydrolyzing such proteins [11]. Therefore, these results suggest that *Jatropha curcas* L. var. Sevangel is a suitable substrate for alcalase and flavourzyme hydrolysis.

Table 1. Hydrolysis degree and bioactivities (antioxidant, antihypertensive, and antidiabetic) with alcalase and flavourzyme of *Jatropha curcas* L. var Sevangel protein extract hydrolysates.

Time (h)	Hydrolysis Degree (ppm)	FRAP (mmol Fe^{2+})	DPPH (mmol Trolox)	ACE-I Inhibition (%)	DPP-IV Inhibition (%)
Alcalase					
0	1277.25 ± 119.26 ^{a}	15.45 ± 3.31 ^{a}	18.11 ± 1.71 ^{a}	87.34 ± 0.62	20.50 ± 1.02 ^{a}
2	4041.38 ± 50.89 ^{bc}	18.80 ± 1.82 ^{a}	46.17 ± 0.86 ^{b}	80.57 ± 5.25	40.87 ± 2.04 ^{b}

Table 1. *Cont.*

Time (h)	Hydrolysis Degree (ppm)	FRAP (mmol Fe^{2+})	DPPH (mmol Trolox)	ACE-I Inhibition (%)	DPP-IV Inhibition (%)
4	3802.28 ± 267.04 [b]	19.19 ± 1.23 [a]	56.17 ± 1.14 [c]	83.19 ± 4.63	32.07 ± 0.19 [ab]
6	4437.48 ± 345.70 [c]	28.33 ± 0.55 [b]	57.01 ± 0.34 [cd]	81.64 ± 0.03	68.86 ± 8.27 [c]
8	4514.77 ± 163.79 [c]	24.87 ± 0.60 [b]	59.70 ± 0.30 [d]	91.70 ± 1.24	43.10 ± 2.57 [b]
Flavourzyme					
0	859.86 ± 13.28 [a]	14.77 ± 1.44 [a]	10.35 ± 0.90 [a]	81.00 ± 0.93 [a]	28.02 ± 1.75 [a]
2	2090.29 ± 83.90 [b]	14.68 ± 0.12 [a]	16.72 ± 0.95 [b]	80.79 ± 0.62 [a]	39.59 ± 3.35 [b]
4	2901.40 ± 73.30 [c]	14.51 ± 0.12 [a]	22.95 ± 0.37 [c]	80.57 ± 0.31 [a]	24.59 ± 0.84 [a]
6	3435.16 ± 59.31 [d]	18.26 ± 0.84 [b]	26.64 ± 0.52 [d]	86.46 ± 1.85 [b]	52.75 ± 2.23 [c]
8	3843.34 ± 333.33 [d]	20.73 ± 0.96 [b]	24.70 ± 1.00 [cd]	88.43 ± 0.31 [b]	50.17 ± 1.51 [c]

FRAP: ferric-reducing antioxidant power; DPPH: 2,2-diphenyl-1-picrylhydrazyl; ACE-I: angiotensin I-converting enzyme; DPP-IV: dipeptidyl peptidase IV. The DPPH and FRAP results are expressed in 100 mL of hydrolysate. All the results are expressed as the mean ± standard deviation. Different letters between rows for each enzyme system indicate significant differences ($p \leq 0.05$). The table shows that maximum values obtained for the bioactivities of both the alcalase and flavourzyme systems correspond to 6 h of hydrolysis, except for DPPH (4 h) in the alcalase system. There was no statistical difference in ACE inhibition for the alcalase system.

2.2.2. Separation of Peptides by Tris-Glycine-SDS-PAGE

Gel electrophoresis showed that the protein isolate of *Jatropha curcas* L. var. Sevangel presents a complex protein profile of 15 bands between 2 and 50 KDa (Figure 1). The large number of low-molecular-weight bands at 6 h in both hydrolysis systems suggests an extensive hydrolysis, consequently producing small peptides. The low number of electrophoretic bands at time 0 and 2 h was caused by a low degree of hydrolysis (Table 1).

In the electrophoresis gel, bands with molecular weights related to globulins and glutelins, ranging from 15 to 50 KDa, can be observed, as reported by León-Villanueva et al. [7], and are observed to degrade as the hydrolysis time increases. This is closely related to the specificity of the enzymes used in producing the hydrolysis of the PEJ proteins. There is evidence of peptides in *Jatropha curcas* seed with a molecular weight between 693 and 1342 Da with bioactivities such as immunomodulatory, antimalarial, and antimicrobial [12]. Gel electrophoresis of PEJA and PEJF samples showed bands corresponding to peptides smaller than 10 kDa in both systems studied (Figures 1 and 2). Evidence shows that peptides smaller than 10 kDa have antioxidant, antihypertensive, and antidiabetic properties [13]. The accumulation of peptides ≤ 10 KDa was higher in the alcalase system (PEJA) compared to the flavourzyme system (PEJF) (Figures 3 and 4). This is associated with the high catalytic capacity due to the wide range of amino acids that can be recognized by the alcalase enzyme generating hydrolysates with small peptides. The accumulation of low-molecular-weight peptides reported in both systems (PEJA and PEJF) in the present study is higher than that reported by Marrufo-Estrada et al. [6] in a protein isolate of a toxic genotype of *Jatropha curcas* in systems with alcalase and sequential systems with pepsin–pancreatin at 60, 90 and 120 min of hydrolysis. These results suggest that the hydrolysis time, the enzyme/protein ratio and the non-toxic genotype of *Jatropha curcas* influence the degree of hydrolysis.

According to the presence of antioxidant and antihypertensive bioactivities, the peptides of interest are equal to and/or less than 10 KDa [14,15]. Therefore, during enzymatic hydrolysis, an increase in hydrolysis can be observed from the initial time. At the initial time (0 h), 2 h, 4 h, 6 h, and 8 h for the alcalase system, we reported 11.4%, 15.9%, 18.6%, 15.9%, and 27.6%, respectively, in bands ≤ 10 KDa. In the case of the flavourzyme system, 34.3%, 22.0%, 17.7%, 11.2%, and 25.1% were reported for times 0 h, 2 h, 4 h, 6 h, and 8 h, respectively (Figures 3 and 4). No relationship was observed between 6 h, the time with the highest bioactivity in both systems, and the highest concentration of peptides ≤ 10 KDa.

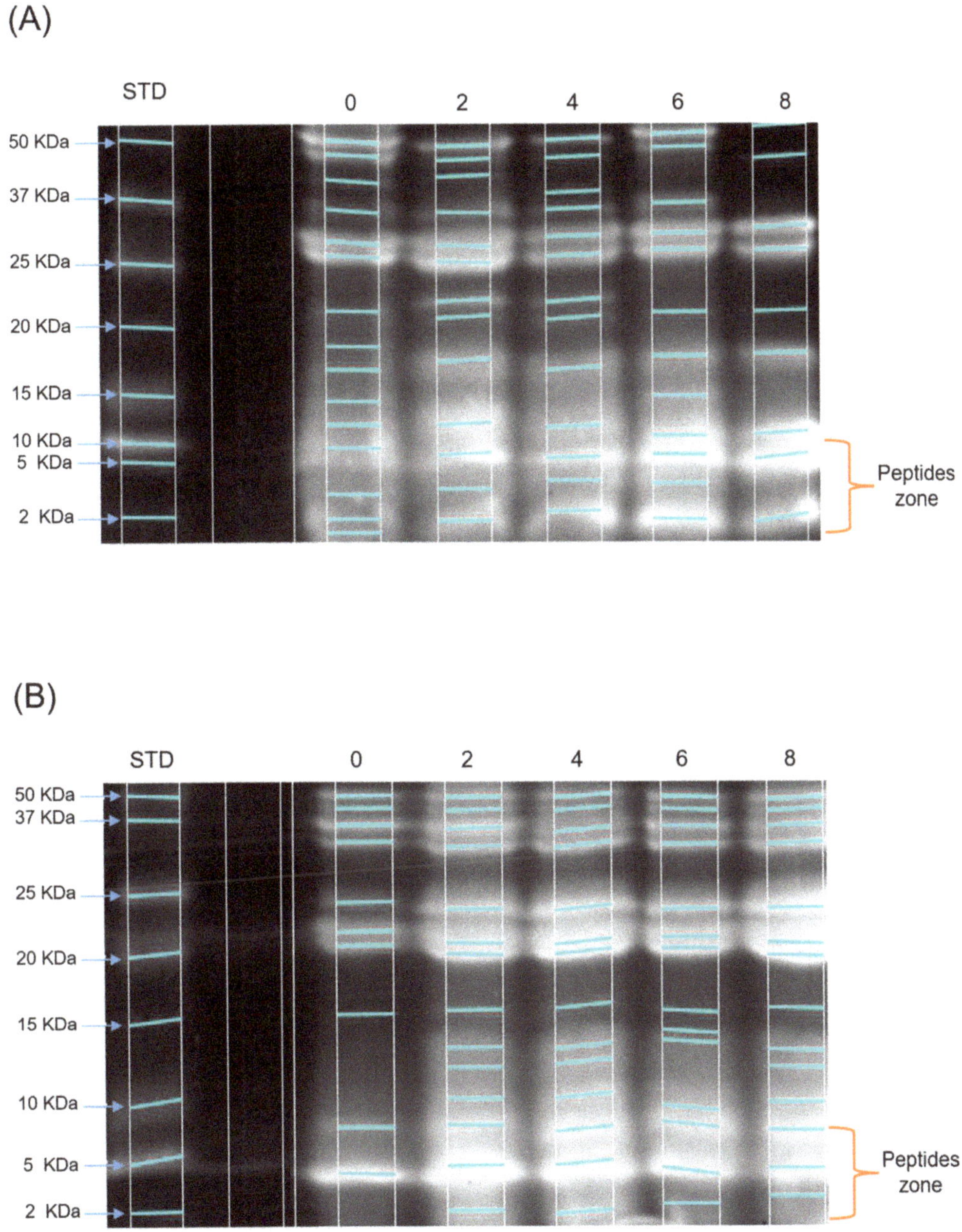

Figure 1. Peptide separation by Tris-Tricine-SDS-PAGE in a protein extract of *Jatropha* hydrolyzed with alcalase (**A**) and a protein extract of *Jatropha* hydrolyzed with flavourzyme (**B**). STD: peptides standard. Hydrolysis time (0–8 h). On the left side of A and B, the molecular mass range of the peptides is observed from 2 to 50 KDa. The blue lines indicate the bands detected in each lane of the electrophoresis gel. The peptide zones of interest in this study are in the range of 2–10 KDa.

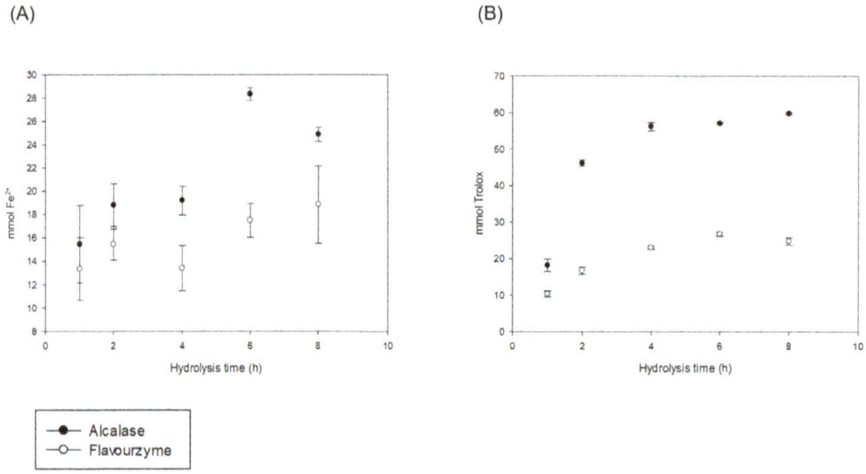

Figure 2. Antioxidant activity by FRAP (**A**) and DPPH (**B**) methods with alcalase and flavourzyme of hydrolysates of a protein extract of *Jatropha curcas* L. var. Sevangel. Results are expressed in 100 mL as mean ± standard error. FRAP: ferric-reducing antioxidant power; DPPH: 2,2-diphenyl-1-picrylhydrazyl hydrolysis time (0–8 h). This figure shows that the alcalase system had higher antioxidant activity than the flavourzyme system at all hydrolysis times, especially at 6 h for DPPH and 4 h for FRAP.

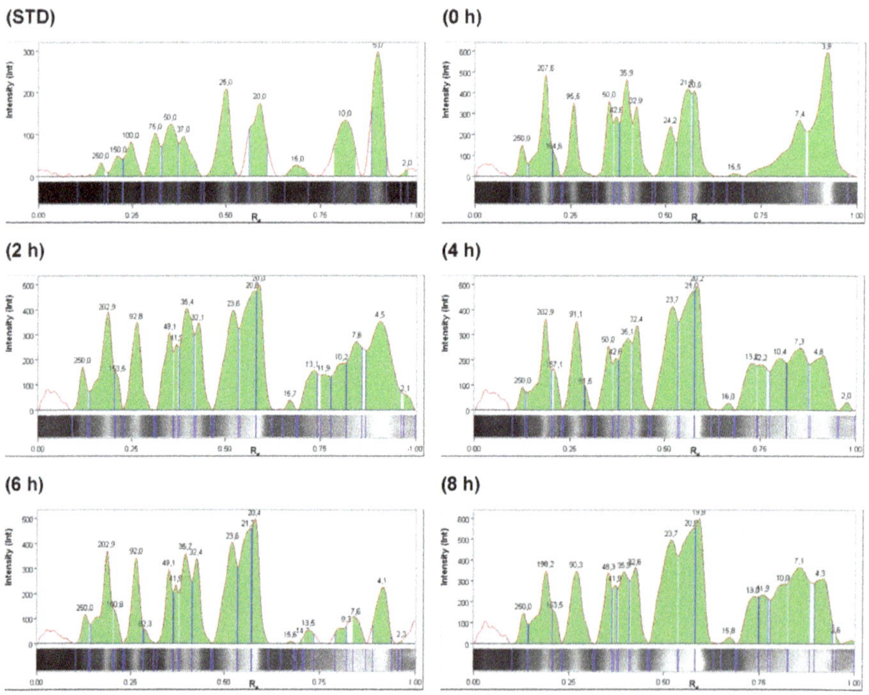

Figure 3. Electropherogram profile at 0 h, 2 h, 4 h, 6 h, and 8 h in *Jatropha* protein extract hydrolyzed with alcalase. STD: peptide standard. The green area in the figure represents the molecular weight concentration of the peptides; for more information see the Data Availability Statement. This figure shows an increase in the concentrations of various peptides ≤ 10 KDa for the initial time (0 h).

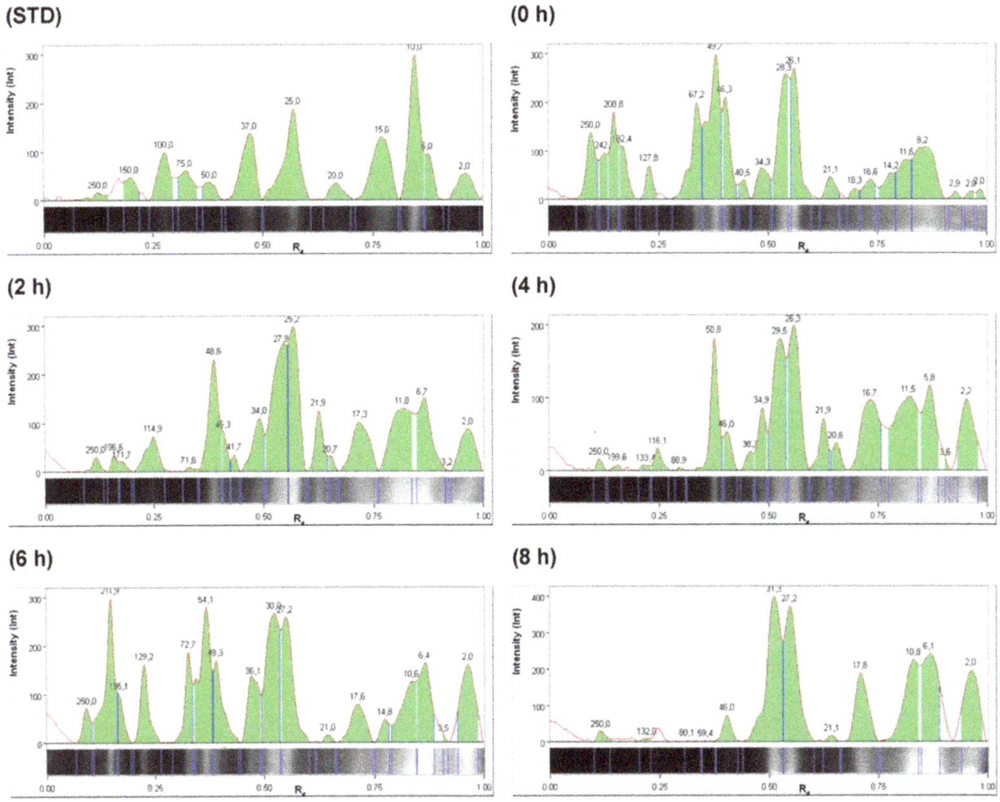

Figure 4. Electropherogram profile at 0 h, 2 h, 4 h, 6 h, and 8 h in *Jatropha* protein extract hydrolyzed with flavourzyme. STD: peptide standard. The green area in the figure represents the molecular weight concentration of the peptides; for more information see the Data Availability Statement. This figure shows an increase in the concentrations of various peptides $\leq$ 10 KDa for the initial time (0 h).

2.3. Antioxidant Activity

Oxidative stress generates many health disorders, such as anti-inflammatory diseases related to tissue damage, cancer, atherosclerosis, diabetes mellitus, and neurodegenerative diseases [13]. The FRAP test is based on the reductive power of the protein hydrolysates in both systems, which was determined by the ability to reduce Fe^{3+} to Fe^{2+}, which indicates the antioxidant capacity by electron donation [16]. On the other hand, the free radical-scavenging activity in the hydrolysis systems was determined using DPPH, a stable free radical, to evaluate the antioxidant activity [17].

The results are presented in Table 1 and Figure 2, where the antioxidant properties are observed in the control times. Subsequently, a linear increase occurs concerning the hydrolysis time, increasing to 6 h in both hydrolysis systems ($p \leq 0.05$), except for DPPH (4 h) in the alcalase system. Gallegos-Tintoré et al. [18] hydrolyzed a *Jatropha curcas* protein extract with alcalase for 60 min. They observed similar behavior in terms of the antioxidant properties, obtaining an increase in antioxidant activity in the final hydrolysis phase.

These results are consistent with other studies of enzymatic hydrolysis in plant proteins, where it has been found that as the degree of hydrolysis increases, the antioxidant activities of the hydrolysates increase [13]. The PEJA samples were the hydrolysates that obtained higher antioxidant activity concerning PEJF. This is due to the high selectivity and specificity in the cleavage during protein hydrolysis, obtaining a lower molecular weight and its accumulation during hydrolysis [13]. This antioxidant activity is because peptides with a molecular weight of less than 3 kDa present high antioxidant activity [14].

Similarly, Marrufo-Estrada et al. [6] showed that the highest antioxidant capacity in a protein hydrolysate of *Jatropha curcas* (toxic genotype) was found in a sequential hydrolysis system with pepsin and pancreatin. This is related to an increased degree of hydrolysis in this system compared to the alcalase system.

2.4. Antihypertensive Activity

Table 1 shows the results obtained for the ACE inhibitory activity in both hydrolysis systems. PEJA showed an ACE inhibition of 81.64–91.70% with no difference between the hydrolysis times ($p \geq 0.05$). In the flavourzyme system, the greatest increase in ACE inhibition was observed at 6 h of hydrolysis with 86.46% ($p \leq 0.05$). These results suggest that the protein concentrate of *Jatropha curcas* L. var. Sevangel cake has antihypertensive activity per se. This differs from the data reported by Marrufo-Estrada et al. [6] in relation to a toxic genotype, as they found an increase at 2 h of hydrolysis with the alcalase system. This is possibly due to the differences between the varieties and climatic conditions among *Jatropha curcas* varieties.

On the other hand, PEJF obtained an ACE inhibition of 80.57–88.43%. However, 6 and 8 h showed an ACE inhibition of 86.46% and 88.43%, respectively, with no statistical difference ($p \geq 0.05$). Therefore, at 6 h of hydrolysis with flavourzyme, the highest values of ACE inhibition were obtained.

The observed ACE-I inhibitory activity was higher than that reported for a *Jatropha curcas* L. hydrolysate with alcalase for 1 h (34.87%) [15]. It was even higher than that reported for amaranth hydrolysates for 4 h with alcalase and flavourzyme with 49.49 and 39.77%, respectively [19].

The high ACE inhibitory activity presented in both hydrolysis systems shows the efficiency of both enzymes in the production of antihypertensive peptides. Flavourzyme is an enzyme mixture used to produce a mixture of peptides of varying molecular weight, high molecular weight (>10 kDa), and low molecular weight (<1 kDa) [11]. Peptides with a molecular weight between 5 and 10 kDa have shown higher ACE inhibitory activity [15]. Similarly, peptides ranging from 5 to 10 kDa were observed in the electrophoresis gels in the present study (Figure 1).

Alcalase, considered a serine endopeptidase, exhibits broad selectivity and specificity in the catalyzed hydrolysis of proteins to produce peptides with hydrophobic characteristics at the C-terminal [13]. It is known that C-terminal peptides can interact at the ACE active site, resulting in ACE inhibition [6].

2.5. Antidiabetic Capacity

The action of the peptides generated from the hydrolysis with alcalase and flavourzyme on the inhibition of DPP-IV was evaluated (Table 1). At the beginning of the hydrolysis, values of 20.50 and 28.02% were obtained for alcalase and flavourzyme, respectively. In the flavourzyme system, it was observed that as the proteolytic activity increased, the inhibition of DPP-IV increased up to 6 h. The maximum values were reached at 6 h for the two hydrolysis systems evaluated, presenting 68.86 and 52.72% for alcalase and flavourzyme, respectively. Alcalase and flavourzyme can generate antidiabetic peptides in a protein concentrate of *Jatropha curcas* L. var. Sevangel. Hydrophobic sequences with molecular weights less than 1 kDa are highly likely to exhibit antidiabetic activity, similar to peptides with antihypertensive effects [20].

The initial values in terms of the inhibitory activity against DPP-IV agree with those of León-Villanueva et al. [7], who reported a protease with antidiabetic activity in stored *Jatropha curcas* cake.

The generation of bioactive peptides with alcalase and flavourzyme that exhibit inhibitory activity against DPP-IV has previously been reported in other hydrolyzed grains, such as lupine, brewer's spent grain, oat protein, soybean paste, and rye protein [21–25].

Sharma et al. [26] obtained a DPP-IV inhibition of 51.51 ± 0.28% from soluble corn distillates with sequential hydrolysis by alcalase and flavourzyme. These values are lower than those reported at 6 h with alcalase and similar to the values obtained with flavourzyme in *Jatropha curcas*. *Jatropha curcas* may be a promising source for obtaining bioactive peptides with antidiabetic activity.

3. Materials and Methods

3.1. Sample

Seeds of *Jatropha curcas* L. var. Sevangel were provided in January 2023 by the Centro de Desarrollo de Productos Bióticos (CEPROBI-IPN) located in Yautepec, Morelos, Mexico. After extracting the oil, the seeds were air-dried and mechanically compressed (7111.5 psi, 80 °C). The resulting residues were ground, sieved, and later defatted using the Bligh–Dyer methodology [27] to obtain *Jatropha curcas* cake. Subsequently, the sample was stored in a container at room temperature until protein extraction.

3.2. Protein Extraction

Protein extraction was performed following the methodology of Ahluwalia et al. [9] with the following conditions: temperature of 60 °C, solubilization pH of 11.0, precipitation pH of 4.41, and an extraction time of 0.78 h. The protein extract of *Jatropha curcas* L. var. Sevangel was freeze-dried (0.045 mBar; −52 °C) and stored at 4 °C until use. The freeze-dried extract was referred to as PEJ. The percent dry matter recovered (Equation (1)) and protein yield (Equation (2)) were calculated from the freeze-dried sample of PEJ according to the following formulas (Equations (1) and (2)):

$$\text{Dry matter}(\%) = \frac{\text{Dry matter weight of protein precipitate}}{\text{Initial seed weight on dry basis}} \times 100 \quad (1)$$

$$\text{Protein yield}(\%) = \frac{\text{DME}(\text{g}) \times \text{protein content extract}(\%)}{\text{ICW}(\text{g}) \times \text{cake protein content}(\%)} \times 100 \quad (2)$$

where:

DME = Dry matter extract

ICW = Initial cake weight

3.3. Enzymatic Hydrolysis

Enzymatic hydrolysis was performed following the methodology of Islas-Martínez et al. [25]. Firstly, 10 g of PEJ and 0.1% xanthan gum (m/v) was taken and diluted in phosphate buffer (0.1 M, pH = 7.5) and then pasteurized (90 °C for 10 min). The PEJ was hydrolyzed by the alcalase (>2.4 U/g, Hanson units; Sigma-Aldrich, USA, MA) (PEJA) and flavourzyme (>500 U/g; Sigma-Aldrich, USA, MA) (PEJF) systems at a total protein/enzyme mass ratio of 100:2.5 in both cases. The PEJ was hydrolyzed for 8 h at 60 °C and 130 rpm with oscillating agitation for both reaction systems (alcalase and flavourzyme), and samples were taken every 2 h. Then, each collected sample was heated at 85 °C for 10 min to stop the reaction. Finally, the samples were centrifuged at 10,000 rpm for 10 min at 4 °C, and the supernatant was separated and stored at −18 °C for use in subsequent analyses.

3.4. Proteolytic Capacity

The proteolytic capacity was determined by the TNBS technique, and the peptides that were released in the enzymatic hydrolysis were separated using Tris-Glycine polyacrylamide gel electrophoresis (SDS-Tris-Glycine-PAGE).

3.4.1. Free Amino Groups by the TNBS Method

Determination of the hydrolysis degree was performed by the 2,4,6-trinitrobenzene sulfonic acid (TNBS) test according to the methodology of Sashidhar et al. [28], with some modifications. The PEJ samples (0.250 mL) were mixed with 2 mL of 0.21 M phosphate buffer solution at pH 8.2 and 2 mL of 0.1% TNBS reagent (Sigma-Aldrich, St. Louis, MO-USA). The resulting mixes were incubated at 50 °C for 60 min, protected from light. Four mL of 0.1 M HCl was added to stop the reaction, and its absorbance was read at 340 nm. The concentration of free amino groups was obtained from a calibration curve performed with glycine at concentrations of 0–200 ppm.

3.4.2. Tris-Glycine Polyacrylamide Gel Electrophoresis (Tris-Glycine-SDS-PAGE)

The method proposed by Pérez-Escalante et al. [29] was performed. Electrophoresis was performed on a 15% separating T-gel and 4% for a concentration T-gel from a 30% T-solution (acrylamide/bisacrylamide 37.5:1 and 2.7% cross-linker, Bio-Rad, Hercules, CA, USA) and analyzed with Gel-Doc EZ (Image Lab 6.1) imaging system software (Bio-Rad, Hercules, CA, USA).

3.5. *Antioxidant Activity*

The antioxidant activity was evaluated using two different methods, as described below.

3.5.1. Ferric-Reducing Power

The antioxidant activity was evaluated using Benzie and Strain's methodology [16]. A FRAP preparation was obtained at a 10:1:1 ratio of 0.3 M sodium acetate buffer at pH 3.6, TPTZ (Sigma-Aldrich, St. Louis, MO, USA), and ferric chloride at 20 mM. Subsequently, 250 μL of PEJA and PEJF samples were mixed with 1 mL of FRAP solution to 10 mL volumetric capacity with distilled water and incubated at 37 °C for 15 min. The absorbance was measured at 593 nm, and the results were compared with an iron (II) sulfate calibration curve at 200 mM. The antioxidant activity was expressed as micromole equivalents of iron (II) sulfate per 100 mL (mmol E Fe II/100 mL).

3.5.2. Radical Scavenging Properties by DPPH

The antiradical activity was determined by Brand-Williams et al.'s [17] technique. A methanolic solution of DPPH was prepared (0.1 mM dissolved in methanol). Firstly, 100 μL of the PEJA or PEJF sample was added to 2.9 mL DPPH solution and kept for 50 min. Finally, the absorbance of the supernatant was measured at 515 nm and expressed as mg Trolox equivalents/L (mg ET/100 mL).

3.6. *Antihypertensive Activity*

The antihypertensive activity was assessed by the angiotensin-converting enzyme (i-ACE) inhibitory effect, according to Cushman et al. [30]. First, 200 μL of substrate hippuryl-histidyl-leucine (HHL) (Sigma-Aldrich, St. Louis, MO, USA) and 20 μL of rabbit lung angiotensin-converting enzyme reconstituted in buffer to achieve a concentration of 0.1 U/mL (EC 3. 4 15.1, 0.1 U/mg; Sigma-Aldrich, St. Louis, MO, USA) were added to 80 μL of 5 mM sodium borate solution, at pH 8.2, in an of 0.3 M sodium chloride solution to obtain a final concentration of 5 mM of the substrate. Subsequently, 80 μL of the PEJA or PEJF sample replaced the buffer and was mixed with 200 μL of HHL and 20 μL of ACE. The reaction was carried out for 80 min at 37 °C, and the enzyme was inactivated with 1 mL of 0.1 M HCl. The hippuric acid formed was extracted with 1.7 mL ethyl acetate and diluted with deionized water to measure its absorbance at 220 nm. The organic extraction was performed three times, and 800 μL of the organic layer was separated and evaporated by heating at 80 °C for 1 h in the same dry bath. The extracted hippuric acid was reconstituted with 500 μL of deionized water. The latter volume was mixed with 300 μL of pyridine and 150 μL of benzene sulfonyl chloride, and the absorbance at 410 nm was recorded in a UV–vis spectrophotometer. The inhibitory activity of ACE was calculated by the following formula (Equation (3)):

$$\text{Inhibitory activity}(\%) = \frac{A_C - A_S}{A_C - A_B} \times 100 \tag{3}$$

where:

A_C = Hippuric acid formed during the action of ACE without an inhibitor

A_B = Unreacted hippuryl-histidyl-leucine that was extracted with ethyl acetate

A_S = Hippuric acid formed after the action of ACE in the presence of an inhibitory substance

3.7. Antidiabetic Capacity

The antidiabetic capacity was determined by the DPP-IV inhibitory activity [31], with some modifications. A 100 μL sample of PEJA or PEJF added to 100 μL of Gly-Pro-p-nitroanilide at 1.6 mM in Tris-HCl buffer (0.1 M, pH = 8) was pre-incubated at 37 °C in a dry bath for 10 min, and added then to 200 μL of DPP-IV diluted in Tris-HCl (0.01 U/mL). After 60 min, the reaction was stopped by adding 400 μL of 0.1 M potassium carbonate solution. Finally, the absorbance was measured at 405 nm, and the DPP-IV inhibition (DI) was calculated by the following equation (Equation (4)):

$$\text{Inhibitory DPP} - \text{IV}(\%) = \frac{A_{100} - (A_S - A_{SC})}{A_{100}} \times 100 \quad (4)$$

where:

A_{100} = Absorbance at 405 nm of the enzyme reaction without hydrolysate.

A_S = Absorbance at 405 nm of the enzymatic reaction with hydrolysate.

A_{SC} = Absorbance at 405 nm of hydrolysate where the enzyme and substrate were replaced by Tris-HCl buffer pH = 8 and potassium carbonate.

3.8. Statistical Analysis

All the experiments were performed in triplicate and analyzed by one-way ANOVA. Tukey's contrast test determined significant differences at a significance of 0.05. All the statistical tests were analyzed with Statgraphics Centurion XVI.I software.

4. Conclusions

The enzyme systems proposed for a non-toxic genotype of *Jatropha* (*J. curcas* L var. Sevangel) were shown to have antioxidant, antihypertensive, and antidiabetic bioactivity. However, the best results were obtained using alcalase. Previous studies highlighted *J. curcas* as a source of peptides showing antioxidant and antihypertensive activity. The generation of bioactive peptides from the *Jatropha curcas* protein concentrate showed its nutritional and pharmaceutical potential for treating chronic degenerative diseases, such as cancer, diabetes, and hypertension. However, this is the first report of its antidiabetic activity. Regarding multi-bioactivity, the alcalase hydrolysate performed better than the flavourzyme hydrolysate and the cereals reported in other studies. These findings are important for obtaining the sequencing of peptides with multi-bioactivities. For all these reasons, the by-product of *Jatropha curcas* is emerging as a functional food due to its high protein content, which can contribute to treatments for diabetes, blood hypertension, and the reduction of free radicals.

Author Contributions: All the authors contributed to the study's conception and design. Conceptualization, methodology, and supervision were performed by M.-C.D. and M.-S.J.C. Project administration, data collection, data, and formal analysis were performed by C.-L.E., G.-R.M.A. and P.-E.E. Funding acquisition, experimental laboratory data collection, and validation tools were performed by M.-C.D. and P.-F.J.G. The first draft of the manuscript was written by O.E.J. and all the authors commented on previous versions. All authors have read and agreed to the published version of the manuscript.

Funding: E.J.O. gratefully acknowledges the Consejo Nacional de Humanidades, Ciencia y Tecnologías (CONAHCYT, Mexico) for the scholarship received.

Data Availability Statement: The data provided from the gel electrophoresis (image reports and electropherograms) can be found at the following link: https://drive.google.com/drive/folders/1Wx5FI4KXogn3vZ70X651y8OjsZRmlfsO?usp=sharing (accessed on 23 May 2024).

Acknowledgments: The authors would like to thank CEPROBI-IPN for their support in obtaining samples for this study.

Conflicts of Interest: The authors declare no conflicts of interest.

References

1. Mitra, S.; Ghose, A.; Gujre, N.; Senthilkumar, S.; Borah, P.; Paul, A.; Rangan, L. A review on environmental and socioeconomic perspectives of three promising biofuel plants Jatropha curcas, *Pongamia pinnata* and *Mesua ferrea*. *Biomass Bioenergy* **2021**, *151*, 106173. [CrossRef]
2. Ramadan, M.F. Bioactive Phytochemicals from Jatropha (*Jatropha curcas* L.) Oil Processing Byproducts. In *Bioactive Phytochemicals from Vegetable Oil and Oilseed Processing By-Products*; Springer: Berlin/Heidelberg, Germany, 2022; pp. 1–19.
3. Olloqui, E.J.; Castañeda-Ovando, A.; Evangelista-Lozano, S.; Alanís-García, E.; Ramírez-Moreno, E.; Valadez-Vega, C.; Añorve-Morga, J. Measurement of nutrients and minor components of a non-toxic variety of Jatropha curcas. *J. Food Meas. Charact.* **2022**, *16*, 1029–1037. [CrossRef]
4. Patil, S.M.; Sujay, S.; Tejaswini, M.; Sushma, P.P.; Prithvi, S.; Ramu, R. Bioactive peptides: Its production and potential role on health. *Innov. Food Sci. Emerg. Technol.* **2020**, *7*, 167–182.
5. Cruz-Casas, D.E.; Aguilar, C.N.; Ascacio-Valdés, J.A.; Rodríguez-Herrera, R.; Chávez-González, M.L.; Flores-Gallegos, A.C. Enzymatic hydrolysis and microbial fermentation: The most favorable biotechnological methods for the release of bioactive peptides. *Food Chem. Mol. Sci.* **2021**, *3*, 100047. [CrossRef] [PubMed]
6. Marrufo-Estrada, D.M.; Segura-Campos, M.R.; Chel-Guerrero, L.A.; Betancur-Ancona, D.A. Defatted *Jatropha curcas* flour and protein isolate as materials for protein hydrolysates with biological activity. *Food Chem.* **2013**, *138*, 77–83. [CrossRef]
7. León-Villanueva, A.; Huerta-Ocampo, J.A.; Barrera-Pacheco, A.; Medina-Godoy, S.; de la Rosa, A.P.B. Proteomic analysis of non-toxic *Jatropha curcas* byproduct cake: Fractionation and identification of the major components. *Ind. Crops Prod.* **2018**, *111*, 694–704. [CrossRef]
8. León-Villanueva, A.; Espinosa-Alonso, L.G.; Udenigwe, C.C.; Valdez-Morales, M.; Valdez-Ortiz, A.; Barba de la Rosa, A.P.; Medina-Godoy, S. Chemical and functional characterization of major protein fractions extracted from nontoxic *Jatropha curcas* byproduct meals. *J. Am. Oil Chem. Soc.* **2022**, *99*, 511–523. [CrossRef]
9. Ahluwalia, S.; Bidlan, R.; Shrivastav, A.K.; Goswami, R.K.; Singh, P.; Sharma, J.G. Optimization of protein extraction from detoxified Jatropha seed cake using response surface methodology and amino acid analysis. *Int. J. Environ. Sci. Technol.* **2020**, *17*, 1087–1100. [CrossRef]
10. Liu, B.; Li, N.; Chen, F.; Zhang, J.; Sun, X.; Xu, L.; Fang, F. Review on the release mechanism and debittering technology of bitter peptides from protein hydrolysates. *Compr. Rev. Food Sci. Food Saf.* **2022**, *21*, 5153–5170. [CrossRef]
11. Merz, M.; Eisele, T.; Berends, P.; Appel, D.; Rabe, S.; Blank, I.; Stressler, T.; Fischer, L. Flavourzyme, an enzyme preparation with industrial relevance: Automated nine-step purification and partial characterization of eight enzymes. *J. Agric. Food Chem.* **2015**, *63*, 5682–5693. [CrossRef]
12. Juca, L.T.; Ramos, V.M.; de Freitas, D.T.C.; Monteiro-Moreira, C.O.A. Peptides from the genus Jatropha: Beyond isolation. *Curr. Chem. Biol.* **2017**, *11*, 100–109. [CrossRef]
13. Tacias-Pascacio, V.G.; Morellon-Sterling, R.; Siar, E.H.; Tavano, O.; Berenguer-Murcia, A.; Fernandez-Lafuente, R. Use of Alcalase in the production of bioactive peptides: A review. *Int. J. Biol. Macromol.* **2020**, *165*, 2143–2196.
14. Lv, R.; Dong, Y.; Bao, Z.; Zhang, S.; Lin, S.; Sun, N. Advances in the activity evaluation and cellular regulation pathways of food-derived antioxidant peptides. *Trends Food Sci. Technol.* **2022**, *122*, 171–186. [CrossRef]
15. Segura-Campos, M.R.; Peralta-González, F.; Castellanos-Ruelas, A.; Chel-Guerrero, L.A.; Betancur-Ancona, D.A. Effect of *Jatropha curcas* peptide fractions on the angiotensin I-converting enzyme inhibitory activity. *BioMed Res. Int.* **2013**, *2013*, 541947. [CrossRef]
16. Benzie, I.F.; Strain, J.J. The ferric reducing ability of plasma (FRAP) as a measure of "antioxidant power": The FRAP assay. *Anal. Biochem.* **1996**, *239*, 70–76. [CrossRef]
17. Brand-Williams, W.; Cuvelier, M.E.; Berset, C.L.W.T. Use of a free radical method to evaluate antioxidant activity. *LWT-Food Sci. Technol.* **1995**, *28*, 25–30. [CrossRef]
18. Gallegos-Tintoré, S.; Torres-Fuentes, C.; Martínez-Ayala, A.L.; Solorza-Feria, J.; Alaiz, M.; Girón-Calle, J.; Vioque, J. Antioxidant and chelating activity of *Jatropha curcas* L. protein hydrolysates. *J. Sci. Food Agric.* **2011**, *91*, 1618–1624. [CrossRef]
19. Ayala-Niño, A.; Rodríguez-Serrano, G.M.; González-Olivares, L.G.; Contreras-López, E.; Regal-López, P.; Cepeda-Saez, A. Sequence identification of bioactive peptides from amaranth seed proteins (*Amaranthus hypochondriacus* spp.). *Molecules* **2019**, *24*, 3033. [CrossRef]
20. Berraquero-García, C.; Rivero-Pino, F.; Ospina, J.L.; Pérez-Gálvez, R.; Espejo-Carpio, F.J.; Guadix, A.; García-Moreno, P.J.; Guadix, E.M. Activity, structural features and in silico digestion of antidiabetic peptides. *Food Biosci.* **2023**, *55*, 102954. [CrossRef]
21. Chirinos, R.; Cerna, E.; Pedreschi, R.; Calsin, M.; Aguilar-Galvez, A.; Campos, D. Multifunctional in vitro bioactive properties: Antioxidant, antidiabetic, and antihypertensive of protein hydrolyzates from tarwi (*Lupinus mutabilis* Sweet) obtained by enzymatic biotransformation. *Cereal Chem.* **2021**, *98*, 423–433. [CrossRef]
22. Ribeiro-Oliveira, R.; Martins, Z.E.; Sousa, J.B.; Ferreira, I.M.; Diniz, C. The health-promoting potential of peptides from brewing by-products: An up-to-date review. *Trends Food Sci. Technol.* **2021**, *118*, 143–153. [CrossRef]

23. Fuentes, L.R.; Richard, C.; Chen, L. Sequential alcalase and flavourzyme treatment for preparation of α-amylase, α-glucosidase, and dipeptidyl peptidase (DPP)-IV inhibitory peptides from oat protein. *J. Funct. Foods* **2021**, *87*, 104829. [CrossRef]
24. Zhang, M.; Zhu, L.; Zhang, H.; Wang, X.; Liu, T.; Qi, X.; Wu, G. Identification of novel dipeptidyl peptidase-4 inhibitory peptides from pea proteins: A combined in silico and in vitro study. *Food Biosci.* **2023**, *56*, 103374. [CrossRef]
25. Islas-Martínez, D.; Ávila-Vargas, Y.N.; Rodríguez-Serrano, G.M.; González-Olivares, L.G.; Pérez-Flores, J.G.; Contreras-López, E.; Olloqui, E.J.; Pérez-Escalante, E. Multi-Bioactive Potential of a Rye Protein Isolate Hydrolysate by Enzymatic Processes. *Biol. Life Sci. Forum* **2023**, *26*, 38. [CrossRef]
26. Sharma, S.; Pradhan, R.; Manickavasagan, A.; Tsopmo, A.; Thimmanagari, M.; Dutta, A. Corn distillers solubles by two-step proteolytic hydrolysis as a new source of plant-based protein hydrolysates with ACE and DPP4 inhibition activities. *Food Chem.* **2023**, *401*, 134120. [CrossRef]
27. Bligh, E.G.; Dyer, W.J. A rapid method of total lipid extraction and purification. *Can. J. Biochem. Physiol.* **1959**, *37*, 911–917. [CrossRef]
28. Sashidhar, R.B.; Capoor, A.K.; Ramana, D. Quantitation of ϵ-amino group using amino acids as reference standards by trinitrobenzene sulfonic acid: A simple spectrophotometric method for the estimation of hapten to carrier protein ratio. *J. Immunol. Methods* **1994**, *167*, 121–127. [CrossRef]
29. Pérez-Escalante, E.; González-Olivares, L.G.; Cruz-Guerrero, A.E.; Galán-Vidal, C.A.; Páez-Hernández, M.E.; Álvarez-Romero, G.A. Size exclusion chromatography (SEC-HPLC) as an alternative to study thrombin inhibition. *J. Chromatogr. B* **2018**, *1074*, 34–38. [CrossRef]
30. Cushman, D.W.; Cheung, H.S.; Sabo, E.F.; Ondetti, M.A. Design of potent competitive inhibitors of angiotensin-converting enzyme. Carboxyalkanoyl and mercaptoalkanoyl amino acids. *Biochemistry* **1977**, *16*, 5484–5491. [CrossRef]
31. Nongonierma, A.B.; Mooney, C.; Shields, D.C.; FitzGerald, R.J. Inhibition of dipeptidyl peptidase IV and xanthine oxidase by amino acids and dipeptides. *Food Chem.* **2013**, *141*, 644–653. [CrossRef]

molecules

Article

Quantification of Trimethylamine-*N*-Oxide and Trimethylamine in Fish Oils for Human Consumption

Dominik Dörfel [1,2,*], Sascha Rohn [2] and Eckard Jantzen [1]

[1] GALAB Laboratories GmbH, Am Schleusengraben 7, 21029 Hamburg, Germany; eckard.jantzen@galab.de
[2] Department of Food Chemistry and Analysis, Institute of Food Technology and Food Chemistry, Technical University Berlin, Gustav-Meyer-Allee 25, 13355 Berlin, Germany; rohn@tu-berlin.de
* Correspondence: dominik.doerfel@galab.de

Abstract: Supplementing fish oil is one of the strategies to reduce the risk of cardiovascular disease, the leading cause of death around the world. Contradictorily, fish oil may also contain trimethylamine-*N*-oxide, a recently emerged risk factor for cardiovascular disease, as well as one of its precursors, trimethylamine. A method suitable for routine quantification of trimethylamine-*N*-oxide and trimethylamine in fish oil with a quick and easy liquid extraction without derivatization has been developed. Liquid chromatography with tandem mass spectrometry detection was employed along with a zwitterionic hydrophilic interaction liquid chromatography column and a gradient elution with eluents containing 50 mmol/L of ammonium formate. An internal standard (triethylamine) was used for quantification by mass spectrometry with an external calibration. The assay proved high linearity in the ranges of 10 to 100 ng/mL and 100 to 1000 ng/mL for trimethylamine-*N*-oxide and trimethylamine, respectively. The lowest limit of quantification was determined to be 100 μg/kg for trimethylamine and 10 μg/kg for trimethylamine-*N*-oxide, with the limit of detection at 5 μg/kg and 0.25 μg/kg, respectively. Accuracy ranged from 106–119%. Precision was below 7% the relative standard deviation for both analytes. The method was successfully applied for the determination of trimethylamine-*N*-oxide and trimethylamine contents in nine commercially available liquid fish oils and three commercially available fish oil capsules, showing that trimethylamine and trimethylamine-*N*-oxide are not present in highly refined fish oils.

Keywords: trimethylamine-*N*-oxide; trimethylamine; fish oil; HILIC-MS/MS; cardiovascular disease; liquid extraction

1. Introduction

According to the World Health Organization, cardiovascular diseases (CVD) are the leading cause of death globally, taking an estimated 17.9 million lives each year [1]. One popular way to reduce risk for CVD is supplementing fish oil, as several studies have shown a correlation between fish oil consumption and a reduced risk of suffering from CVD [2,3]. Hence, according to the United States National Institute of Health, fish oil is one of the most common non-vitamin and non-mineral dietary supplements used by Americans [4,5]. The main beneficial compounds in fish oil are omega-3 polyunsaturated fatty acids, shaping the membranes of the cardiovascular system [2,3]. However, especially fish oils from marine fish can also contain undesirable compounds such as trimethylamine (TMA) and trimethylamine-*N*-oxide (TMAO), as well as further biogenic amine derivatives. TMAO is a zwitterionic organic molecule that recently emerged as a candidate risk factor for CVDs, being associated with atherosclerosis, heart failure, hypertension, and other CVDs [6,7]. It is introduced into the human bloodstream either by direct consumption or through conversion of TMA by hepatic flavin monooxygenases [8,9]. While one source of TMA is the transformation of choline and carnitine by the human gut microbiota in the large intestine, readily available TMA from food is also absorbed by intestinal cells and quickly enters the portal blood for subsequent conversion to TMAO in the liver [9]. Furthermore, TMAO from food has also been shown to be absorbed in the gut and to quickly enter the bloodstream [10]. In mammalian kidneys, TMAO is accumulated to counteract the destabilization of macromolecular structures like proteins and nucleic acids by urea, as well as to offset its inhibitory effects on functions such as ligand binding [11]. In marine organisms, TMAO acts as an organic osmolyte for maintaining cell volume [11]. After the harvest of fish and shellfish, bacteria chemically reduce TMAO, consequently increasing the levels of TMA [12]. Hence, fish, shellfish, and the products thereof are the main dietary sources of TMAO and TMA, with concentrations of TMAO from below 5 mg/kg up to 3200 mg/kg and concentrations for TMA ranging from below 2 mg/kg up to 550 mg/kg being reported for the main traded fish species in Hong Kong [13].

Comprehensive analysis of TMAO and its precursors such as TMA in foodstuffs is required for exposure estimations in humans. However, TMAO and TMA, although structurally quite similar, possess different characteristics relevant for their analysis, especially regarding their volatility. TMA is a highly volatile (boiling point: 3 °C) organic amine. Therefore, it is primarily analyzed by headspace gas chromatography (HS-GC) in combination with mass spectrometry (MS) [14,15]. TMAO, on the other hand, is non-volatile and, therefore, rarely analyzed by GC-MS. The most popular method for their simultaneous determination in foodstuffs is capillary electrophoresis, as proposed for fish extracts by Timm and Jorgensen [16]. This method is fast, but requires expensive specialized equipment, and reproducible detector responses are hard to obtain [17]. Thus, a new method for the determination of dimethylamine, TMA, and TMAO in aquatic products, using ion chromatography with non-suppressed conductivity detection after extraction with trichloroacetic acid, was proposed by Li et al. [17]. However, the required equipment is not necessarily less specialized, although being less expensive. Hefni et al. proposed hydrophilic interaction liquid chromatography (HILIC) with mass spectrometry (MS) detection for the simultaneous quantification of TMA and TMAO along with other methylamines in clinical and food samples [18]. This method was applied to eggs and meatballs and has the inherent disadvantage of requiring a laborious derivatization step for TMA detection, which increases the analysis time and the use of resources and makes this method more prone to errors. Lastly, an ultra-high performance liquid chromatography (UHPLC)-MS method was applied for the quantification of TMA and TMAO in hydrogen peroxide-altered fish samples [19].

While plenty of methods are discussed for the determination of TMA and TMAO in fish, there does not yet exist a method for the quantification of TMA and TMAO in significantly lipophilic matrices. However, similar disadvantages as described for the other methods need to be also overcome for lipophilic matrices. Additionally, extraction from significantly lipophilic matrices may require different extraction conditions and solvents from the ones proposed in the studies published [17–19]. Furthermore, the analysis of TMA and TMAO is of importance to estimate their impact in fish oil supplements on circulating levels of TMAO in the bloodstream and, thus, potential adverse effects on human health.

Consequently, the present study aimed at developing and validating a quick and simple derivatization-free liquid–liquid extraction method followed by hydrophilic interaction liquid chromatography tandem-MS (HILIC-MS/MS) separation for analyzing TMA and TMAO in fish oils (and supplements, i.e., capsules, containing these). To obtain an overview of the quality and range of concentrations, nine commercially available liquid fish oils and three commercially available fish oil capsules were exemplarily analyzed for their TMA and TMAO contents.

2. Results and Discussion

The results obtained were primarily planned and are discussed regarding the method's aptitude for quick and easy derivatization-free analysis of TMA and TMAO in fish oils for human consumption.

2.1. Detection Method Optimization

Detection for all analytes was optimal in positive ion mode as the responses were higher than in negative ion mode. The precursor ions, product ions, the quantifier and qualifier, and the optimal CE and CAV are given in Table 1. The dwell time was set to 10 ms for all transitions. Retention times were 0.9 min for triethylamine (TEA), 1.2 min for TMA, and 1.2 min for TMAO. Hence, the liquid chromatography tandem-mass spectrometry (LC-MS/MS) method can even be reduced to as little as three minutes, if a higher sample throughput is required. However, doing so would decrease the column cleanup during the run and, thereby, possibly the lifetime of the column itself. Despite co-elution, MS/MS detection enabled selective detection and, thus, quantification of TMA and TMAO.

Table 1. Optimized MS/MS parameters for TMA, TMAO, and TEA.

Compound	Precursor Ion [*m*/*z*]	Quantifier Ion [*m*/*z*]	Qualifier Ion [*m*/*z*]	Quantifier CE [V]	Quantifier CAV [V]
TEA	102	58	74	24	8
TMA	60	44	28	24	8
TMAO	76	58	59	25	5

m/*z*: mass-to-charge ratio, CE: collision energy, CAV: cell accelerator voltage, TEA: triethylamine, TMA: trimethylamine, TMAO: trimethylamine-*N*-oxide.

2.2. Method Development

The recovery rates for TMAO for all three extraction solvents ranged from 94 to 99%. For TMA, eluent A and 1% formic acid in methanol resulted in 89% and 96% recovery rates, respectively. The recovery rate for samples in 0.5 M trichloroacetic acid was 336%. As the recovery rates were considered acceptable within a range of 70–120%, according to U.S. Food and Drug Administration (FDA) guidance [20], trichloroacetic acid was excluded from further consideration. Furthermore, regarding peak symmetries, the use of eluent A resulted in a very good symmetry, while the use of methanol with 1% formic acid showed a prevalence for peak shoulder formation. Additionally, unlike with 1% formic acid in methanol, extraction with eluent A did not require the preparation of an additional solution, as eluent A needs to be prepared for the subsequent HILIC-MS/MS analysis. Thus, extraction with eluent A showed better peak symmetries and an overall reduced analysis time, rendering it the most advantageous extraction solvent of the three ones tested. In the next step, the sample cleanup was investigated. Therefore, two samples were extracted with eluent A in duplicate. One of each duplicate sample was subsequently extracted with the same amount of n-hexane by thoroughly mixing. Afterwards, 1 mL of the eluent A phases of each sample was transferred to a 1.5 mL glass vial and dried in an oven. All samples were then weighed, and the net weight of the residue was calculated by subtracting the tare of the glass vials. The average weight of the residue without additional n-hexane extraction was 1.08 $\pm$ 0.09 mg/mL. The average weight of the residue after additional extraction with n-hexane was 1.04 $\pm$ 0.13 mg/mL. The difference in these values was below the measurement certainty of the scale applied. Thus, no significant improvement in sample cleanup resulted from a second extraction step with n-hexane. Hence, this step was not adopted for the final method. Lastly, the necessity of conducting a matrix calibration was investigated by calculating the recovery rates of a matrix calibration measured against an external calibration with an internal standard. Except for the 2 ng/mL level for TMAO, all matrix calibration levels yielded recovery rates from 88–105% for both analytes in both blank samples. The mean values were 96% and 95% for TMA with standard deviations of 6% and 4%, respectively, as well as 89% and 102% for TMAO with standard deviations of 8% and 2%, respectively. Hence, all results were well within the ranges of 70–120% accuracy and <15% precision, as given by the FDA guidelines. Therefore, the external calibration was considered equivalent to the matrix calibration. The application of an external calibration further reduced the time of work required and, thus, the overall analysis time. In conclusion, eluent A showed the best extraction properties, considering extraction efficiency, peak symmetry, and overall handling. Also, further extraction with n-hexane did not result in a significant improvement of the sample cleanup, indicating that eluent A did not extract notable amounts of lipophilic compounds. Furthermore, external calibration with an internal standard was shown to be equivalent to matrix calibration.

2.3. Method Validation

Validation data for TMA and TMAO are shown in Tables 2–4. Linearity was confirmed in the ranges of 100–1000 ng/mL for TMA and 10–100 ng/mL for TMAO. The coefficients of determination (R^2) for both compounds were higher than 0.995 and are given in Table 2 along with the slope and intercept of the acquired calibration curves. Also, the lack-of-fit test and visual inspection of residual plots passed. Thus, a high linearity was proven. The lowest limit of quantification (LLOQ) values were 100 μg/kg for TMA and 10 μg/kg for TMAO, while the limit of detection (LOD) and limit of quantification (LOQ) values were 5 μg/kg and 10 μg/kg for TMA, as well as 0.25 μg/kg and 0.75 μg/kg for TMAO, respectively (Table 3). Chromatograms of a standard mix at the LLOQ are shown in Figure 1.

In comparison with the capillary electrophoresis method, as proposed by Timm and Jørgensen [16], this method showed increased sensitivity by lowering the linear range from approximately 1.5 μg/mL–150 μg/mL for both analytes to 10–100 ng/mL for TMAO and 100–1000 ng/mL for TMA, the LOD from ~1 mg/L for both analytes to 0.25 μg/kg for TMAO and 5 μg/kg for TMA, and the LOQ from approximately 3 mg/L for both analytes to 0.75 μg/kg for TMAO and 10 μg/kg for TMA. Similarly, this method showed a superior LOD compared to the ion exchange chromatography method proposed by Li et al. [17], lowering the LOD of TMA from 0.08 mg/L to 5 μg/kg and the LOD of TMAO from 0.10 mg/L to 0.25 μg/kg. Hefni et al. reported the LOD for TMA and TMAO to be 2.9 ng/mL and 4.13 ng/mL, respectively [18]. However, the reported value refers to the extract only. When calculating the LOD in relation to the employed food source, LOD values of 116 μg/kg for TMA and 165 μg/kg for TMAO result. Accuracy for the presented method was between 113 and 119% for TMA with intraday precision ranging from 1–3% and inter-day precision at 4–7% (Table 4). The determination of TMAO showed an accuracy of 106–113% with intra-day and inter-day precisions between 1–3% and 3–6%, respectively (Table 4). The precision results were within the acceptable range of ± 15% standard deviation, as well as ± 20% standard deviation for the LLOQ, as recommended by the FDA guideline. The obtained values for precision were in line with the previously reported values by Timm and Jørgensen [16], Li et al. [17], Hefni et al. [18], and Dal Bello et al. [19], who obtained precision values ranging from approximately 3 to 11% for both compounds. However, accuracy was only reported by Dal Bello et al. [19] and Hefni et al. [18] in the form of recovery and compared well to the results obtained with the newly developed method, giving values ranging from 75.8 to 102.5% for TMAO and 86.0 to 97.9% for TMA [17,18]. In the present study, carry-over was found to be below 1% for both analytes, as well as the internal standard and, thus, below the acceptable threshold of 20% of the response at the LLOQ for the analytes and 5% for the internal standard. Hence, the developed method showed good accuracy and precision, as well as high sensitivity and linearity with little carry-over. The method validation showed that the presented method is well-suited for the analysis of TMA and TMAO in oils for human consumption also in comparison with methods for other matrices published before.

Table 2. Validation results for HILIC-ESI-MS/MS analysis of TMA and TMAO in oil.

Compound	R^2	Linear Range [ng/mL]	Slope	Intercept
TMA	0.9984	100–1000	0.039	0.002
TMAO	0.9986	10–100	31.915	0.253

R^2: coefficient of determination, TMA: trimethylamine, TMAO: trimethylamine-*N*-oxide.

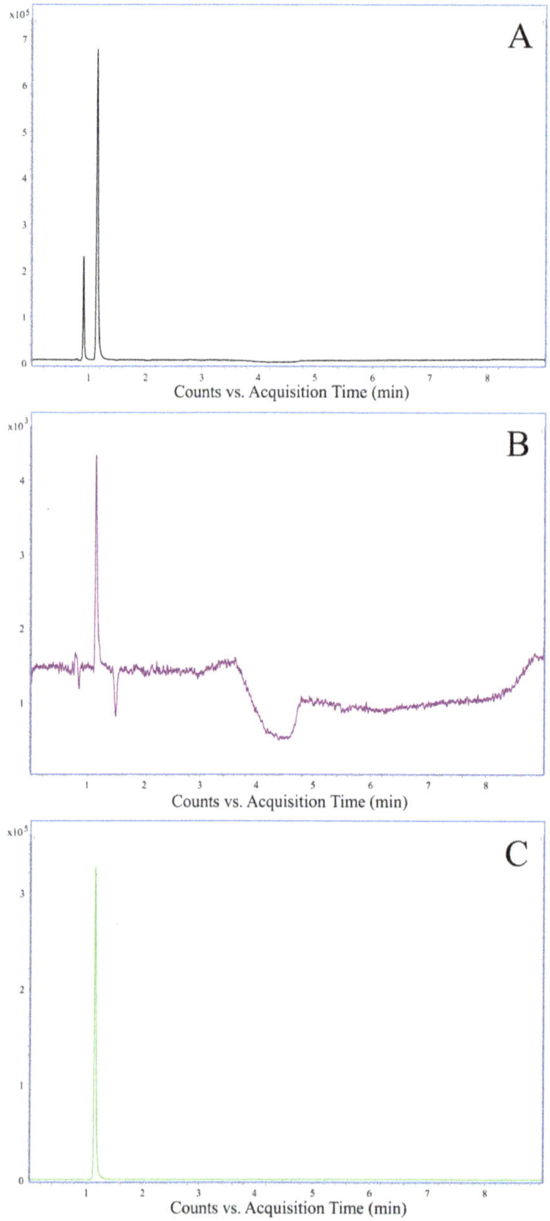

Figure 1. Chromatograms of a standard mixture at the LLOQ. (**A**) Total ion chromatogram; (**B**) chromatogram of the quantifier transition of TMA; (**C**) chromatogram of the quantifier transition of TMAO.

Table 3. Validation data for HILIC-ESI-MS/MS analysis of TMA and TMAO in oil.

Compound	LOD [μg/kg]	LOQ [μg/kg]	LLOQ [μg/kg]	Carry-Over [%]
TMA	5	10	100	0.41
TMAO	0.25	0.75	10	0.70

LOD: limit of detection, LOQ: limit of quantification, LLOQ: lowest limit of quantification (the lowest concentration of analytes, which can be quantitatively measured with suitable accuracy and precision), TMA: trimethylamine, TMAO: trimethylamine-*N*-oxide.

Table 4. Validation data for HILIC-ESI-MS/MS analysis of TMA and TMAO in oil.

Compound	Accuracy [%]				Intra-Day Precision RSD [%]				Inter-Day Precision RSD [%]			
	Q	L	M	H	Q	L	M	H	Q	L	M	H
TMA	113	115	117	119	2	3	1	1	7	4	4	5
TMAO	106	109	113	113	3	2	1	1	6	4	3	3

Blank oil samples were spiked at four different levels of 500 ng (Q), 1000 ng (L), 2500 ng (M), and 4000 ng (H) of TMA, as well as 50 ng (Q), 100 ng (L), 250 ng (M), and 400 ng (H) of TMAO (n = 5). RSD: relative standard deviation, TMA: trimethylamine, TMAO: trimethylamine-*N*-oxide.

2.4. Analysis of Commercially Available Fish Oils

Nine liquid fish oil samples and three fish oil capsules were investigated exemplarily for their TMA and TMAO contents to have an impression of the range and variety present in commercially available fish oils. The results are shown in Table 5. TMA and TMAO were not detectable in any of the liquid fish oil samples. Similar results were found for the fish oil capsules, as TMA and TMAO were found to be below the LLOQ in all three samples. However, TMA was found in two of the samples with contents higher than the LOD, but lower than the LLOQ. TMAO was detectable above the LOQ and below the LLOQ in one sample. Exemplary chromatograms of the results of one fish oil with TMA and TMAO contents above the LOD are shown in Figure 2. All samples were spiked with TMA and TMAO at the LLOQ level, and the resulting recoveries ranged from 81 to 104% for TMA and 86 to 110% for TMAO (Table 5). Overall, no significant amounts of TMA and TMAO were found in any of the fish oils analyzed in the present study, even though high concentrations of up to 2200 mg TMAO/kg fish and 99 mg TMA/kg fish have been reported for cod [13]. This is most likely due to the processing applied during fish oil production. TMA and TMAO possess a strong fishy odor [21]. Hence, they are most likely removed during processing to ensure sensory acceptance by the customer. Off-flavor attributes like the ones originating from TMA and TMAO are still a concern for many customers, as they result in so-called "fish burps" [22]. Originally, these off-flavors were masked by encapsulating the oils [23]. Besides fish oil supplementation, encapsulation aims also at providing fish oils as ingredients for the fortification of products such as yoghurt, goat cheese, and other products [24–26]. Consequently, refining processes are necessary [27]. Usually, one of the processing steps is deodorization, where odorous compounds are removed by steam distillation or other means, although researchers are working on gentler options to remove odors, which require less energy than high-temperature steam distillation [27]. However, residual TMA and TMAO might be present, as the removal rates of some of the processing methods are significantly lower [27]. Furthermore, the refinement process is rarely complete, as sensory evaluation of fish oil still shows a fishy odor even after deodorization due to the incomplete deodorization. This results in volatile compounds still being present in the marketed products [28]. A further important fact to consider is that the raw materials used for fish oil production originate from a plethora of sources. While cod liver oil is the prevalent source for fish oil in Germany, in other regions of the world, fish oil is also produced from different species [29]. Also, whereas the German consumer market does not embrace strong fishy flavors, other countries indulge in delicacies like surströmming (Swedish sour herring) or Icelandic hakarl (fermented or cured shark), which are famous for their overpowering fishy odor [30].

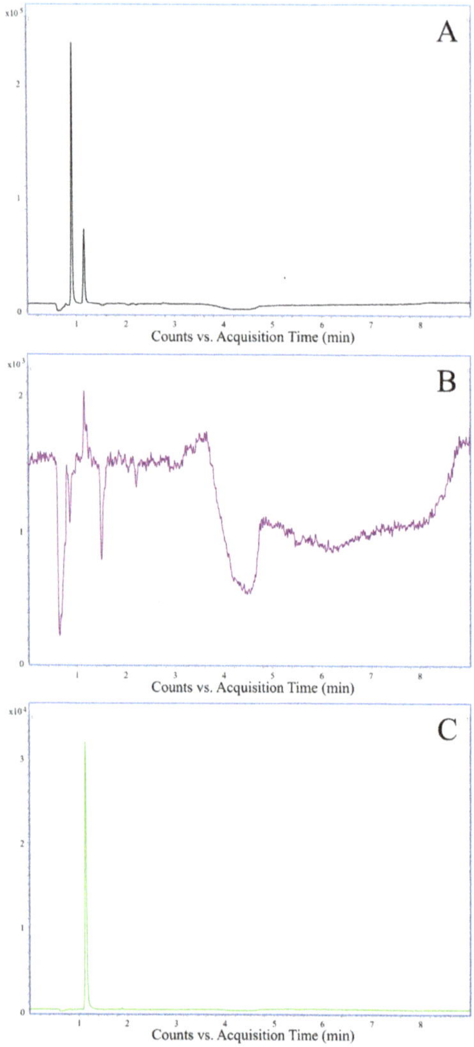

Figure 2. Chromatograms of a fish oil sample with analyte concentrations below the LOQ. (**A**) Total ion chromatogram; (**B**) chromatogram of the quantifier transition of TMA; (**C**) chromatogram of the quantifier transition of TMAO.

Table 5. Results of TMA and TMAO quantification in nine liquid fish oil samples and three fish oil capsules.

Sample	TMA Content [µg/kg]	Recovery Rate [%]	TMAO Content [µg/kg]	Recovery Rate [%]
Fish oil liquid 1	n.d.	97	n.d.	96
Fish oil liquid 2	n.d.	81	n.d.	96
Fish oil liquid 3	n.d.	104	n.d.	96
Fish oil liquid 4	n.d.	101	n.d.	94
Fish oil liquid 5	n.d.	103	n.d.	99
Fish oil liquid 6	n.d.	101	n.d.	97
Fish oil liquid 7	n.d.	104	n.d.	95

Table 5. *Cont.*

Sample	TMA Content [µg/kg]	Recovery Rate [%]	TMAO Content [µg/kg]	Recovery Rate [%]
Fish oil liquid 8	n.d.	104	n.d.	101
Fish oil liquid 9	n.d.	95	n.d.	86
Fish oil capsule 1	n.d.	100	n.d.	109
Fish oil capsule 2	16 *	102	n.d.	110
Fish oil capsule 3	23 *	102	1 *	107

Fish oil samples were spiked with 500 ng of TMA and 50 ng of TMAO. * Concentrations are below the lowest limit of quantification (LLOQ), but higher than the absolute limit of quantification (LOQ). TMA: trimethylamine, TMAO: trimethylamine-*N*-oxide, n.d.: not detectable.

3. Materials and Methods

3.1. Chemicals

TEA hydrochloride (98%) and TMAO (95%) were purchased from Sigma-Aldrich Chemie GmbH (Schnelldorf, Germany). TMA hydrochloride (for synthesis) was acquired from Merck KGaA (Darmstadt, Germany). Trichloroacetic acid (100%), formic acid (98%), acetonitrile (MeCN), and water of LC-MS grade were obtained from VWR International GmbH (Darmstadt, Germany). Ammonium formate (>99%, for LC-MS) was acquired from Carl Roth GmbH & Co. KG (Karlsruhe, Germany). Hydrochloric acid (>37%) was obtained from Honeywell Deutschland Holding GmbH (Offenbach, Germany). Methanol (>99.95%) and hexane (>95%) were purchased from Th. Geyer GmbH & Co. KG (Renningen, Germany). Syringe filters Chromafil Xtra RC-20/25 were acquired from Macherey-Nagel GmbH & Co. KG (Düren, Germany).

3.2. Sample Material

Organic olive (*Olea europaea*) oil and fish oil capsules were acquired from a local supermarket. Blank fish oil samples for method development, i.e., fish oil where TMA and TMAO have been removed through processing steps, were provided by NORSAN GmbH (Berlin, Germany). A total of nine fish oils of different origins for quantification of TMA and TMAO were purchased online. Two of these samples were marketed for children (as mentioned on the declaration). All nine liquid fish oil samples were cod or cod liver oil (as mentioned on the declaration), primarily. One of the samples catering to children also contained around 20% olive oil (as mentioned on the declaration). No flavoring was added to three liquid fish oil samples, while four samples contained lemon flavoring and two samples contained orange flavoring. Vitamin E was added to all samples, with vitamin D3 added to five samples and vitamin A added to one sample. The fish oil capsules contained sea fish oil with one sample also declaring <5% salmon oil. Vitamin E was also added to all fish oil capsules. The number and type of fish oil samples were chosen to represent the easily obtainable fish oil supplements on the market.

3.3. Sample Preparation

Samples were stored in a refrigerator at 4–8 °C until use. Next, 5 ± 0.05 g of sample material was weighed into 15 mL screw cap tubes, and 5 mL of extraction solvent was added. The mixture was then shaken vigorously for 5 min before centrifugation (3494× *g*, 5 min). The supernatant was membrane-filtered before injection into the UHPLC electrospray ionization (ESI) tandem-MS (MS/MS) system.

3.4. UHPLC-ESI-MS/MS Analysis

UHPLC-ESI-MS/MS was performed on an Agilent Technologies 1260 Infinity II LC system equipped with an Agilent Technologies 6495C triple quadrupole mass spectrometer (Agilent Technologies Deutschland GmbH, Waldbronn, Germany). After extensive method development, the amines were separated on a Poroshell 120 HILIC-Z column (150 mm × 2.1 mm, 2.7 µm) in combination with a Poroshell 120 HILIC-Z guard column

(5 mm × 2.1 mm, 2.7 μm) obtained from Agilent Technologies Deutschland GmbH (Waldbronn, Germany). The column was heated to 40 °C in a column heater. The mobile phase consisted of two eluents: 90:10 (*v*/*v*) ACN–water (A) and water (B) to both of which 50 mM ammonium formate and 2.5% formic acid were added. The elution program was started with 100% eluent A and held for 2 min. The percentage of eluent B was then linearly raised to 50% over 3 min. Within 2 min, the percentage of eluent B was reduced to 0%, and the column was then equilibrated for another 2 min. The mobile phase flow was set constant at 0.5 mL/min. The injection volume was set to 1 μL. UHPLC-ESI-MS/MS data were acquired and processed by the use of the MassHunter QQQ Quantitative Analysis software version B.08.00 (Agilent Technologies Deutschland GmbH, Waldbronn, Germany).

3.5. Stock Solutions, Calibration Standards, and Quality Control Sample Preparation

Next, 10 g/L stock solutions in 1 M hydrochloric acid were prepared for each analyte and stored at −20 °C for a maximum of four weeks. Olive oil was used as a quality control sample, because it does not naturally contain TMA or TMAO. Calibration standard solutions were made in a range from 10 ng/mL to 100 ng/mL for TMAO and from 100 ng/mL to 1000 ng/mL for TMA. TEA was added as an internal standard to each calibration solution to reach a final concentration of 50 ng/mL. For accuracy and precision measurements, blank samples were spiked with standard solution in eluent A. Concentration levels for spiked samples were 50 ng, 100 ng, 250 ng, and 400 ng for TMAO and 500 ng, 1000 ng, 2500 ng, and 4000 ng for TMA. Then, 250 ng of TEA was added to every sample as the internal standard. All standards were prepared freshly every day from the stock solutions.

3.6. Detection Method Optimization

For optimization of the ESI-MS/MS detection of the analytes, 1 μL of 100 ng/mL standard solutions was injected directly into the MS/MS system for each analyte and step. Firstly, the optimal polarity was determined by performing a full scan in positive and negative ion mode and the comparison of the resulting peaks in the spectra, which overlapped with the calculated masses. Then, a product ion scan was conducted to look for the most intense product ions by comparing mass spectral intensity. Subsequently, the collision energy (CE) and cell accelerator voltage (CAV) were optimized by alternating the values in multiple-reaction-monitoring (MRM) mode and selecting the values resulting in high peak areas and signal-to-noise ratios (S/N).

3.7. Extraction Method Development

Three extraction solvents (0.5 M trichloroacetic acid, eluent A, and 1% formic acid in methanol) were investigated for the best extraction efficiency. Trichloroacetic acid (TCA, 0.5 M) was chosen, as it is often used for amine extraction from fish samples [31]. Formic acid 1% is traditionally used for other analytes containing amine groups and was chosen to reduce the extraction solvent's elution strength. The latter is also the reason for using eluent A as an extraction solvent, as 100% eluent A is the starting condition for the liquid chromatographic method. All three extraction solvents created a two-phase system after addition to the fish oil. For every extraction solvent, two samples of a salmon oil sample with a fishy odor, indicative of the presence of TMA, were weighed into screw cap tubes. For each extraction solvent, one sample was spiked. The samples extracted with eluent A and 1% formic acid in methanol were spiked with 2500 ng of TMA and 250 ng of TMAO, while the sample to be extracted with trichloroacetic acid was spiked with 25,000 ng of TMA and 2500 ng of TMAO. The higher concentration for samples extracted with trichloroacetic acid is necessary due to peak splitting being prevalent in purely aqueous solutions, requiring a 1:10 dilution step before injection. Hence, TCA as the extraction solvent would result in higher limits of detection and quantification than 1% formic acid in methanol and eluent A. All samples were measured against an external calibration, consisting of 10 equidistant points ranging from 10 to 100 ng/mL for TMAO and 100 to 1000 ng/mL for TMA. To evaluate the extraction efficiency of the extraction solvents, the difference between the measured analyte content of the spiked and non-spiked samples was divided by the known amount of analyte spiked. The peak symmetries and overall handling of the different extraction solvents were also taken into consideration. After the best-suited extraction solvent was determined, sample cleanup was investigated. Therefore, 2 mL of the extract obtained with the best extraction solvent was subsequently extracted with 2 mL of n-hexane to extract lipophilic compounds. Then, 1 mL of the extract gained after extraction with n-hexane was placed into a 1.5 mL glass vial and dried in an oven at 70 °C. The same was performed with the extract obtained before extraction with n-hexane. Both samples were analyzed gravimetrically (n = 2). Lastly, it was investigated whether a calibration by standard addition is required or if an external calibration with the use of an internal standard would suffice. For this, 20 g of two different blank sample materials was extracted with 20 mL extraction solvent each, and the extracts were spiked with five equidistantly chosen amounts of the standard, resulting in concentrations ranging from 2 to 10 ng/mL for TMAO and from 100 to 500 ng/mL for TMA. These samples were then measured against a calibration consisting of eluent A spiked with standards resulting in the same concentration ranges. This experiment was evaluated by calculating the measured amounts and dividing them by the known amounts of added analyte.

3.8. Method Validation

The analysis of TMAO and TMA in different edible oils was validated to obtain the calibration model, accuracy and precision, LOD. and LOQ, as well as carry-over according to the guidance of bioanalytical method validation published by the FDA with modifications where necessary [19]. The linearity of the method was confirmed by the analysis of a ten-point standard curve (n = 3) ranging from 10 ng/mL to 100 ng/mL for TMAO and from 100 ng/mL to 1000 ng/mL for TMA. The accuracy and precision values were determined fivefold at every concentration level. Precision was determined intra-day (n = 5) and inter-day (n = 5), with inter-day samples being analyzed on three different days by three different coworkers of the lab. The LOD and LOQ were determined by spiking blank samples with multiple low analyte concentrations. The LOD and LOQ for TMA were defined as the concentration resulting in a S/N of 3 and 10, respectively. This was not possible for TMAO, as a very small, but constant peak was detected in every sample. Thus, the LOD and LOQ for TMAO were defined as the lowest value to exceed the blank peak area by factors of 3 and 10, respectively. Carry-over was determined by injecting a solvent blank after the highest calibration level and dividing the resulting peak areas by the areas of the LLOQ.

3.9. Analysis of Commercially Available Fish Oils

Liquid fish oils and fish oil capsules were stored at 4–8 °C until processing. Liquid fish oils were vigorously shaken and transferred into screw cap tubes for analysis. Fish oil capsules were cut open, and their contents were squeezed into screw cap tubes. Then, 5 ± 0.05 g of each sample was weighed into the screw cap tubes twice. For each sample, one aliquot was spiked with 50 ng of TMAO, 500 ng of TMA, and 250 ng of TEA.

4. Conclusions

A reliable and highly sensitive HILIC-ESI-MS/MS method for the quantification of TMA and TMAO without derivatization and with a quick and easy sample preparation was developed. This method shows an improved sensitivity compared to the capillary electrophoresis method proposed by Timm and Jørgensen, as well as the ion chromatography with suppressed conductivity detection method proposed by Li et al. [16,17]. The capillary electrophoresis method is more time consuming and cannot be run unattended over a long period of time, for example overnight. Thus, its use in service laboratories is less economical than the presented method. Additionally, the developed method requires less time and resources than the method proposed by Hefni et al. [18], as it does not need a derivatization step and does not employ standard addition for quantification of TMA and

TMAO. Furthermore, by employing LC with MS/MS detection, no additional specialized equipment is required. Also, this method is the only one tailored specifically to be used with significantly lipophilic matrices such as oils for human consumption and fish oils in particular. Thus, this method is well suited for the analysis of TMA and TMAO in oils, also with regard to routine analysis in service laboratories. Also, when an even higher sample throughput is required, the method length may be reduced from nine to as little as three minutes, thus saving even more time and resources. Hence, this method will enable quick and reliable detection of TMA and TMAO.

The applicability of this method for TMA and TMAO exposure estimation has been further proven exemplarily by analysis of fish oil samples. The analysis of nine commercially available liquid fish oils did not detect any TMA or TMAO. The analysis of three commercially available fish oil capsules resulted in values of less than 100 µg/kg TMA and less than 10 µg/kg TMAO. Hence, commercially available fish oil, when processed to the newest technological standards, is unlikely to contribute to the circulating TMA and TMAO in human blood. Nonetheless, the presence of residual TMA and TMAO in some of the present samples showed that regular analysis of these compounds as a part of the quality control process may be reasonable to reduce the risk of adverse health effects for consumers. It will be helpful for exposure estimation and presents as a reasonable parameter to control as part of the manufacturer's quality assurance process. However, no regulation limiting the concentrations of TMA and TMAO in foodstuffs has been established to this date.

Author Contributions: Conceptualization, D.D.; methodology, D.D., E.J. and S.R.; formal analysis, D.D.; investigation, D.D.; resources, E.J.; supervision, E.J. and S.R.; validation, D.D. and S.R.; visualization, D.D.; writing—original draft preparation, D.D.; writing—review and editing, S.R. and E.J. All authors have read and agreed to the published version of the manuscript.

Funding: The project is supported by funds of the Federal Ministry of Food and Agriculture (BMEL) based on a decision of the Parliament of the Federal Republic of Germany via the Federal Office for Agriculture and Food (BLE) under the innovation support program (FKZ: 28-1-A5.01B-19).

Institutional Review Board Statement: Not applicable.

Informed Consent Statement: Not applicable.

Data Availability Statement: The raw data supporting the conclusions of this article will be made available by the authors on request.

Acknowledgments: Many thanks are given to Svenja Badekow and Kim Hanisch for their help with the analysis of the inter-day precision samples. We would also like to recognize the contributions of Markus Schröder for data interpretation.

Conflicts of Interest: GALAB Laboratories GmbH is an independent service laboratory for external quality control, especially with regard to food analysis. Services include standard methods, as well as methods tailored for individual specifications and requests. Part of the daily business is the development of new methods for new target compounds. The authors declare that they have no known competing financial interests or personal relationships that could have appeared to influence the work reported in this paper.

References

1. World Health Organization. Cardiovascular Diseases (CVDs). Available online: https://www.who.int/news-room/fact-sheets/detail/cardiovascular-diseases-(cvds) (accessed on 17 August 2023).
2. Artham, S.M.; Patel, D.; Lavie, C.J.; Milani, R.V.; O'Keefe, J.H. Impact of Specific Diets and Nutritional Supplements on Cardiovascular Diseases. In *Handbook of Cardiovascular Behavioral Medicine*, 1st ed.; Waldstein, S.R., Kop, W.J., Suarez, E.C., Lovallo, W.R., Katzel, L.I., Eds.; Springer Nature: Berlin, Germany, 2022; Volume 1, pp. 331–355.
3. Sidhu, K.S. Health benefits and potential risks related to consumption of fish or fish oil. *RTP Regul. Toxicol. Pharmacol.* **2003**, *38*, 336–344. [CrossRef]
4. National Institutes of Health, Office of Dietary Supplements. Omega-3 Fatty Acids. Available online: https://ods.od.nih.gov/factsheets/Omega3FattyAcids-HealthProfessional/#:~:text=Fish%20oil%20is%20one%20of,EPA%20[45,46] (accessed on 17 August 2023).

5. Clarke, T.C.; Black, L.I.; Stussman, B.J.; Barnes, P.M.; Nahin, R.L. Trends in the use of complementary health approaches among adults: United States, 2002–2012. *Natl. Health Stat. Rep.* **2015**, *79*, 1–16.
6. Velasquez, M.; Ramezani, A.; Manal, A.; Raj, D. Trimethylamine N-Oxide: The Good, the Bad and the Unknown. *Toxins* **2016**, *8*, 326. [CrossRef]
7. Zhen, J.; Zhou, Z.; He, M.; Han, H.-X.; Lv, E.-H.; Wen, P.-B.; Liu, X.; Wang, Y.-T.; Cai, X.-C.; Tian, J.-Q.; et al. The gut microbial metabolite trimethylamine N-oxide and cardiovascular diseases. *Front. Endocrinol.* **2023**, *14*, 1085041. [CrossRef] [PubMed]
8. Thomas, M.S.; Fernandez, M.L. Trimethylamine N-Oxide (TMAO), Diet and Cardiovascular Disease. *Curr. Atheroscler. Rep.* **2021**, *23*, 12. [CrossRef]
9. Cho, C.E.; Caudill, M.A. Trimethylamine-N-Oxide: Friend, Foe, or Simply Caught in the Cross-Fire? *TEM Trends Endocrinol. Metab.* **2016**, *28*, 121–130. [CrossRef] [PubMed]
10. Cho, C.E.; Taesuwan, S.; Malysheva, E.B.; Tulchinsky, N.F.; Yan, J.; Sutter, J.L.; Caudill, M.A. Trimethylamine-N-oxide (TMAO) response to animal source foods varies among healthy young men and is influenced by their gut microbiota composition: A randomized controlled trial. *Mol. Nutr. Food Res.* **2016**, *61*, 1600324. [CrossRef] [PubMed]
11. Yancey, P.H. Organic osmolytes as compatible, metabolic and counteracting cytoprotectants in high osmolarity and other stresses. *J. Exp. Biol.* **2005**, *208*, 2819–2830. [CrossRef]
12. Dalgaard, P. Qualitative and quantitative characterization of spoilage bacteria from packed fish. *Int. J. Food Microbiol.* **1995**, *26*, 319–333. [CrossRef]
13. Chung, S.W.C.; Chan, B.T.P. Trimethylamine oxide, dimethylamine, trimethylamine and formaldehyde levels in main traded fish species in Hong Kong. *Food Addit. Contam. B Surveill.* **2009**, *2*, 44–51. [CrossRef]
14. Dehaut, A.; Duthen, S.; Grard, T.; Krzewinski, F.; N'Guessan, A.; Brisabois, A.; Duflos, G. Development of an SPME-GC-MS method for the specific quantification of dimethylamine and trimethylamine: Use of a new ratio for the freshness monitoring of cod fillets. *J. Sci. Food Agric.* **2016**, *96*, 3787–3794. [CrossRef]
15. Duflos, G.; Coin, V.M.; Cornu, M.; Antinelli, J.-F.; Malle, P. Determination of volatile compounds to characterize fish spoilage using headspace/mass spectrometry and solid-phase microextraction/gas chromatography/mass spectrometry. *J. Sci. Food Agric.* **2006**, *86*, 600–611. [CrossRef]
16. Timm, M.; Jørgensen, B.M. Simultaneous determination of ammonia, dimethylamine, trimethylamine and trimethylamine-N-oxide in fish extracts by capillary electrophoresis with indirect UV-detection. *Food Chem.* **2002**, *76*, 509–518. [CrossRef]
17. Li, F.; Liu, H.; Xue, C.; Xin, X.; Xu, J.; Chang, Y.; Xue, Y.; Yin, L. Simultaneous determination of dimethylamine, trimethylamine and trimethylamine-n-oxide in aquatic products extracts by ion chromatography with non-suppressed conductivity detection. *J. Chromatogr. A* **2009**, *31*, 5924–5926. [CrossRef]
18. Hefni, M.E.; Bergström, M.; Lennqvist, T.; Fagerström, C.; Witthöft, C.M. Simultaneous quantification of trimethylamine N-oxide, trimethylamine, choline, betaine, creatinine, and propionyl-, acetyl-, and L-carnitine in clinical and food samples using HILIC-LC-MS. *Anal. Bioanal. Chem.* **2021**, *413*, 5349–5360. [CrossRef]
19. Dal Bello, F.; Aigotti, R.; Zorzi, M.; Giaccone, V.; Medana, C. Multi-Analyte MS Based Investigation in Relation to the Illicit Treatment of Fish Products with Hydrogen Peroxide. *Toxics* **2020**, *8*, 2. [CrossRef]
20. Food and Drug Administration. Guidance for Industry, Bioanalytical Method Validation. U.S. Department of Health and Human Service, Food and Drug Administration, Center for Drug Evaluation and Research, Center for Biologics Evaluation and Research, November 2022, ICH. Available online: https://www.fda.gov/media/162903/download (accessed on 17 August 2023).
21. Prabhakar, P.K.; Vatsa, S.; Srivastav, P.P.; Pathak, S.S. A Comprehensive Review on Freshness of Fish and Assessment: Analytical Methods and Recent Innovations. *Int. Food Res. J.* **2020**, *133*, 109157. [CrossRef]
22. Walker, R.; Decker, E.A.; McClements, D.J. Development of food-grade nanoemulsions and emulsions for delivery of omega-3 fatty acids: Opportunities and obstacles in the food industry. *Food Funct.* **2015**, *6*, 41–54. [CrossRef]
23. Cleland, L.G.; James, M.J.; Proudman, S.M. Fish oil: What the prescriber needs to know. *Arthritis Res. Ther.* **2005**, *8*, 202. [CrossRef] [PubMed]
24. Ghorbanzade, T.; Jafari, S.M.; Akhavan, S.; Hadavi, R. Nano-encapsulation of fish oil in nano-liposomes and its application in fortification of yogurt. *Food Chem.* **2017**, *216*, 146–152. [CrossRef] [PubMed]
25. Hadnadev, M.; Kalic, M.; Krstonosic, V.; Jovanovic-Ljeskovic, N.; Erceg, T.; Skrobot, D.; Dapcevic-Hadnadev, T. Fortification of chocolate with microencapsulated fish oil: Effect of protein wall material on physicochemical properties of microcapsules and chocolate matrix. *Food Chem. X* **2023**, *17*, 100583. [CrossRef] [PubMed]
26. Hughes, B.H.; Perkins, L.B.; Calder, B.L.; Skonberg, D.I. Fish Oil Fortification of Soft Goat Cheese. *J. Food Sci.* **2012**, *77*, S128–S133. [CrossRef] [PubMed]
27. Yi, M.; You, Y.; Zhang, Y.; Wu, G.; Karrar, E.; Zhang, L.; Zhang, H.; Jin, Q.; Wang, X. Highly Valuable Fish Oil: Formation Process, Enrichment, Subsequent Utilization, and Storage of Eicosapentaenoic Acid Ethyl Esters. *Molecules* **2023**, *28*, 672. [CrossRef] [PubMed]
28. Song, G.; Dai, Z.; Shen, Q.; Peng, X.; Zhang, M. Analysis of the Changes in Volatile Compound and Fatty Acid Profiles of Fish Oil in Chemical Refining Process. *Eur. J. Lipid Sci. Technol.* **2018**, *120*, 1700219. [CrossRef]
29. Shepherd, C.J.; Jackson, A.J. Global fishmeal and fish-oil supply: Inputs, outputs and markets. *J. Fish Biol.* **2013**, *83*, 1046–1066. [CrossRef]

30. Skåra, T.; Axelsson, L.; Stefánsson, G.; Ekstrand, B.; Hagen, H. Fermented and ripened fish products in the northern European countries. *J. Ethn. Foods* **2015**, *2*, 18–24. [CrossRef]
31. Tiris, G.; Yanikoglu, R.S.; Ceylan, B.; Egeli, D.; Tekkeli, E.K.; Önal, A. A review of the currently developed analytical methods for the determination of biogenic amines in food products. *Food Chem.* **2022**, *398*, 133919. [CrossRef]

molecules

MDPI

Review

A Review of Phytochemical and Pharmacological Studies on *Galium verum* L., Rubiaceae

Margarita Koleva Petkova [1,*], Neli Hristova Grozeva [1,*], Milena Tankova Tzanova [1] and Mima Hristova Todorova [2]

1 Department of Biological Sciences, Faculty of Agriculture, Trakia University, 6000 Stara Zagora, Bulgaria; milena.tsanova@trakia-uni.bg
2 Department of Plant Breeding, Faculty of Agriculture, Trakia University, 6000 Stara Zagora, Bulgaria; mima.todorova@trakia-uni.bg
* Correspondence: margarita.petkova@trakia-uni.bg (M.K.P.); n.grozeva@trakia-uni.bg (N.H.G.)

Abstract: *Galium verum* (Yellow Bedstraw) is a rhizomatous perennial herb belonging to the Rubiaceae family. It is native to Eurasia and Africa but has also been introduced to southern Canada and the northern U.S. Widely used in traditional medicine, *G. verum* has been recognized for its diuretic, anti-inflammatory, antimicrobial, analgesic, and anticancer properties. Phytochemical studies have shown that the plant is rich in significant bioactive compounds, such as flavonoids, phenolic acids, iridoids, anthraquinones, phytosterols, coumarins, and tannins. Research suggests that *G. verum* exhibits strong antioxidant activity, protecting cells from oxidative stress and inflammation. Its antimicrobial potential has been demonstrated against various bacterial and fungal pathogens, supporting its traditional use in wound healing and infection treatment. Moreover, modern studies indicate its cytotoxic effects on cancer cells, suggesting potential applications in oncology. Additionally, its hepatoprotective and neuroprotective properties highlight its promise for treating metabolic and neurodegenerative disorders. Despite its well-known therapeutic potential, further studies are required to fully clarify its mechanisms of action and ensure its safety for medicinal use. Given the variety of bioactive compounds found in *G. verum* and their pharmacological benefits, this review emphasizes the importance of this species as a valuable medicinal plant, encouraging further scientific research for its application in pharmacology.

Keywords: antioxidants; biological activity; flavonoids; *Galium verum* L.; Rubiaceae; iridoids; pharmacology; phenols; phytochemistry

1. Introduction

In official and traditional medicine, various medicinal plants have been used from antiquity for disease prevention and therapeutic purposes [1]. Plants are a natural source of bioactive substances, many of which have beneficial pharmacological effects for humans [2]. According to Delprete et al., the Rubiaceae family is one of the largest angiosperm families with a large number of species distributed throughout the world, including deserts and high mountains [3]. The overall phytochemical composition of Rubiaceae plants lends to their potential as sources of bioactive compounds [4]. This family has attracted significant attention from researchers due to its diverse pharmacological applications. Many studies detect flavonoids, iridoids, triterpenes, phytosterols, anthraquinones, and others. Heitzman et al. claimed that plants in the Rubiaceae family are widely used in traditional medicine for their diverse therapeutic effects, including antioxidant, antiviral, antibacterial, and

 https://doi.org/10.3390/molecules30081856

anti-inflammatory properties [5]. Additionally, these plants exhibit activity against cardiovascular and central nervous system diseases. The Rubiaceae family also has significant economic importance. For instance, species in the Ixoroideae subfamily are rich in caffeine, a compound that acts as a stimulant for the central nervous system, as well as a diuretic, bronchodilator, and antimigraine agent, as highlighted by Martins et al. [6]. Quinine, a compound isolated from *Cinchona calisaya* Wedd. in the Cinchonoideae subfamily, was the only antimalarial drug for over 200 years, and it has the highest quinine concentrations identified to date [7,8]. The discovery of quinine was revolutionary as it also paved the way for the development of synthetic drugs to treat malaria, which greatly reduced the mortality caused by malaria. The use and importance of natural quinine is still significant and even increasing [9].

Belonging to the Rubiacaeae family and the Rubioideae subfamily is the genus *Galium*, also known as *Bedstraw,* which is pharmacologically significant and is the most species-rich genus within the tribe Rubieae [10–12].

The genus *Galium* comprises approximately 667 species globally, with one-third occurring in Europe [13,14]. Furthermore, approximately 300 species within this genus have been identified as having medicinal properties [5]. These activities are attributed to their rich content of bioactive compounds such as phenolic compounds (including flavonoids) [15–41], phenolic acids [16,22,23,25,35], iridoids [42–50], anthraquinones [41,51–54], terpenoids (including saponins) [33,47,55–59], yellow pigments [52], essential oils [56,58], vitamin C [19,60], phytosterols [61,62], and enzymes [63].

The species of the genus *Galium* possess a wide range of biological activities, including immunomodulatory [32,64], anticancer [65,66], antihaemolytic [67], hepatoprotective [68], diuretic [69], antioxidant [15,23,31,39,70–73], apoptotic [74–76], anti-inflammatory [38,40,77,78], sedative [79], astringent [35,79], wound healing [73,80], enzyme activating [81], and antimicrobial effects [23,73,82–84].

Galium verum L. (commonly known as Yellow or Lady's Bedstraw or Eniovche in Bulgarian) is one of the most widespread species of the genus *Galium*. It is rich in phytochemical compounds with significant biological activity, making it one of the most versatile medicinal plants traditionally used for the prevention and treatment of many diseases due to its anti-inflammatory, anticancer, hepatoprotective, diuretic, cardioprotective, and astringent properties [21,35,65–72,75–77,79–86]. This species has deep roots in Bulgarian traditional medicine, and there is even a holiday named after it, celebrated every year on June 24th. Its name is Eniovden, and it is also known as Midsummer—the longest day of the year. On this day, it is believed that the herbs have the greatest power, and according to tradition, women should go out early in the morning to collect them [87].

The aim of this review is to provide an objective assessment of the available data on the phytochemical composition of *Galium* species, particularly *G. verum,* and the pharmacological effects of the identified classes of metabolites. The goal is to highlight the therapeutic benefits of this medicinal plant and to achieve a more comprehensive understanding of the genus. Such efforts will help identify areas where further research is needed, stimulate more in-depth clinical trials, and potentially lead to the discovery of new pharmacological effects. The final result suggests the rational utilization of *Galium* species as a valuable source of bioactive substances.

2. Materials and Methods

This review was compiled using a comprehensive search strategy that included collecting data from journals and books published between 1971 and 2025, sourced from databases such as EBSCOhost, Web of Science, ScienceDirect, Scopus, Scimago Journal, PubMed, PubChem, ResearchGate, and Elsevier. The search criteria aimed to identify studies that reported quantitative and qualitative determination and biological activity of phytochemical compounds derived from *Galium* species. Studies on the mechanisms of action of phytochemicals that have been proven to be present in *Galium* species but have not been specifically studied in them were also included. Inclusion criteria involved articles related to the phytochemistry of *Galium* species, along with the corresponding biological and pharmacological activities. Exclusion criteria comprised studies that lacked experimental confirmation and chemical characterization.

The two-dimensional chemical structures included in this review were prepared using the software package Revvity ChemDraw, version 23.1.2 (PerkinElmer Informatics, 2023).

The phytochemical compounds included in this review were selected, as they are the most frequently studied in *Galium* species by researchers and are proven to affect organisms at the cellular level through the mechanisms of biological activities they exhibit. A tabular format was chosen to summarize the information obtained, making it easily accessible and understandable.

3. Results and Discussion

3.1. *Phytochemical Composition and Biological Activity of Galium Species*

The pharmacological properties of Rubiaceae plants are largely attributed to the content of various phytochemical compounds with diverse biological effects. While these effects are of significant scientific interest, they remain incompletely researched.

The genus *Galium* has been used in traditional medicine for ages due to its therapeutic properties [5,77,79,80,82].

Many studies have focused on the potential of specific *Galium* species, known for their therapeutic properties in ethnomedicine, such as diuretic, sedative, wound healing, and immunomodulatory [73,79–81]. Similar compounds are detected within the genus, which often demonstrate potent biological activity, determining their mechanisms of action in biological systems. Table 1 summarizes the presence of different phytochemical groups of compounds in some *Galium* species.

As presented in Table 1 the phytochemical composition of the *Galium* genus varies significantly among species; however, flavonoids and iridoids are the most commonly reported bioactive compounds. Aerial parts of the plants are richer in flavonoids, while the roots contain higher concentrations of iridoids [28].

Galium verum and *G. aparine* were found to be the richest in flavonoids, such as quercetin, rutin, and luteolin, while *G. mollugo]* and *G. odoratum* contained more kaempferol and diosmetin [17,19,28,62].

The high content of flavonoids and polyphenols correlates with the strong antioxidant activity of *Galium* species [19,20,22,26,40,78,88], which determine their anticancer [84], immunomodulatory [31], and antimicrobial effects [25,73].

Iridoid compounds are isolated from many *Galium* species and are known to contribute to antioxidant, anti-inflammatory, and anticancer properties of plant-derived products [23,30,37,89,90]. Asperuloside is the most consistently found iridoid across all species of the genus, with *G. verum* and *G. mollugo]* being the richest sources [43–47]. Other iridoids like monotropein, loganin, and geniposidic acid are more species specific and are used for taxonomic markers [46].

Anthraquinones found in *Galium* species exhibit antimicrobial and anticancer properties [6,54]. Phytosterols help reduce blood cholesterol and exhibit antitumor activity [54,61,62]. Saponins exhibit antifungal and antimicrobial potential [55,57].

Most widely used in modern and traditional medicine for their antioxidant, antibacterial, antifungal, and antiparasitic properties are *G. verum*, *G. aparine*, *G. mollugo]*, and *G. odoratum* [28,91].

Table 1. Phytochemistry of *Galium* species.

Species	Phytochemical Group of Compounds	Compounds	Reference
G. aparine	Flavonoids	Astragalin; Hyperoside; Isorhamnetin 3-O-rhamnoglucoside; Isorhamnetin-3-O-rutinoside; Isoquercitrin; Kaempferol; Kaempferol-3-O-β-D-glucopyranosyl-7-O-α-L-rhamnopyranoside; Kaempferol-7-O-α-L-rhamnopyranoside; Luteolin; Nicotiflorin; Quercetin; Quercetin glycoside; Quercetin-3-O-β-D-glucopyranoside; Rutin	[23,28,37,42,54]
	Polyphenols	Caffeic acid; Chlorogenic acid; Coumaric acid; Cryptochlorogenic acid; Dicaffeoylquinic acid isomer; Ferulic acid; Gallic acid; Neochlorogenic acid; p-Coumaric acid; p-Hydroxybenzoic acid; Protocatechuic acid	[23,37,41]
	Iridoids	10-Desacetylasperulosidic acid; Asperuloside; Asperulosidic acid; Deacetylasperulosidic acid; Geniposide; Monotropein; Scandoside	[37,41,42,46,54]
	Anthraquinones	Emodin; Rhein	[41,54]
	Terpenoids	Betulin; Euscaphic acid; Lupeol; Oleanolic acid; Tormentic acid; Ursolic acid	[57]
	Phytosterols	β-Sitosterol; Campesterol	[62]
G. mollugo]	Flavonoids	Astragalin; Catechin; Cosmosiin; Cynaroside; Diosmetin; Diosmetin 7-O-β-D-glucopyranoside; Diosmetin 7-O-β-D-xylopyranosyl-1,6-β-D-glucopyranoside; Diosmetin isomer; Epicatechin; Hesperidin; Hispidulin; Hyperozide; Isorhamnetin; Isorhamnetin 3-O-α-L-rhamnopyranosyl-1,6-β D-glucopyranoside; Isorhoifolin; Kaempferol; Kaempferol-O-glucoside; Luteolin; Quercetin; Quercetin-3-O-β-D-glucopyranoside; Quercitrin; Rutin	[23,37,50,54]
	Polyphenols	Caffeic acid; Chlorogenic acid; Complicatus; Cryptochlorogenic acid; Ferulic acid; Gallic acid; p-Coumaric acid; Coumaric acid	[23,28,37,50,54]
	Iridoids	10-Desacetyl asperulosidic acid; 10-Hydroxyloganin; 10-Hydroxymorroniside; Asperulosidic acid; Asperuloside; Deacetylalpinoside; Deacetyl-daphylloside; Deacetylasperulosidic acid; Daphylloside; Galioside; Gardenosidic acid; Geniposidic acid; Loganin; Mollugoside; Monotropein; Scandoside; Scandoside methyl ester; Secogalioside; 6-Acetylscandoside; 6-O-epi-Acetyl scandosid	[37,42,50,54]
	Phytosterols	β-Sitosterol; Campesterol	[62]
G. odoratum	Flavonoids	Kaempferol; Quercetin; Quercitrin; Rutin	[23,40]
	Polyphenols	Caffeic acid; Chlorogenic acid; p-Coumaric acid; Ferulic acid	[23,40,54]
	Iridoids	10-Deacetyl asperulosidic acid; Asperulosidic acid; Asperuloside; Deacetyl asperuloside; Geniposidic acid; Monotropein; Scandoside	[40,46,54]
	Phytosterols	β-Sitosterol; Campesterol	[54,62]
G. verum	Flavonoids	Apigenin; Apigetrin; Astragalin; Catechin; Chrysin; Cynaroside; Diosmin; Diosmetin; Epicatechin; Fisetin; Hesperidin; Hyperoside; Isorhoifolin; Isorhamnetin; Isoquercetin; Isoquercitrin; Kaempferol; Luteolin; Quercetin; Quercitrin; Rutin	[16–18,20–23,25,28,29,35–37,47,48,50,52,54,84]
	Polyphenols	Caffeic acid; Chlorogenic acid; Coumarinic acid; p-Coumaric acid; Ferulic acid; Gallic acid;	[16,20,22,23,25,35,37,50,84]
	Iridoids	Asperuloside; Asperulosidic acid; Daphylloside; Deacetyl-asperulosidic acid; Deacetyl-asperuloside; Geniposidic acid; Loganin; Monotropein; Scandoside	[37,46,50,54]
	Anthraquinones	Physcion; 1,3-Dihydroxy-2-methylanthraquinone (Rubiadin)	[53]
	Terpenoids	α-Terpineol; Betulalbuside A; Betulin; Borneol; Camphor; Euscaphic acid; Germacrene D; Lupeol; Oleanolic acid; Rubifolic acid; Squalene; Tormentic acid; Ursolic acid; Uvaol	[54,57]
	Phytosterols	β-Sitosterol; Campesterol; Stigmasterol	[61,62]

Galium verum blossoms and herb, *G. aparine* herb, and *G. mollugo]* herb are a valuable source of phenolics, iridoids, and volatile phytochemicals long known to mankind for their therapeutic properties [28,37].

Natural products of *G. aparine* such as flavonoids, terpenoids, and steroids also have different pharmacological properties, including antioxidant and antitumor activity [74]. As a natural antioxidant *G. aparine* is used in the treatment of various diseases such as diabetes, cancer, and hypertension [92].

By virtue of their antioxidant properties, *G. verum* and *G. aparine* are traditionally used in Europe and the Balkans as diuretics, blood purifiers, and liver detoxifiers, consumed as tea for kidney and liver disorders and urinary tract infections. Externally, they are applied as wound healers for eczema, ulcers, and burns [28,32,33,35,69,73,77,79,93]. Antioxidant properties of *Galium* species are also utilized in derma cosmetics [14].

Galium mollugo has moderate antioxidant activity and exhibits antibacterial properties [33,46]. It is externally used for skin irritations and inflammations as it showed strong anti-inflammatory potential, likely due to its high iridoid content, and it is internally used as a diuretic and digestive aid [33,46].

Due to its antioxidant, neuroprotective, and anti-inflammatory properties, *G. odoratum* is recognized for antispasmodic, sedative, and anticoagulant effects and is used for digestive support [23,33,46,62,93].

3.2. Phytochemical Composition, Biological Activity, and Pharmacological Effects of G. verum

Galium verum is one of the most significant herbs in ethnomedicine and has recently attracted the attention of scientists for its diverse biological activities and its rich phytochemical profile. Research on the phytochemistry of *G. verum* supports its traditional use and potential medicinal application. The latest studies on the composition of the species overlap with older ones, with some documenting the content of substances unknown to the species. As a source of phenolic compounds, such as flavonoids and phenolic acids, iridoids, anthraquinones, and other bioactive compounds, *G. verum* has been used for its antioxidant [33,34,37], anti-inflammatory [38,54,71,72], immunomodulatory [32], diuretic [69,79,80], sedative [79,82], wound healing [35,80], anticancer [65,66,84], antiseptic [82], and antibacterial [84] properties for treating kidney and liver diseases [33] and cardiovascular diseases [86], and it is applied externally for healing wounds, ulcers, and rashes [35,80,82].

The phytochemical compounds isolated from *G. verum* and determined, and their biological activities (where information is available) are illustrated in Table 2.

Table 2. Chemical structure and biological activity of phytochemicals isolated from *Galium verum*.

№	Phytochemical Compound	Molecular Formula	2D Chemical Structure *	Biological Activity	Ref.
			Flavonoids		
1	Apigenin	$C_{15}H_{10}O_5$	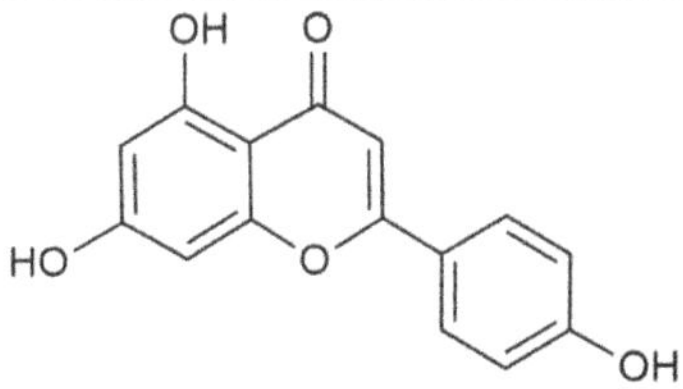	Antioxidant	[22,36,84]
2	Apigetrin (Cosmosiin, Apigenin 7-glucoside)	$C_{21}H_{20}O_{10}$	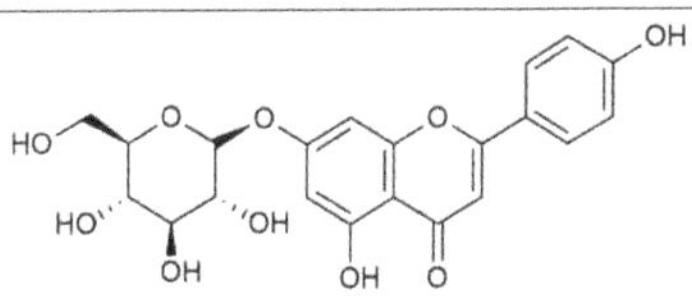		[22,28]

Table 2. *Cont.*

№	Phytochemical Compound	Molecular Formula	2D Chemical Structure *	Biological Activity	Ref.
3	Astragalin (Kaempferol 3-O-glucoside)	$C_{21}H_{20}O_{11}$	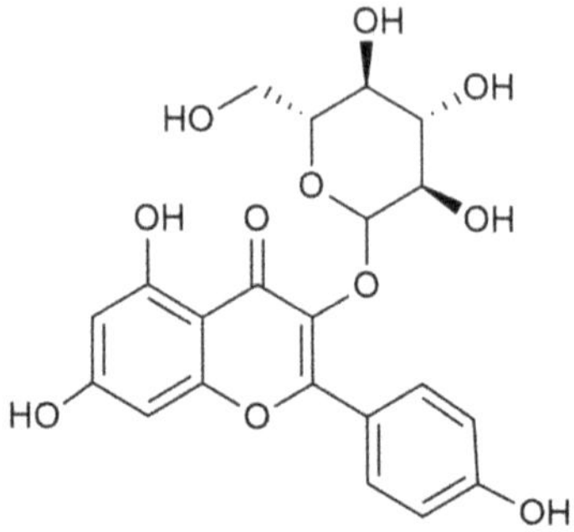		[47]
4	(+)-Catechin (Cianidanol)	$C_{15}H_{14}O_6$	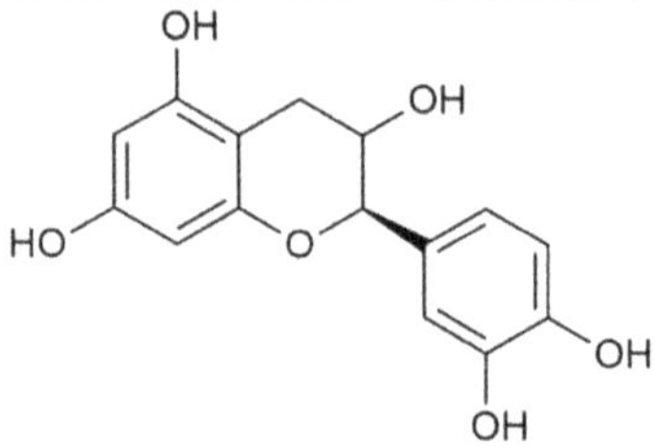	Antioxidant Anti-inflammatory Antimicrobial	[25]
5	Chrysin	$C_{15}H_{10}O_4$	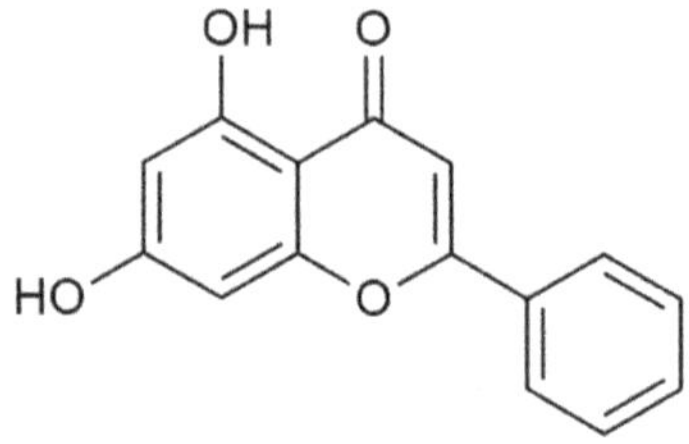		[25]
6	Cynaroside (Luteolin 7-O-glucoside)	$C_{21}H_{20}O_{11}$	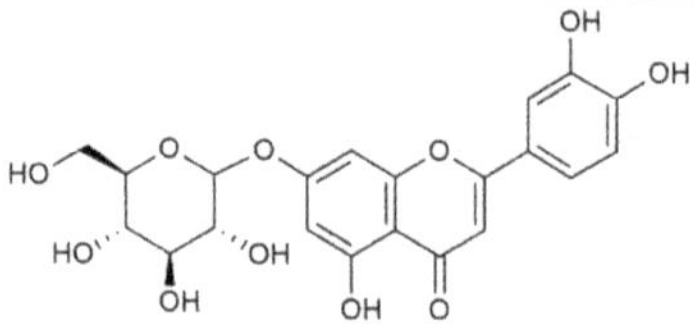		[28]
7	Diosmin	$C_{28}H_{32}O_{15}$	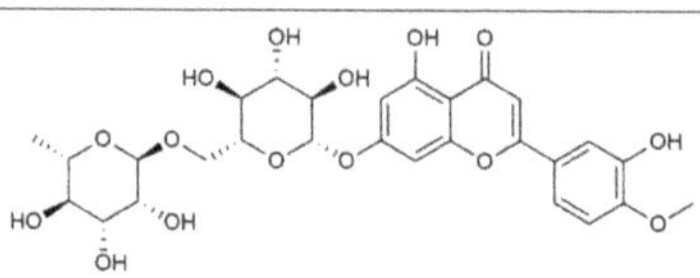	Anti-thrombotic	[29]
8	Diosmetin	$C_{16}H_{12}O_6$	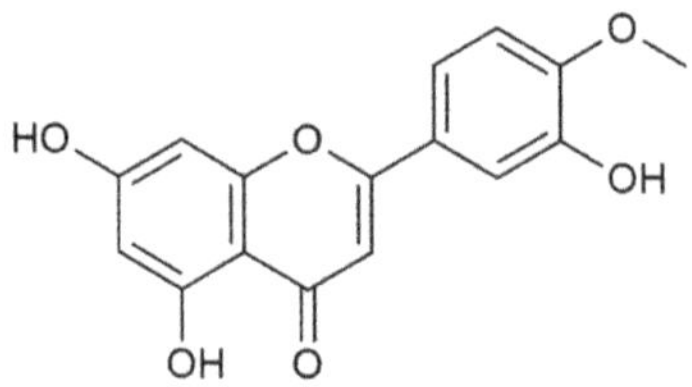	Anticancer Antiapoptotic	[17,18,21]

Table 2. *Cont.*

№	Phytochemical Compound	Molecular Formula	2D Chemical Structure *	Biological Activity	Ref.
9	(-)-Epicatechin	$C_{15}H_{14}O_6$	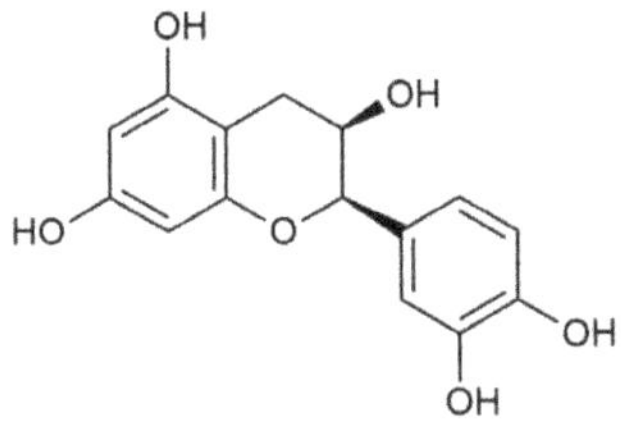		[25,84]
10	Fisetin	$C_{15}H_{10}O_6$	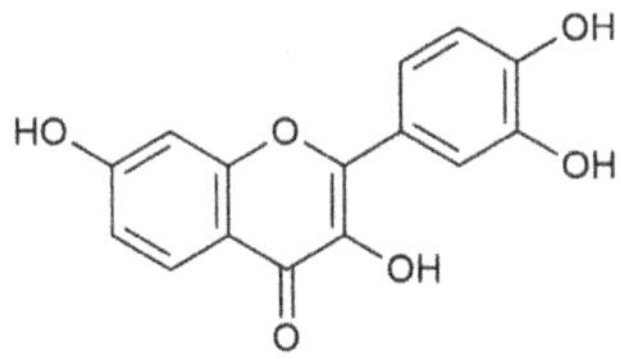		[25]
11	Hesperidin	$C_{28}H_{34}O_{15}$	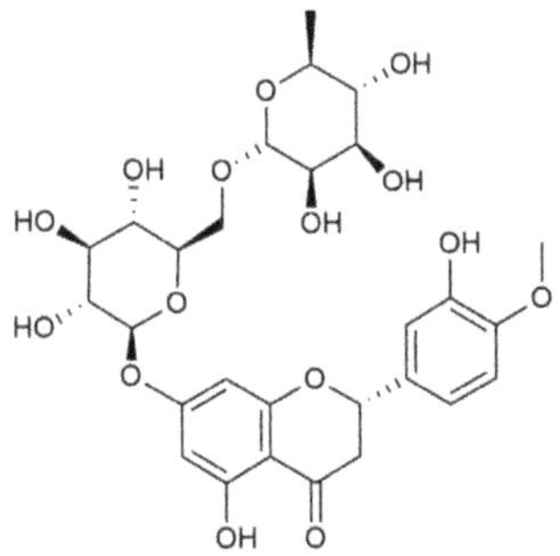		[25]
12	Hyperoside	$C_{21}H_{20}O_{12}$	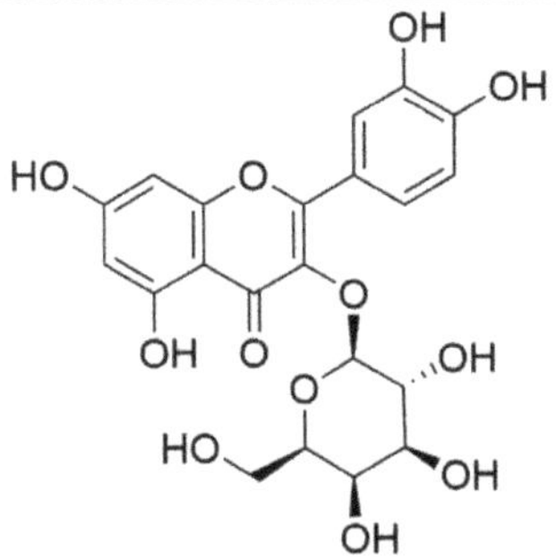		[16,36]
13	Isorhoifolin (Apigenin 7-O-rutinoside)	$C_{27}H_{30}O_{14}$	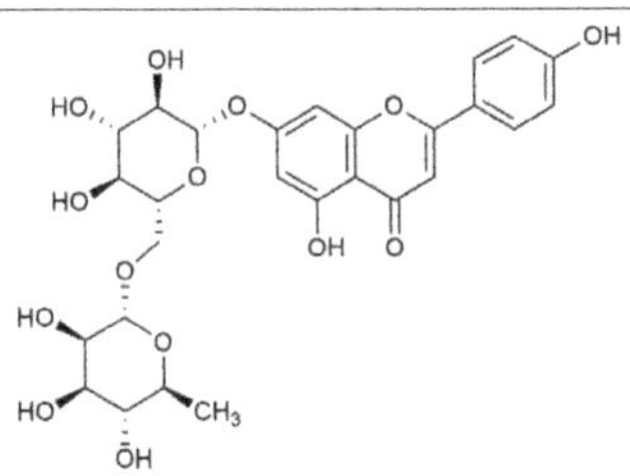		[28]

Table 2. *Cont.*

№	Phytochemical Compound	Molecular Formula	2D Chemical Structure *	Biological Activity	Ref.
14	Isorhamnetin	$C_{16}H_{12}O_7$	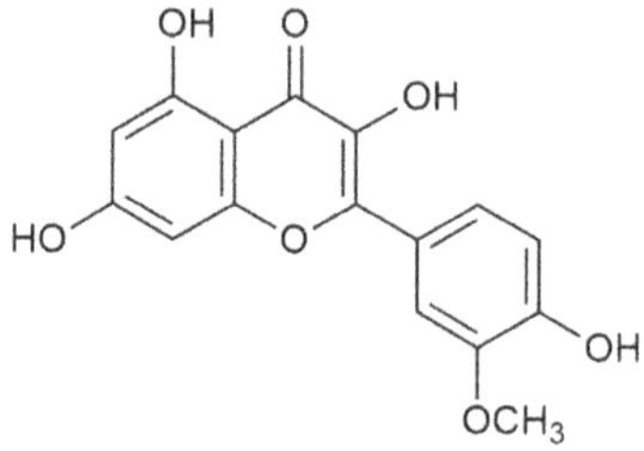		[18]
15	Isoquercetin	$C_{21}H_{20}O_{12}$	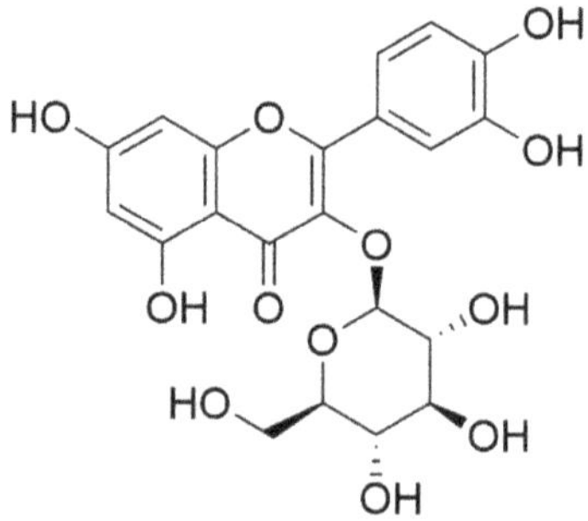		[36]
16	Isoquercitrin	$C_{21}H_{20}O_{12}$	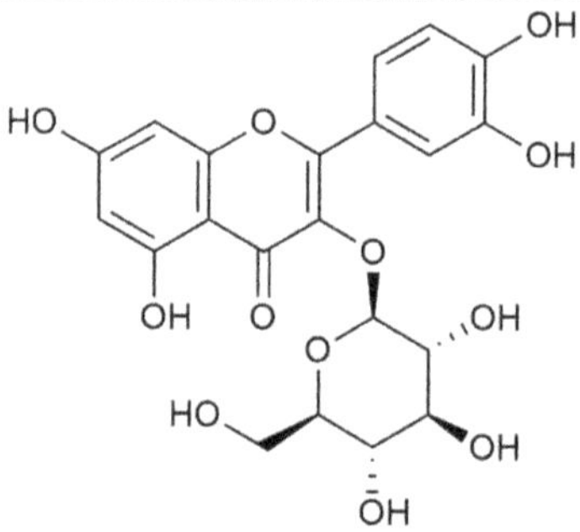	Anticancer	[23,25,84]
17	Kaempferol	$C_{15}H_{10}O_6$	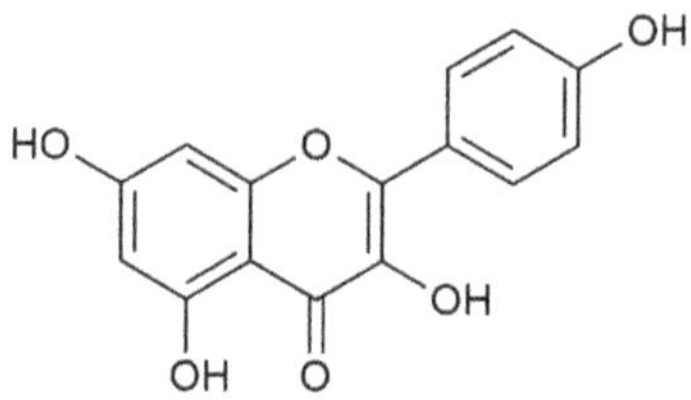	Antioxidant	[22,23]
18	Luteolin	$C_{15}H_{10}O_6$	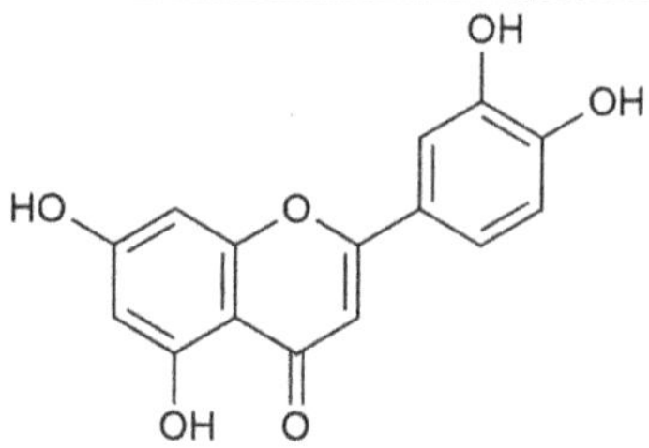	Antioxidant	[20,22,84]

Table 2. *Cont.*

№	Phytochemical Compound	Molecular Formula	2D Chemical Structure *	Biological Activity	Ref.
19	Quercetin	$C_{15}H_{10}O_7$	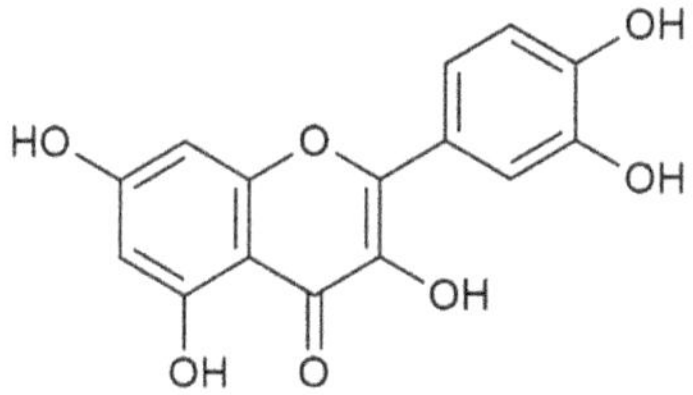	Anti-hypertensive Anti-inflammatory	[22,35,36]
20	Quercitrin	$C_{21}H_{20}O_{11}$	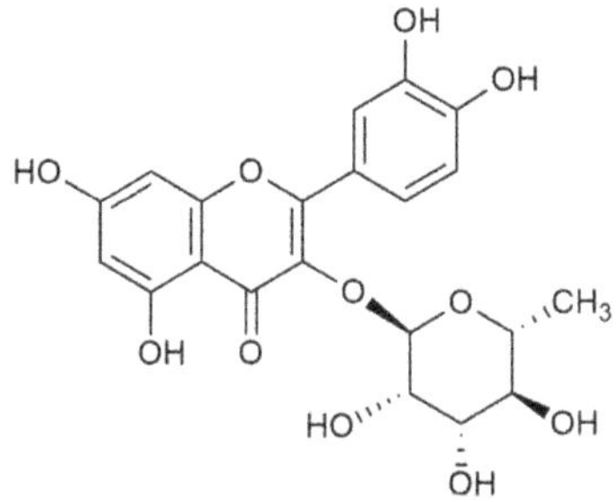	Antioxidant Antimicrobial	[16,23,35,36]
21	Rutin	$C_{27}H_{30}O_{16}$	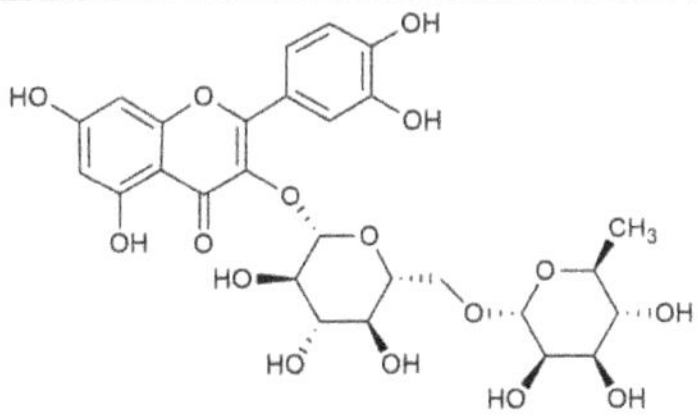	Antioxidant Anticancer Antimicrobial	[16,20,22,35,36,47,84]
			Phenolic acids		
22	Caffeic acid	$C_9H_8O_4$	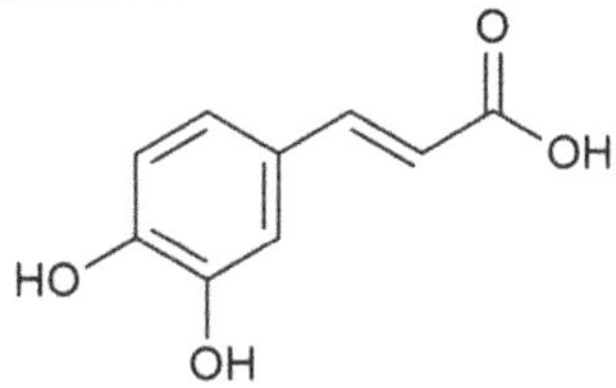	Antioxidant	[16,20,22,25]
23	Chlorogenic acid	$C_{16}H_{18}O_9$	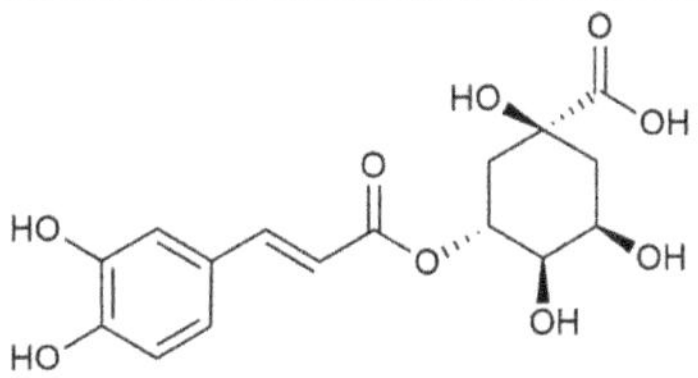	Antioxidant Anticancer Antimicrobial	[16,22,23,25,35]
24	Coumarinic acid	$C_9H_8O_3$	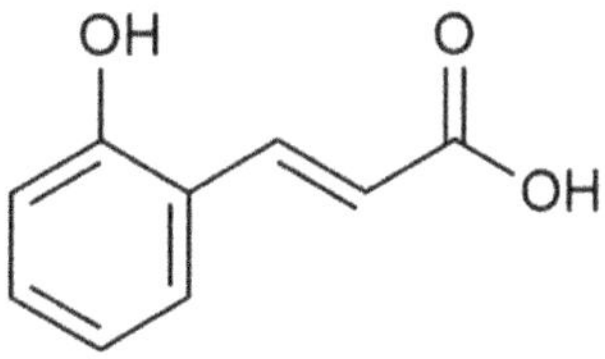		[22]

Table 2. *Cont.*

№	Phytochemical Compound	Molecular Formula	2D Chemical Structure *	Biological Activity	Ref.
25	p-Coumaric acid	$C_9H_8O_3$	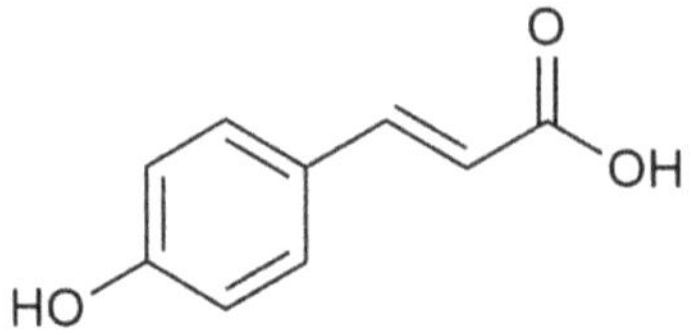	Antioxidant	[22,23,25,35,84]
26	Ferulic acid	$C_{10}H_{10}O_4$	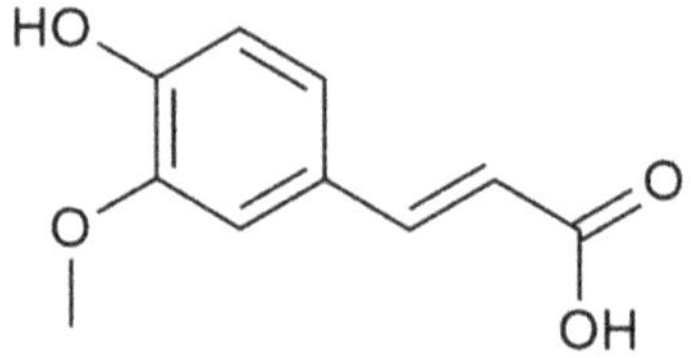		[22,23,25,84]
27	Gallic acid	$C_7H_6O_5$	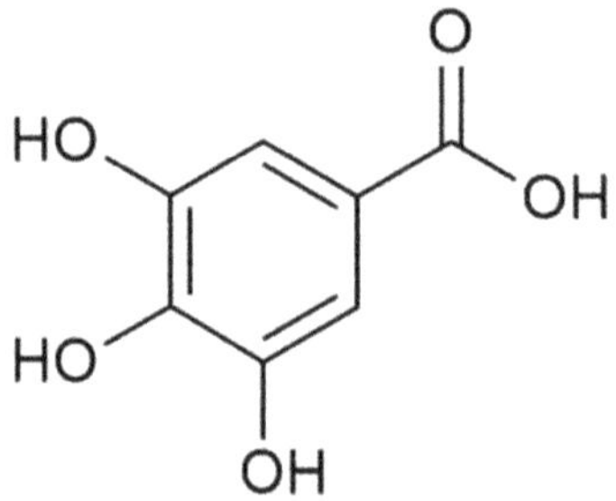		[35]
			Iridoid glycosides		
28	Asperuloside	$C_{18}H_{22}O_{11}$	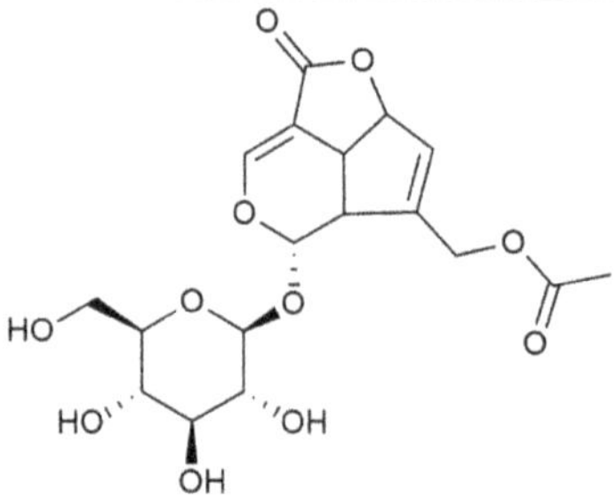	Antioxidant Anticancer Anti-inflammatory	[46–48]
29	Asperulosidic acid	$C_{18}H_{24}O_{12}$	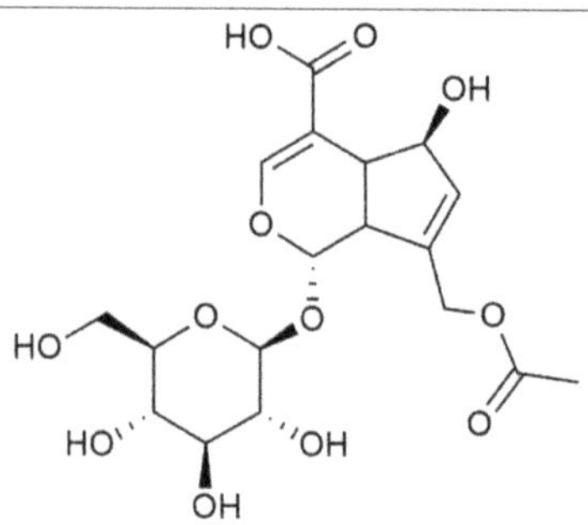		[46–48]

Table 2. *Cont.*

№	Phytochemical Compound	Molecular Formula	2D Chemical Structure *	Biological Activity	Ref.
30	Daphylloside	$C_{19}H_{26}O_{12}$	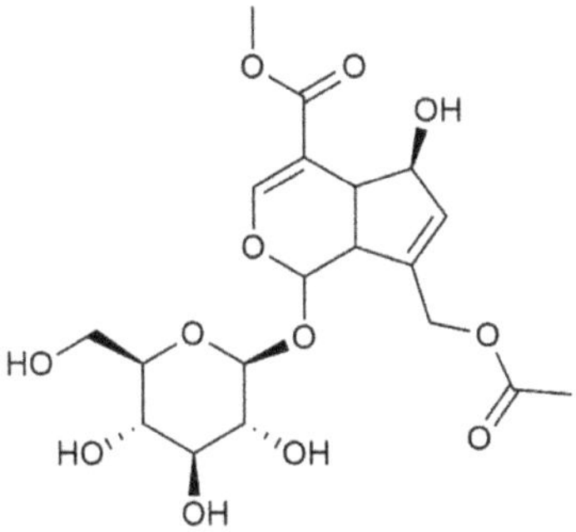	Hepatoprotective	[47]
31	Deacetylasperulosidic acid	$C_{16}H_{22}O_{11}$	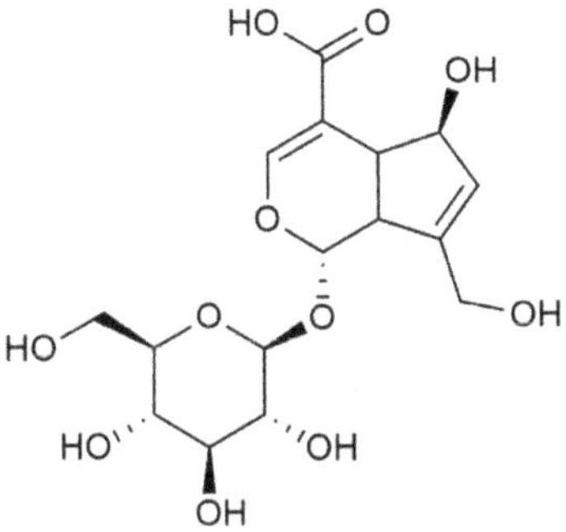		[46,47]
32	Deacetylasperuloside	$C_{16}H_{20}O_{10}$	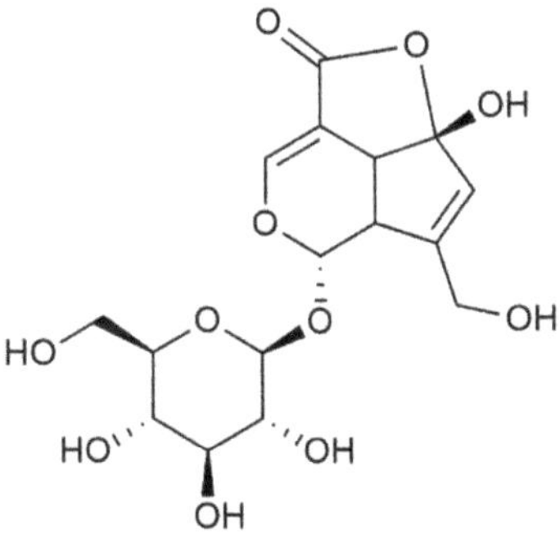		[48]
33	Geniposidic acid	$C_{16}H_{22}O_{10}$	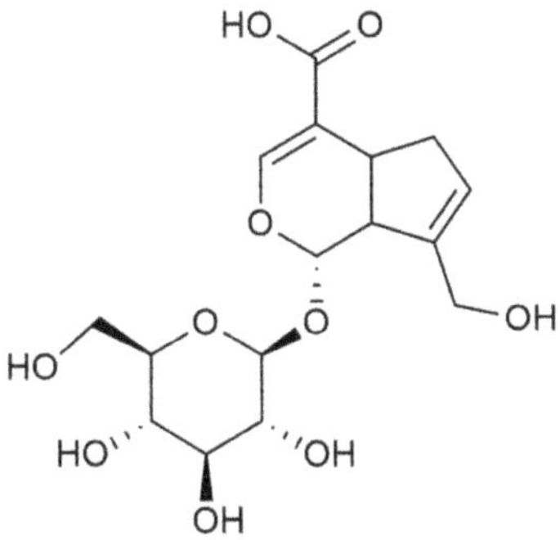		[44,45]

Table 2. *Cont.*

№	Phytochemical Compound	Molecular Formula	2D Chemical Structure *	Biological Activity	Ref.
34	Loganin	$C_{17}H_{26}O_{10}$	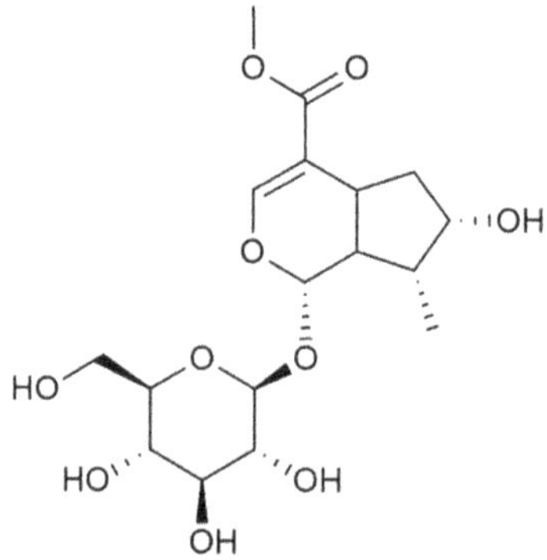		[46]
35	Monotropein	$C_{16}H_{22}O_{11}$	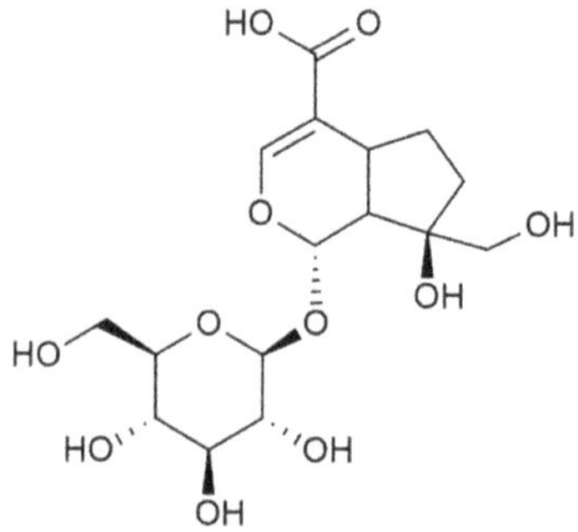		[46,47]
36	Scandoside	$C_{16}H_{22}O_{11}$	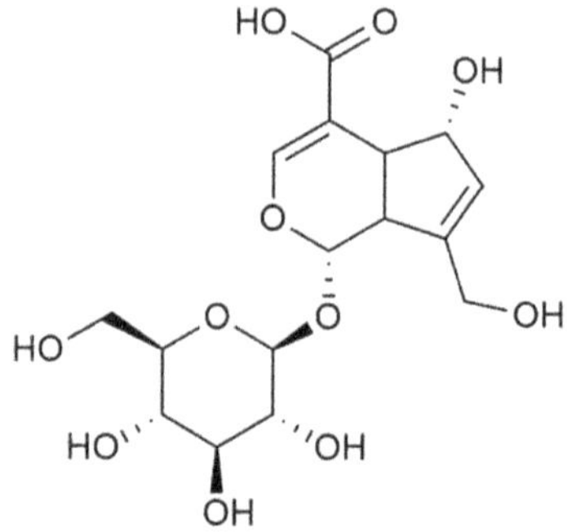		[46,48]
			Anthraquinones		
37	Physcion	$C_{16}H_{12}O_{5}$	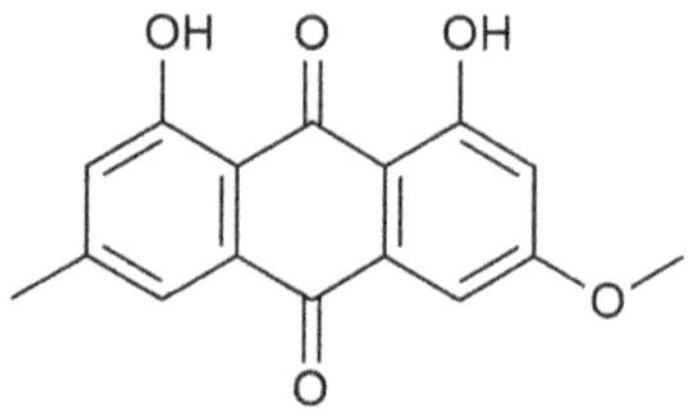		[53]

Table 2. *Cont.*

№	Phytochemical Compound	Molecular Formula	2D Chemical Structure *	Biological Activity	Ref.
38	Rubiadin (1,3-dihydroxy-2-methylanthraquinone)	$C_{16}H_{12}O_5$	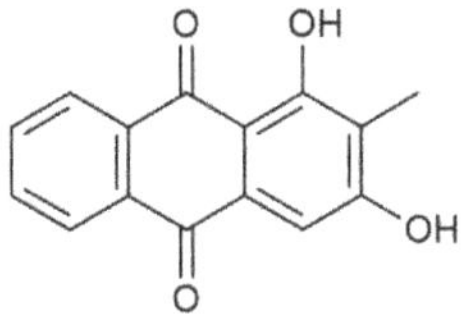		[53]
			Terpenoids		
39	α-Terpineol	$C_{10}H_{18}O$	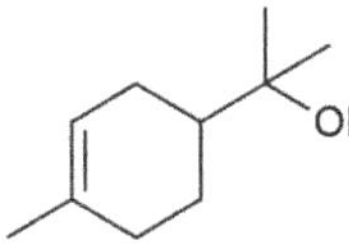		[56,58]
40	Betulalbuside A	$C_{16}H_{28}O_7$	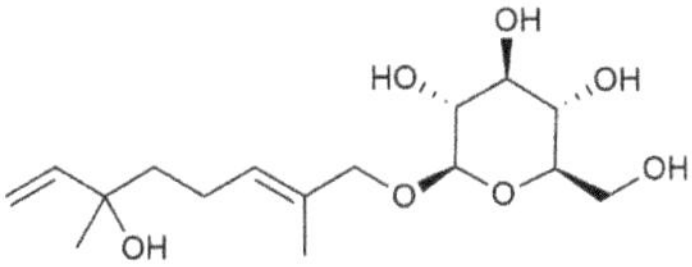		[47]
41	Betulin	$C_{30}H_{50}O_2$	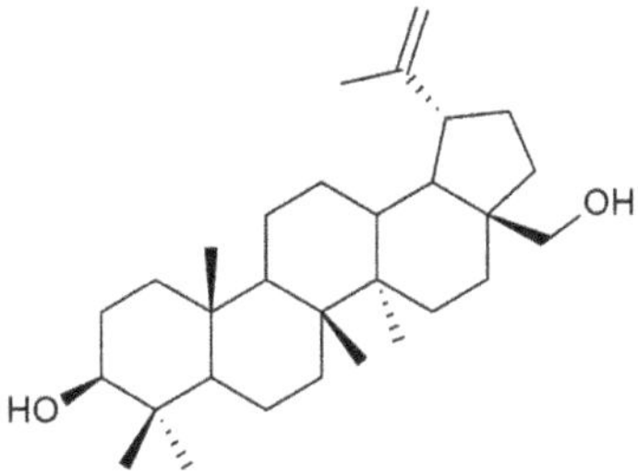		[57]
42	Borneol	$C_{10}H_{18}O$	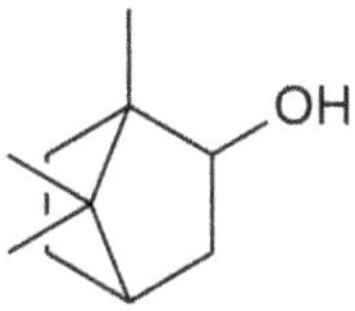		[56,58]
43	Camphor	$C_{10}H_{16}O$	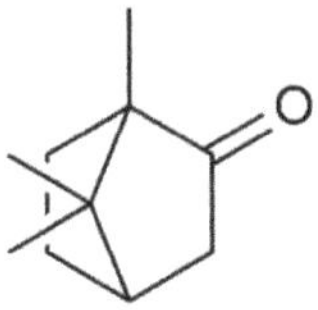	Antioxidant Cytotoxic Antimicrobial	[56,59]
44	Euscaphic acid	$C_{30}H_{48}O_5$	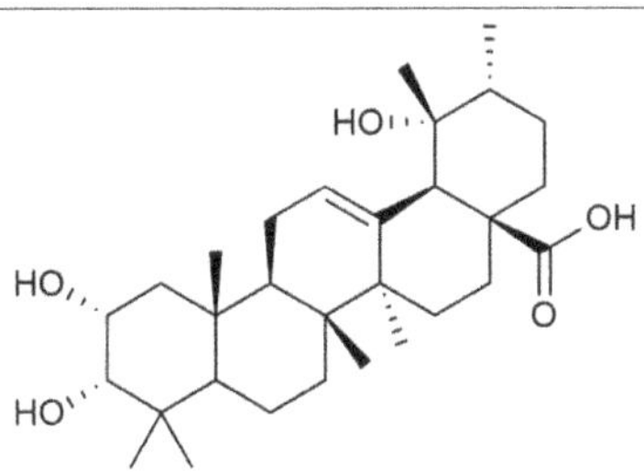		[57]

Table 2. *Cont.*

№	Phytochemical Compound	Molecular Formula	2D Chemical Structure *	Biological Activity	Ref.
45	Germacrene D	$C_{15}H_{24}$	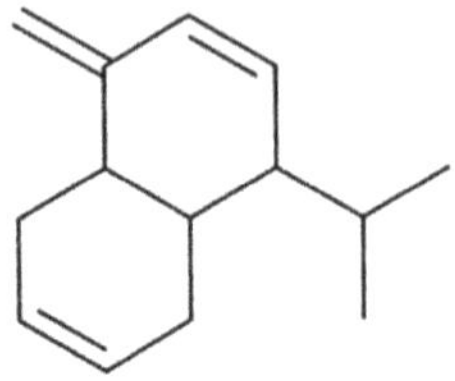	Antioxidant Antimicrobial	[58]
46	Lupeol	$C_{30}H_{50}O$	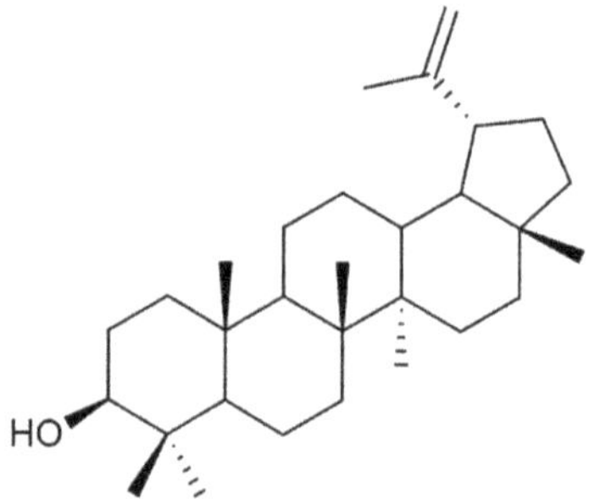		[57]
47	Oleanolic acid	$C_{30}H_{48}O_3$	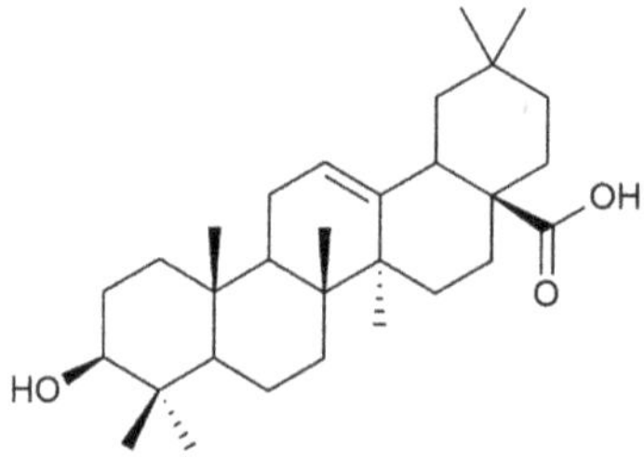		[57]
48	Rubifolic acid	$C_{30}H_{48}O_4$	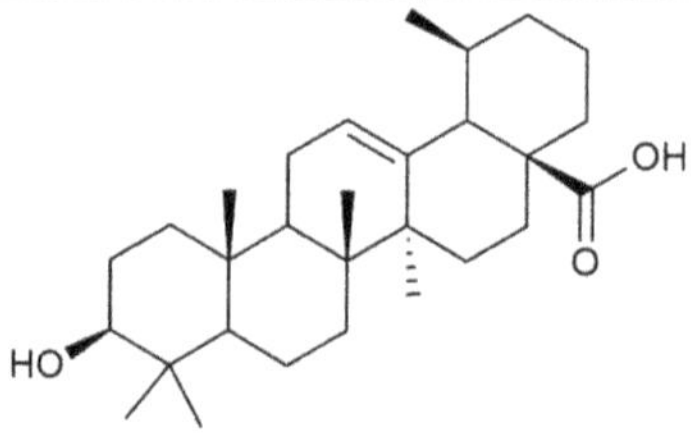		[18,32]
49	Squalene	$C_{30}H_{50}$	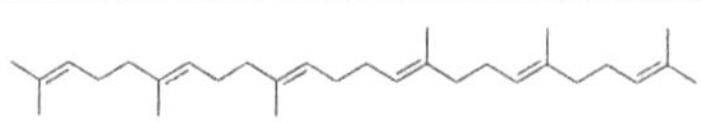	Antioxidant Cytotoxic Antimicrobial	[56,58,59]
50	Tormentic acid	$C_{30}H_{48}O_5$	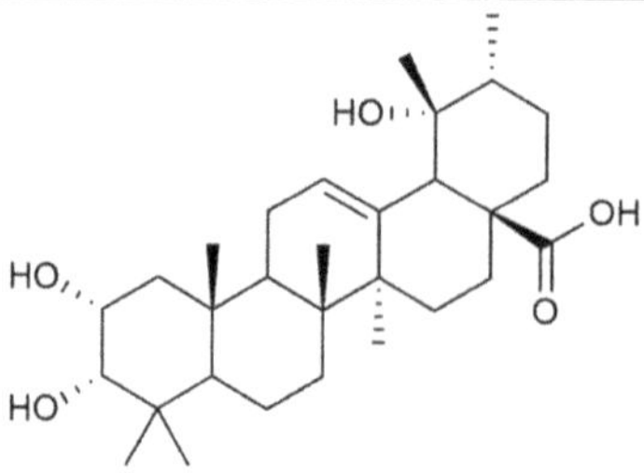		[57]

Table 2. *Cont.*

№	Phytochemical Compound	Molecular Formula	2D Chemical Structure *	Biological Activity	Ref.
51	Ursolic acid	$C_{30}H_{48}O_3$	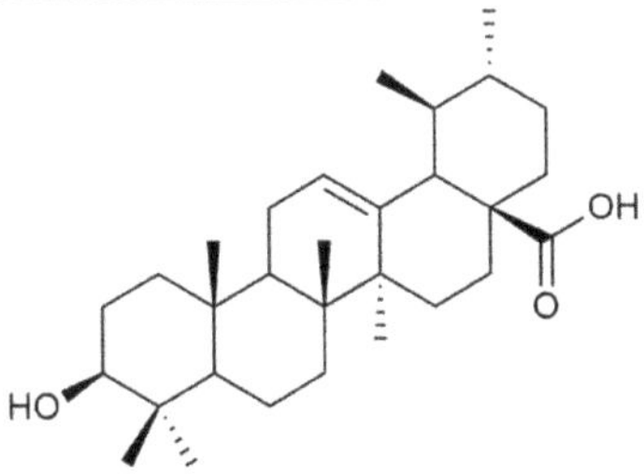		[18,32,57]
52	Uvaol	$C_{30}H_{50}O_2$	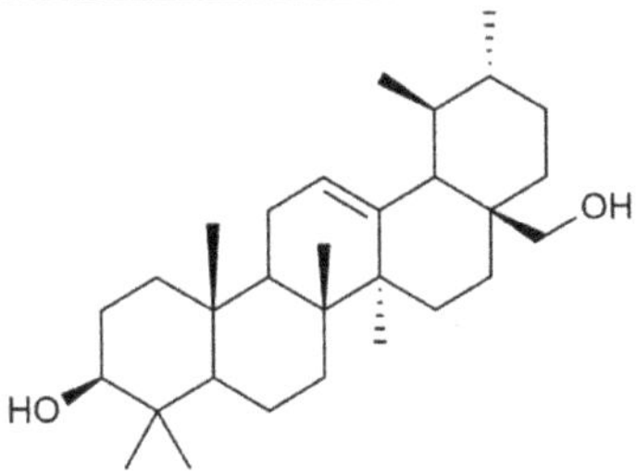		[57]
			Phytosterols		
53	β-sitosterol	$C_{29}H_{50}O$	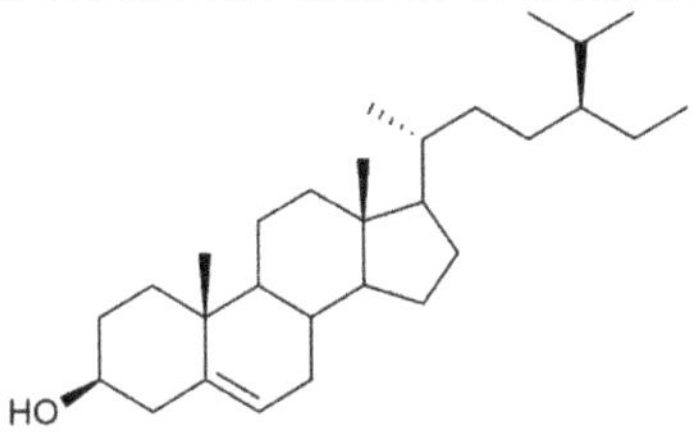	Antioxidant Anticancer Anti-inflammatory	[62]
54	Campesterol	$C_{28}H_{48}O$	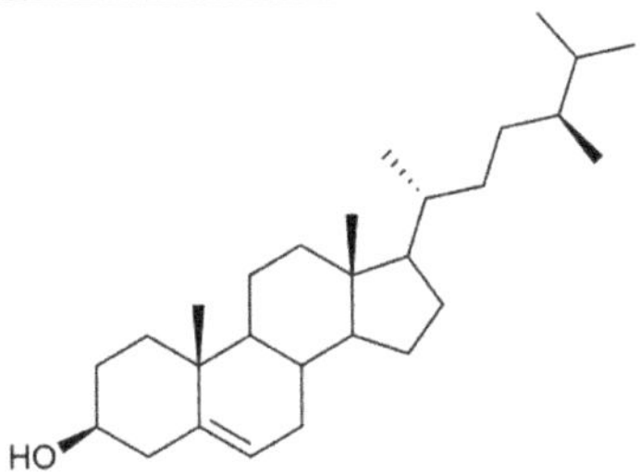	Anticancer	[61,62]
55	Stigmasterol	$C_{29}H_{48}O$	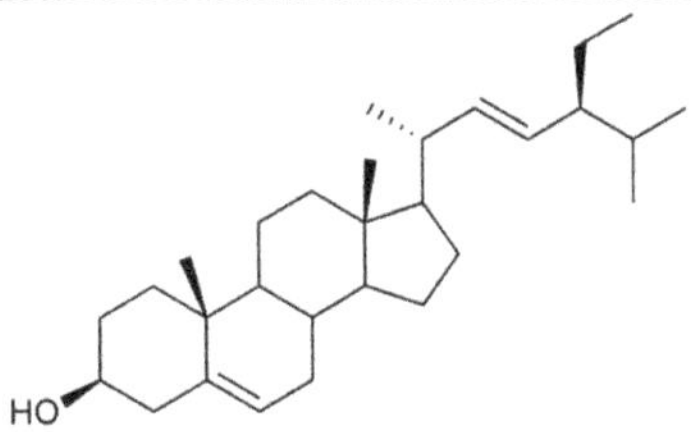		[61]

* Two-dimensional chemical structures, drawn with ChemDraw Software.

As shown in Table 2. numerous phytochemical compounds have been reported in the content of *G. verum*. Many of them correlate with certain biological activity. To understand how these compounds contribute to the healing properties of the species, a more detailed review of the available research for each group of bioactive compounds and the correlating pharmacological effects will be discussed in the subsections below.

3.2.1. Content of Phenolic Compounds (Flavones, Flavonols, Flavone Glycosides, Flavonol Glycosides, Phenolic Acids) and Antioxidant Activity

The extraction of phenolic compounds from medicinal plants has attracted growing interest due to their significant antioxidant properties and widespread presence in plants [94–96]. Antioxidants have protective roles against the harmful effects of various drugs and chemicals. They can mitigate oxidative stress, a key factor in cellular damage, thereby offering potential therapeutic strategies to counteract toxicity induced by pharmaceuticals and environmental agents [97]. They also have the potential to mitigate the effects of oxidative stress in aging and related diseases [98].

The antioxidant activity of *G. verum* mainly relies on its rich phenolic content. Polyphenols possess potent antioxidant properties, modulating enzyme and cellular receptor activity, regulating nitric oxide levels, inducing apoptosis, scavenging free radicals, and inhibiting cell proliferation and angiogenesis [99–102]. These mechanisms underline their preventive effects, including anti-inflammatory, antimicrobial, cardioprotective, and other health-promoting activities. A number of epidemiological data indicate that these activities may be effective against neurodegenerative diseases, cardiovascular conditions, and disorders linked to oxidative stress [103–105].

Mavi et al. were among the first to examine the antioxidant activity of *G. verum* [15]. Using various methods, a connection between the reducing power of plant extracts and the total phenolic content was identified. As extract concentrations increased, so did their phenolic content, reducing power. Despite a relatively low total phenolic content detected, *G. verum* exhibited strong antioxidant activity, including DPPH (2,2-diphenyl-1-picrylhydrazyl) radical scavenging activity and peroxidation inhibition, suggesting that its phenolic compounds are powerful antioxidants.

Tămaş et al. conducted comparative phytochemical research of *G. verum L.* and *G. mollugo]* L. [16]. Using TLC, it was established that these species contained five flavonoid compounds: hyperoside (12), quercitrin (20), rutin (21), caffeic (22), and chlorogenic acid (23). The amounts of the identified compounds were different for the species studied. *G. verum* contained higher amounts of hyperoside, while *G. molugo* contained higher amounts of rutin. The total content of flavonoids was also different, with over three times higher amounts for *G. verum*.

Zhao et al. conducted a detailed analysis of the phenolic composition of *G. verum* [17,18]. Their research identified several phenolic compounds, including diosmetin (8), isorhamnetin (14), kaempferol (17), and quercetin (19).

Lakić et al. conducted a comparative study of two *G. verum* populations in Serbia and found significant differences in flavonoid content, chlorophyll levels, and radical-scavenging activity based on geographical and environmental factors [19]. The following indicators were determined in the study: total phenolic and flavonoid content; chlorophyll "a" and "b" content; and antioxidant activity by several methods: DPPH radical scavenging activity, OH radical scavenging activity, H_2O_2 scavenging activity, and lipid peroxidation. The researcher found higher values of phenolic content (4.57–5.16 mg GAE/g dm) (GAEs—gallic acid equivalents), flavonoids, and quercetin equivalents (15.56–17.96 μg QE/g dm) in the population exposed to environmental urban stressors, and on the contrary, higher total content of chlorophyll "a" and "b" in plants from the mountain populations (0.25 mg—chlorophyll "a"; 0.46 mg—chlorophyll "b"), which are exposed to direct sunlight at higher altitudes. This corresponds to the higher IC_{50} values of the DPPH analysis: 8.04 μg/mL for the urban population vs. 3.10 μg/mL for the mountain population. The authors observed a stronger dependence of DPPH radical-scavenging activity on the extract concentration. The same tendencies were determined at the hydroxyl radical scavenging tests. IC_{50} values of 0.05 μg/mL were determined for the samples from the mountain population and 0.54 μg/mL for the urban samples. Reversed, the degree of neutralization of a 50% solution of hydrogen peroxide (H_2O_2) varies from 4.98 μg/mL to 3.80 μg/mL for the mountain and urban samples, respectively. More general conclusions were drawn in the same work. The degree of inhibition of lipid peroxidation varied widely, ranging from 2.07% to 69.39% and from 23.91% to 48.25% for the mountain and urban samples, respectively. Both tested extracts expressed a noticeable inhibitory activity on lipid peroxidation, with the following values established for IC_{50}: 11.70 μg/mL and 19.47 μg/mL, respectively. Lakić et al. concluded that the superior neutralization of DPPH and hydroxyl radicals by mountain plant extracts was due to higher chlorophyll content, while the better hydrogen peroxide scavenging observed in Veternik extracts correlated with higher phenolic and flavonoid levels.

Data from analysis of ethanol extracts from *G. verum* var. *asiaticum* from Korea showed strong antioxidant activity [20]. The researcher explained it by the high content of phenolic compounds such as luteolin (18), rutin (21), and caffeic acid (22). Caffeic acid was identified as the compound with the most significant antioxidant activity.

Zhao et al. discovered that diosmetin (8) isolated from *G. verum* exhibits an anticancer effect [21]. Treated mice with this compound developed a dose-dependent effect on tumor growth, and the degree of inhibition increased with the dose increasing. Diosmetin application protected cells from tumor-induced apoptosis.

Danila et al. conducted a comparative analysis of several medicinal plants, including *G. verum,* from the territory of Romania [22]. The study determined the total phenolic content via spectrophotometry and identified the phenolic compounds' high-performance liquid chromatography (RP-HPLC). Antioxidant activity was determined by DPPH radical scavenging activity and ABTS (2,2′-azino-bis(3-ethylbenzothiazoline-6-sulfonic acid) cation radical scavenging activity. The results showed relatively high total phenolic content and antioxidant activity for *G. verum*. Alcoholic extracts yielded higher phenolic concentrations than aqueous ones, with optimal yields for *G. verum* obtained using 30% ethanol. This approach of comparing the type of extract highlighted the differences between the concentrations of phenolic compounds as a function of the extraction solvent. To determine the phenolic and flavonoid composition of the analyzed plants, the authors developed and validated a new HPLC method. The following phenols were identified: caffeic acid (22), chlorogenic acid (23), coumarinic acid (24), and ferulic acid (26), and the flavonoids kaempferol (17), luteolin (18), quercetin (19), and rutin (21). Chlorogenic acid was the predominant compound, followed by caffeic and coumarinic acids. The researchers concluded that the high phenolic content and antioxidant activity of *G. verum* make it a promising candidate for medical purposes.

Vlase et al. conducted a comparative study of four *Galium* species collected from Romania [23]. Polyphenol and flavonoid content, antioxidant activity, and antimicrobial properties of 70% ethanol extracts further reinforce the medicinal potential of *G. verum*. Using the HPLC-MS/MS method, diverse polyphenolic compounds were identified in *G. verum* extracts, some of which had been previously reported for this species: isoquercitrin (16), kaempferol (17), quercetin (19), quercitrin (20), rutin (21), chlorogenic acid (23), p-coumaric acid (25), and ferulic acid (26). Among these, chlorogenic and ferulic acids were present in minor quantities, while rutin was identified as the predominant compound, with a concentration of 804 mg/100 g of dried plant material. Interestingly, compounds, such as luteolin, caffeic acid, and apigenin, which were identified in prior studies, were not detected in this analysis. This suggests that the polyphenol composition may vary across populations, influenced by ecological factors such as habitat, altitude, and latitude. Additionally, variations may arise from differences in the identification methods, solvents, or extraction techniques used (e.g., with or without ultrasound). In the same study, the total content of polyphenols, flavonoids, and caffeic acid derivatives was quantified using spectrophotometric methods. Among the four species studied, *G. mollugo]* and *G. verum* exhibited the highest levels of these phytochemical compounds. Based on these findings, Vlase et al. suggested that both species hold potential as sources of antioxidants for pharmaceutical applications. Researchers supported this claim with additional studies. Antioxidant activity was measured using the DPPH radical scavenging assay, and the results connected strongly with the total phenolic content. *Galium verum* demonstrated the highest antioxidant potential among the species studied, with an IC_{50} value of 105.43 ± 0.15 μg/mL. The antibacterial activity of the extracts was evaluated using a diffusimetric method. The results indicated varying degrees of inhibitory activity against the tested pathogens, particularly against Gram-positive bacteria, such as *S. aureus* and *L. monocytogenes*. *G. verum* exhibited moderate antibacterial activity but showed limited antifungal activity against *C. albicans*. The comparative study by Vlase et al. highlighted significant differences in the polyphenol content among the four *Galium* species, suggesting that these differences could serve as taxonomic markers for distinguishing species within the genus [23].

The pro-oxidant reactivity of the extracts was evaluated by Moţ et al. [24]. The reactivity was significantly higher than the average for other plant extracts tested with the same method. This increase was attributed to the quercetin present in the *G. verum* extract, which is known for its ability to generate radicals easily. The second stage of the study included an in vitro experiment with female rats. They were exposed to oxidative stress by being kept in complete darkness. The rats treated with *G. verum* extracts showed reduced oxidative damage and restored antioxidant balance compared to untreated groups. This study demonstrated that *G. verum* extract may have the potential to counteract biochemical damage caused by stress and highlighted *G. verum*'s significant potential as a source of antioxidants. Thus, it could be considered for use in pharmaceutical formulations, although further research is necessary to confirm these findings.

Matei et al. conducted further phytochemical studies on *G. verum* and related species [25]. They found that *G. verum* contains a 3-fold higher flavonoid concentration than other species, which explains its notable antioxidant activity. A total of 13 phenolic compounds were identified, including catechin (4), chrysin (5), epicatechin (9), fisetin (10), hesperidin (11), isorhamnetin (14), isoquercitrin (16), quercitrin (20), rutin (21), caffeic acid (22), chlorogenic acid (23), p-coumaric acid (25), and ferulic acid (26). The study developed an HPLC method to quantitatively analyze these compounds in ethanol extracts. It was observed that the type of solvent and extraction method significantly influenced the results, with reflux extraction yielding the most efficient results.

Layali et al. focused their research exclusively on *G. verum* to evaluate its potential for use in traditional medicine and as a functional food source [26]. Plants were collected from Iran, and extracts from the aerial parts were analyzed using four different in vitro systems to measure radical scavenging activity. These methods included DPPH radical scavenging activity, nitric oxide scavenging activity, hydrogen peroxide scavenging rate, and iron-reducing power (rate of conversion of Fe(III) to Fe(II) by electron donation), and the results obtained by another researcher were confirmed [22]. The authors confirmed the well-documented antioxidant potential of flavonoids, attributing their efficacy to the hydroxyl groups responsible for free radical scavenging. These results emphasize the potential health benefits of increasing flavonoid consumption in the diet, as supported by previous studies.

Total phenolic and total flavonoid content in *G. verum* was determined by classical colorimetric methods, developed earlier by Ebrahimzadeh [106,107], and the results obtained were 753 ± 21 mg GAE/g dm and 151.25 ± 8.2 mg QE/g dm. These high values underscore *G. verum*'s potential as a significant source of phenols. DPPH radical scavenging activity increased with higher extract concentrations, yielding an IC_{50} value of 59.6 ± 0.04 μg/mL. For comparison, ascorbic acid and BHA (butylated hydroxyanisole) had IC_{50} values of 8.78 ± 0.21 and 92.9 ± 4.5 μg/mL, respectively. Nitric oxide scavenging activity was exceptionally high, with an IC_{50} of 1.7 ± 0.01 μg/mL, and the extract demonstrated a 92.5% inhibition rate of H_2O_2 at a concentration of 50 μg/mL. Additionally, the extract showed strong iron-reducing capabilities at concentrations of 50–800 μg/mL, comparable to vitamin C at higher concentrations ($p > 0.05$).

Dong et al. further validated the protective effects of flavones derived from *G. verum* using human umbilical vein endothelial cells subjected to oxidative stress induced by hydrogen peroxide [27]. The flavones significantly reduced oxidative damage by enhancing nitric oxide levels. A different approach was taken in the study of Ilyina et al., who explored the relationship between the morphological characteristics of *G. verum* and its flavonoid content [28]. The study revealed correlations between specific morphological traits and the chemical profiles of the species.

The research by Cheng et al. was in a different direction [29]. This research proved the anti-thrombotic effect of diosmin (the aglycone part of diosmetin) extracted from *G. verum* by treating rats. The depletion of the key protein for the prevention of thrombosis, CER350, reduces the stability of microtubules. During the experiments, it was found that diosmin (7) causes protein changes and prevents the protein levels from dropping.

Kuhtinskaja et al. compared four extraction methods for bioactive compounds from two plant species, including *G. verum* [30]. The results did not show a clear advantage of one method. Chlorogenic acid (23) was most effectively extracted from *G. verum* with pressurized hot water, whereas rutin (21) was most efficiently extracted using methanol. Despite slight variations, all tested methods were deemed effective for extracting phenols and iridoids, with hot water extraction being preferred due to its environmental friendliness. In the same study, using HPLC- MS (HPLC with mass detection) identified 14 major compounds in *G. verum* extracts, including flavonols and iridoid glucosides, reaffirming the species' rich phenolic and iridoid content.

In 2018, Farcas et al. used in vitro analyses to evaluate the antioxidant and pro-oxidant activities of the flavonoids contained in *G. verum* [31]. The first stage of the study determined the phytochemical composition of *G. verum* using HPLC. High levels of rutin (21) and chlorogenic acid (23) were identified, confirming their role as anti-stress modulators. The antioxidant activity of the extracts was assessed using the DPPH and TEAC methods (Trolox-equivalent antioxidant capacity), with DPPH showing higher activity levels.

Shynkovenko et al. investigated the phytochemical profile of *G. verum*, with results that were largely consistent with previous studies [32]. Any differences were likely due to variations in habitat conditions and analysis methods. The researchers also examined the immunomodulatory effects of the ethanolic extract of *G. verum* using an in vitro experiment with lymphocytes (immune system cells) from heparinized blood. The study is the first of its kind for *G. verum*. It was found that all the substances tested exhibited a significant stimulating effect on the transformation activity of peripheral blood mononuclear cells. The highest immunomodulatory activity was observed with the 96% ethanol extract, which increased proliferation compared to spontaneous transformation. These findings provide a foundation for further research into the immunomodulatory activity of *G. verum* extracts.

Friščić et al. studied the bioactive components and antioxidant potential of eight species of the genus *Galium* in Croatia [33]. Qualitative phytochemical analysis, spectrophotometric determination of total phenols, flavonoids, and iridoids, and analysis of antioxidant activity using the ABTS and DPPH tests were carried out. The results revealed that *G verum* contains some of the highest levels of total phenolics (86.40 ± 1.74 mg GAE/g dm) and flavonoids (23.11 ± 0.12 mg QE/g dm) and demonstrated strong antioxidant activity. The presence of other bioactive substances further suggests biomedical potential, warranting further in-depth studies.

In the same year, Hanganu et al. published data on three species of the genus *Galium* from Romania [34]. The study was similar to Friščić's study, but different methods of analysis were used. Extraction was performed with 70% ethanol, and antioxidant activity was assessed using the FRAP (ferric ion-reducing antioxidant power) method (using Trolox), the CUPRAC method, and the xanthine oxidase method. The study showed that *G. verum* had the broadest spectrum of extracted chemical compounds, although *G. odoratum* had higher levels of total phenols and flavonoids. All three extracts exhibited strong antioxidant capacity, which was directly correlated with their total phenol and flavonoid content. These findings align with most of the available literature, except for the study by Vlase et al. [23], which reported that *G. verum* had higher flavonoid content and antioxidant potential compared to *G. aparine*.

Vuletic et al. assessed the medicinal properties of *G. verum* in an in vivo experiment with rats [35]. In the first phase of the study, the phytochemical composition of the species was analyzed by the HPLC-DAD (HPLC with diode-array detection) technique. In the second phase, a mucoadhesive gel based on *G. verum* extract was developed and applied to rats, with recurrent aphthous stomatitis induced in a laboratory setting. Similar to previous studies on *G. verum*'s phenolic composition, quercetin (19), quercitrin (20), rutin (21), caffeic acid (22), chlorogenic acid (23), p-coumaric acid (25), and gallic acid (27) were identified. Rutin had the highest amount of 23.81 ± 1.90 mg/g dm. For the in vivo experiment, 60 male rats were used. Ulcers were induced in their oral cavity by applying glacial acetic acid. The rats were divided into three groups: Group 1—negative control (no treatment), Group 2—control treated with a gel base without *G. verum* extract, and Group 3—test group treated with a 20% *G. verum* gel. By the second day of gel application, the test group showed significantly more effective ulcer shrinkage compared to the control groups. This improvement continued throughout the experiment, with the test group achieving 100% ulcer shrinkage by the 6th day, which was twice the shrinkage percentage seen in the control groups. In conclusion, the researchers summarized that treatment with *G. verum* reduced pro-oxidant generation in tissues, which helped limit oxidative stress and accelerated the healing process. These effects are likely due to the synergistic activity of the phenolic compounds present in the *G. verum* extract.

In 2023, Ohindovschi et al. used TLC to identify the phenolic content of hydro-ethanol plant extract obtained from *G. verum* [36]. The chromatographic study revealed the content of apigenin (1), hyperoside (12), isoquercetin (15), quercetin (19), quercitrin (20), and rutin (21), and the following phenolic acids: caffeic (22), chlorogenic (23), p-coumaric (25), and gallic (27).

In the same year, Laanet et al. conducted a study on three species of the genus *Galium*, including *G. verum*, from Estonia [37]. The analysis focused on the content of volatile and non-volatile chemical compounds and antioxidant activity. The sensitive HPLC-MS method and colorimetric tests were used for phytochemical analysis. For antioxidant capacity assessment, the ORAC (Oxygen Radical Absorbance Capacity) method was applied [108]. Volatile compounds were quantified by SPME-GC-MS (solid-phase microextraction with gas chromatography with mass detection). Hexanal, anethole, and β-caryophyllene (≥1%) were detected in all samples. The results from colorimetric tests showed that *G. verum* has high levels of polyphenols (up to 27.2 ± 1.5 mg GAE/g), flavonoids (up to 7.3 ± 0.5 mgQE/g), and iridoids (up to 40.8 ± 2.9 mgEq asperuloside/g). Chromatographic analyses identified individual chemical compounds, revealing differences between the flowers and the whole plant. The flowers contained higher concentrations of certain compounds, with the highest content of asperuloside (28) found in both flower and whole stems. The analysis of antioxidant activity showed that all the studied species exhibit a strong antioxidant capacity (up to 9.3 ± 1.2 mgTE/g). Among the studied species, extracts from *G. verum* flowers stand out for containing the highest amounts of bioactive substances and exhibiting the most pronounced antioxidant potential. The polyphenolic composition is dominated by rutin (21) and chlorogenic acid (23), both known for their antioxidant properties. The rutin content in *G. verum* is the highest among the studied species. The results of the analyses conducted by the researchers show a clear correlation between the total polyphenol content and the antioxidant activity of *G. verum* extracts. The antioxidant properties of plant extracts from the genus *Galium* reveal their potential as future therapeutic agents for treating diseases caused by oxidative stress. Further in-depth studies are necessary to elucidate their mechanisms of action, optimize extraction methods, and assess their clinical efficacy. This will contribute to the development of novel therapies using the antioxidant effect of plant-derived products.

Antoniak et al. studied the antiangiogenic and anti-inflammatory properties of several medicinal plant species, including *G. verum* [38]. The researchers used an in vitro approach, applying ethanol extracts from various species of the genus *Galium*, which are rich in bioactive substances with potential antiangiogenic effects, to endothelial cells from human umbilical cord blood vessels in a controlled environment. They aimed to evaluate the effect of plant extracts on endothelial cell viability, cell proliferation, migration, invasiveness, and the production of angiogenic and angiostatic factors. Prior to the in vitro experiment, the following analyses were conducted: total phenolic content, volatile compounds content determined by GC-MS, and antioxidant activity by the DPPH and FRAP methods. The results for *G. verum* from the spectrophotometric study showed a high phenolic content and fresh weight (58.47 ± 4.40 mg GAE/g FW). Five different volatile compounds in the plant extract (7-ethyl-4-decen-6-one, ascaridole epoxide, 4-hydroxy-benzenepropanoic acid, (E,Z,Z)-2,4,7-tridecatrienal, and estra-1,3,5(10)-trien-17ß-ol) were identified. The tests confirmed the antioxidant properties of all three species studied, indicating that these properties correlate with the high polyphenol content. In vitro experiments showed that ethanolic plant extracts of all three species significantly increased cell invasiveness compared to the control group. However, only two species, including *G. verum*, reduced cell proliferation. These species also exhibited the most pronounced anti-inflammatory activity. Furthermore, the tested extracts reduced the production of proangiogenic platelet-derived growth factor (PDGF) and hepatocyte growth factor (HGF) and thus may affect angiogenesis at various levels. In conclusion, the authors highlighted that the modifying effects of the studied extracts could have beneficial implications for pathological processes related to free radical formation, inflammation, and angiogenesis.

Rashed et al. performed an experiment with rats that demonstrated the antioxidant effect of *G. verum* [39]. The rats were subjected to acute kidney injury, induced by folic acid, and divided into groups. One of the groups was treated with *G. verum* extract orally for seven consecutive days. The results showed improvement in kidney structure and enhanced renal function recovery in the treated group compared to the other groups.

Semenescu et al. reported the content of the following flavonoids: apigenin (1), epicatechin (9), isoquercitrin (16), luteolin (18), and rutin (21), as well as the following phenolic acids: chlorogenic acid (23), p-coumaric acid (25), ferulic acid (26) [84]. The comparative approach of the study suggests that *G. verum* extracts possess promising antioxidant, antimicrobial, and anticancer properties, which strongly depend on the extraction method. The diethyl ether extract demonstrated the highest bioactivity, particularly in terms of antioxidant capacity, antibacterial effects against Gram-positive bacteria, and cytotoxicity against malignant melanoma cells. These findings highlight the importance of extraction methods in optimizing the therapeutic potential of *G. verum* for future biomedical applications.

3.2.2. Content of Iridoid Glycosides

Iridoids are a large group of naturally occurring compounds found in medicinal plants, known for their broad range of pharmacological effects [109–112]. The plants of the genus *Galium* have long been recognized for their rich iridoid content. Research on iridoids began in 1978, when Corrigan et al. studied 12 species of the genus and discovered that they all contained similar iridoids, supporting the idea of a close relationship between species within the genus, which remains accepted today [43]. A few years later, Bojthe-Horvath et al. isolated tricyclic iridoid glycosides from the aerial parts of *G. verum* using spectroscopic and X-ray diffraction methods, marking the first X-ray analysis of such compounds [44,45]. Later research has further supported and expanded these findings, as scientists have used more advanced analysis methods, such as spectrophotometry and liquid and gas chromatography [33,46,47].

Mitova et al. studied 19 species of the genus *Galium* in Bulgaria and used the content of specific iridoid acids to suggest that the iridoid composition of the genus's ancient ancestors underwent early evolutionary changes [46]. These changes led to the formation of three distinct evolutionary lines, each with a specific phytochemical composition. These lines contributed to the differentiation of the species we know today. One of these lines, including *G. verum*, *G. mollugo]*, and *G. humifusum*, resulted in distinct iridoid content, such as iridoid esters, hydroxy and carboxy derivatives of iridoids (like asperuloside), and secoiridoids. The study confirmed a close relationship between *G. verum* and *G. humifusum*, which share similar chemical profiles and likely evolved from a common ancestor.

Demirezer et al. employed spectrophotometric and chromatographic methods to isolate seven types of iridoids from the phytochemical composition of *G. verum*, including asperuloside (28), asperulosidic acid (29), daphylloside (30), deacetyl-asperulosidic acid (31), and monotropein (35) [47].

In a study of *G. verum* var. *asiaticum* in Korea, seven derivatives of iridoid glycosides were reported: asperuloside (28), asperulosidic acid (29), deacetylasperuloside (32), and scandoside (36) [48].

Friščić et al. researched eight species of the genus *Galium* and reported that *G. verum* has the highest iridoid content among them, confirming previous studies [33]. The study found that asperuloside (28) was the most common iridoid. Asperuloside is an iridoid glucoside, which gives a positive blue reaction when tested with the Trim-Hill reagent [113]. The study also indicated that the highest yield of asperuloside is obtained when the plants are fully in bloom, as the inflorescences contain the highest iridoid content. According to the study, although iridoids dominate the composition of *G. verum*, no correlation was found between their quantity and the plant's strong antiradical capacity.

Camero et al. investigated the antiangiogenic effects of iridoids isolated from *G. tunetanum*, some of which are also present in *G. verum*, such as asperuloside (28), asperulosidic acid (29), daphylloside (30), deacetyl-asperuloside (32), geniposidic acid (33), and monotropein (35) [49]. The study applied an in vivo model using the chorioallantoic membrane of a hen's egg with a developed embryo. The iridoids isolated from *G. tunetanum* were applied to the membrane, resulting in the inhibition of microvessel formation compared to the control. The antiangiogenic effect, expressed as a percentage of inhibition compared to the control, reached 67%. This inhibition of angiogenesis could potentially be a promising approach for anticancer therapies.

A study of species in the genus *Galium*, including *G. verum*, conducted in Estonia by Laanet et al., found similar levels of asperulosidic acid (29), which confirmed the thesis on the chemotaxonomic role of iridoids [37]. Hydroacetone extract yielded higher amounts of asperuloside (28), although the hydroethanol extract, which produced slightly lower yields, is considered more suitable for biological applications.

Numerous pharmacological studies confirmed that naturally occurring iridoids in *G. verum* have a wide range of beneficial properties that can be utilized for the therapy and prevention of various diseases. Iridoids, especially asperuloside, can exhibit the following properties: neuroprotective, immunomodulatory, antidiabetic, cardioprotective, antihepatotoxic, hepatoprotective, choleretic, hypoglycemic, hypolipidemic, anti-inflammatory, antispasmodic, antitumor, antiviral, antibacterial, and antifungal [102,103]. Asperuloside has been identified as a key compound responsible for the sedative effects observed in plants of the genus *Galium*. Based on this evidence, Bradic et al. suggest that *G. verum* may be beneficial for managing nervousness and phobias [50]. In addition, iridoids extracted from *Galium* species also exhibit antiangiogenic properties by suppressing the formation of new blood vessels that support tumor growth [38,49]. This makes *Galium* species suitable for application in cancer treatment.

3.2.3. Content of Anthraquinones

Anthraquinones are phytochemicals with notable biological activity that have the ability to affect some physiological processes at the cellular level. Thus, they can exhibit antimicrobial effects on some pathogens and induce apoptosis in cancer cells [46,54,75,76,114,115]. However, their manner of action must be fully elucidated as they exhibit cytotoxicity not only on cancer cells but also on normal ones [65,66].

Studying *G. mollugo]* cells, Heide et al. reported that anthraquinones are located in vacuoles and are present in small amounts [51]. This explains the limited data on these compounds in members of the genus *Galium*.

As early as 1995, Banthorpe et al. [52] were among the first to report information about the identification of anthraquinones in *G. verum*. Zhao et al. [53] confirmed the content of anthraquinones, including physcione (37) and rubiadin (38). Physcion was isolated for the first time from the genus *Galium*. Kanso et al. found that anthraquinones are more abundant in the roots of *G. verum* than in other parts of the plant [54]. The study also highlighted the biological effects of these compounds, such as their antibacterial and anticancer potential. This activity was explained by the inhibitory effect of anthraquinones on nucleic acid synthesis in bacterial cells and their induced destruction [55]. Anthraquinones are highly polar, which gives them a stronger bactericidal effect against drug-resistant bacteria, including both Gram-positive and Gram-negative bacteria.

3.2.4. Content of Terpenoids (Monoterpenoids, Sesquiterpenoids, Triterpenoids, Triterpenoid Saponins) and Volatile Organic Compounds (VOCs)

Terpenoids are among the largest classes of secondary metabolites and are produced in plants, playing a significant role in pharmacology and plant defense along with VOCs. Triterpenoid saponins are known for their broad antifungal and antimicrobial potential and also exhibit a wide range of biological activities, such as anticancer and anti-inflammatory effects. The antimicrobial properties of some species of the genus *Galium* are attributed to the interaction between sterols on bacterial erythrocyte membranes and saponins [116].

In 2006, monoterpene glycosides were reported for the first time in the composition of *G. verum*. The identified compounds were included in betulalbuside A (40) [47]. Later, Ilyina et al. conducted a study on essential oil from flowers of *G. verum* using the GC-MS technique [56]. The detected lipophilic volatile compounds included α-Terpineol (39), borneol (42), camphor (43), squalene (49), and some unknown substances. Phytochemical screening conducted by Friščić et al. confirmed that *G. verum* contains not only flavonoids, tannins, and iridoids but also saponins and triterpenes [33].

Shynkovenko et al. determined the content of triterpene saponins in *G. verum* by the HPLC method [57]. The saponins identified include the ursane type: euscaphic acid (44), tormentic acid (50), ursolic acid (51), and uvaol (52); the oleanane type: oleanolic acid (47); and the lupane type: botulin (41) and lupeol (46). Tava et al. identified a total of more than 70 volatile compounds in the composition of *G. verum* [58]. The largest amounts were detected of germacrene D (45) in the flowers. According to the study, the specific phytochemical composition has a significant ecological role, as it protects the plants from herbivores and aphids in their environment and attracts pollinators.

Ciotlaus et al. conducted a comparative study on the content of volatile organic compounds in fresh and dried *G. verum* plants [59]. The fresh aerial parts contained a total of twenty-eight compounds, while the dried flower contained a total of fifty compounds. The fresh floral bouquet comprised mainly oxygenated monoterpenes, while the dried bouquet contained mainly aldehydes, monoterpenes, alcohols, sesquiterpenes, and acetates.

3.2.5. Phytosterol Content

Phytosterols are an important part of a person's diet, not only because they help reduce blood cholesterol but also because they have been shown to exhibit antitumor activity through several mechanisms: by inducing apoptosis, enhancing immune recognition of cancer cells, and directly inhibiting tumor growth [117,118].

Research on phytosterols in *G. verum* is limited. One of the few studies published on this topic is by Qing-jie et al. [61]. The researchers analyzed the chemical composition of *G. verum* via GC-MS. Some of the components were identified for the first time in *G. verum*. The results showed the presence of β-sitosterol (53), campesterol (54), and stigmasterol (55).

Mocan et al. studied four species of the genus *Galium* and identified two phytosterols, β-sitosterol (53) and campesterol (54), in all of them [62]. The determined amounts were 85.46 ± 1.24 μg/g and 9.86 ± 0.04 μg/g, respectively. This study offers a scientific basis for the traditional uses of *Galium* species because these secondary metabolites might be responsible for the pharmacological effects of *Galium* plants.

Since existing data suggest that the intake of phytosterols, such as stigmasterol and β-sitosterol, can reduce the risk of tumor development, it would be useful to study the mechanism of action of phytosterols found in *G. verum*.

3.2.6. Pharmacological Effects of *G. verum*

The pharmacological properties exhibited by species of the genus *Galium* on biological systems are mainly due to their high antioxidant activity. Integrating antioxidant therapy is of most importance to enhance the safety and efficacy of conventional treatments [97]. The radical scavenging potential [26], antiangiogenic effects [38], and cytotoxicity [65,66] of *Galium* plants contribute to their anticancer effects. Various studies have shown that flavonoids are of leading importance for the anticancer effect of *G. verum*. In two consecutive years, Schmidt et al. conducted an in vitro experiment and proved that the decoction of

G. verum exhibited cytotoxicity and inhibited cancer cell growth. Additionally, the decoction protected the DNA of epithelial cells from primary mucosa against the mutagenic effects of benzo[a]pyrene, a key DNA-damaging agent found in cigarette smoke. These findings support the idea that *G. verum* could be a valuable source for developing herbal medicines aimed at cancer prevention and therapy [65,66].

Khalili et al. determined the antihaemolytic activity of plant extracts of ten known for their antioxidant activity plants [67]. Antihaemolytic activity was examined in the red blood cells of mice. Vitamin C has been selected as a control antioxidant. Nine of the extracts were more potent than vitamin C, of which *G. verum* was the most potent. Hemolysis inhibition was related to the method of extraction and extract concentration. This study proved that *G. verum* could be used as a source of natural antioxidants for the pharmaceutical industry.

The hepatoprotective activity of the extract of *G. verum* was tested on carbon tetrachloride-induced acute hepatitis in rats [68]. The treatment with plant extracts led to the improvement of all assessed biochemical parameters and histopathological analysis. The hepatoprotective effect was comparable with the hepatoprotective activity of the reference drug.

A comparative study of the diuretic activity of the aqueous and alcoholic extracts of *G. verum* was conducted [69]. The extracts were applied to rats according to Berkhin's method [119]. The results demonstrated that a 60% ethanol extract of *G. verum* exhibits the most pronounced diuretic effect. According to this study, the diuretic activity of *G. verum* is based on flavonoids, anthracene derivatives, and terpenoid content.

A series of rat experiments were conducted from 2019 to 2023 to evaluate the biological properties of the methanolic extract of *G. verum* [70–72]. The effects of the methanol extract of *G. verum* were investigated on the redox status of isolated hearts of spontaneously hypertensive rats after ischemia [70]. The results showed that 4-week treatment has the ability to significantly alleviate cardiac oxidative stress in a dose-dependent manner. Other researchers tested the effects of this extract on myocardial ischemia in spontaneously hypertensive rats, too [71]. After four weeks of treatment, it was found that the methanol extract had positive effects on heart function as it decreased the generation of pro-oxidants, thus reducing oxidative damage. In another study, rats were treated with doxorubicin-induced cardiotoxicity, also by the methanol extract of *G. verum* [72]. The extract was proven to increase the activity of the antioxidant defense system and prevent the pathological injuries caused by doxorubicin via a decrease in oxidative stress and apoptosis. The results of these studies overlap and confirm the high cytoprotective effect of methanol extracts prepared from *G. verum*. However, more data are needed to fully clarify the mechanism of action of the extracts of *G. verum*.

Another study demonstrated that the methanol extract of *G. verum* exhibits a cytotoxic effect when applied to colon cancer cells (HT29) [75]. As a result, the level of reactive oxygen species (ROS) increases in the mitochondria of the cancer cells, leading to the induction of apoptosis. Apoptosis is a process of programmed cell death, which occurs naturally and is beneficial to the body, especially in response to changes in environmental factors or the development of tumor cells. When the DNA of these tumor cells is damaged, they stop dividing and eventually die. This study explains the mechanism by which phenolic compounds in *G. verum* work, revealing their therapeutic potential for treating tumor-related diseases.

The studies conducted by Pashapour et al. found a connection between the dose of plant extract and the occurrence of side effects in non-tumor human cells [76]. At high doses above 400 μg/mL, there was an increased induction of apoptosis in normal cells, which decreased their survival rate.

The research of Marković et al. on the ethnobotanical use of plants from the genus *Galium* used an unusual approach [77]. It was performed as a survey among the rural population in four municipalities of Pirot District in Serbia. The people interviewed claimed that infusion from *G. verum* can be used for the treatment of inflammation of the oral cavity, hoarseness, kidney and bladder diseases, diabetes, and fainting, while compression can be applied for skin diseases and irritation.

Other studies conducted using the same method show that the plant has been used for its sedative and wound-healing action and as an enzyme activator [79–81].

3.3. Relationship Between Bioactive Compounds, Biological Activities, and Medicinal Uses

Galium species contain a diverse range of phytochemical compounds, contributing to their wide array of potential applications in medicine and health. Their potential is primarily due to the multiple mechanisms of action they possess. This makes them suitable for therapy and the prevention of various diseases.

These compounds include flavonoids, phenolic acids, iridoids, anthraquinones, saponins, and essential oils. They exhibit significant biological activity and exert numerous beneficial effects on various human body systems, including the central nervous, hepatobiliary, renal, gastrointestinal, and urinary systems. Their therapeutic potential is largely attributed to their preventive actions, including antioxidant, antibacterial, antifungal, anticancer, and immunomodulatory properties.

Polyphenols and flavonoids are known for their strong antioxidant properties. Flavonoids such as quercetin, rutin, kaempferol, and luteolin have the ability to increase reactive oxygen species (ROS) in mitochondria, damaging cellular DNA, which leads to the induction of apoptosis in cancer cells [75,76,94,95,120]. Flavonoids can also exhibit pro-oxidant activity under certain reaction conditions [96]. Their anti-inflammatory properties stem from their ability to inhibit pro-inflammatory cytokines, making them relevant for conditions such as arthritis and cardiovascular diseases [95].

Polyphenols include phenolic acids such as chlorogenic acid, caffeic acid, ferulic acid, and gallic acid. They have the ability to neutralize radicals, regulate nitric oxide, and inhibit cell proliferation [20,32,38,59,99,100]. In addition to antioxidant properties, these compounds also exhibit antimicrobial [23] and hepatoprotective properties [68], making them effective in preventing liver damage and bacterial infections.

Iridoids—asperuloside, loganin, geniposidic acid, and scandoside—may exhibit immunomodulatory, antidiabetic, hepatoprotective, choleretic, neuroprotective, anti-inflammatory, and antibacterial effects, though their exact mechanisms are still not fully understood [68,92]. Asperuloside has been shown to exhibit sedative and antiangiogenic effects in vitro [38,111,112], and loganin has been linked to the reduction in neuroinflammation, which is potentially beneficial for Alzheimer's disease [112].

Anthraquinones, such as rubiadin and physcion, are known for their antimicrobial, anticancer, anti-osteoporotic, hepatoprotective, and neuroprotective activities, making them promising candidates for drug development [121]. They can destroy bacterial cell walls, inhibit nucleic acid and protein synthesis, and interfere with bacterial respiration, leading to a bacteriostatic effect. Furthermore, due to their high polarity, anthraquinones possess antibacterial activity against drug-resistant bacteria, including both Gram-positive and Gram-negative bacteria [109,114,115].

Saponins (betalbuside A), along with other terpenoids (germacrene D) and volatile organic compounds (squalene) from the content of essential oils of *Galium* species, possess antifungal, antiviral, antimicrobial, and antitumor effects, making them useful for application on skin and respiratory infections [32,54,56,58,59].

The high phytosterol content in *Galium* species contributes to their anticancer activity, as phytosterols promote apoptosis in cancer cells, leading to programmed cell death [54,118,122].

Many bioactive compounds found in *G. verum*, such as rutin, kaempferol, quercetin, luteolin, chlorogenic acid, caffeic acid, scandoside, asperuloside, β-sitosterol, and campesterol, have also been reported in other species of the genus and the Rubiaceae family, suggesting a biochemical consistency that may lead to similar pharmacological effects. Flavonoids including quercetin, rutin, and kaempferol are common in other Rubiaceae genera, such as *Morinda* and *Coffea*, where they exert similar antioxidant and anti-inflammatory properties [6]. Iridoids, including asperuloside and loganin, are reported in Morinda citrifolia, where they exhibit neuroprotective effects similar to those in *Galium* species [6]. Anthraquinones, such as rubiadin, are present in Rubia cordifolia, another Rubiaceae plant known for its antimicrobial and anticancer properties [4]. Saponins identified in *G. verum* are structurally related to saponins found in other medicinal plants used for immune modulation [6,56,57]. Figure 1 represents the summarized results of our research.

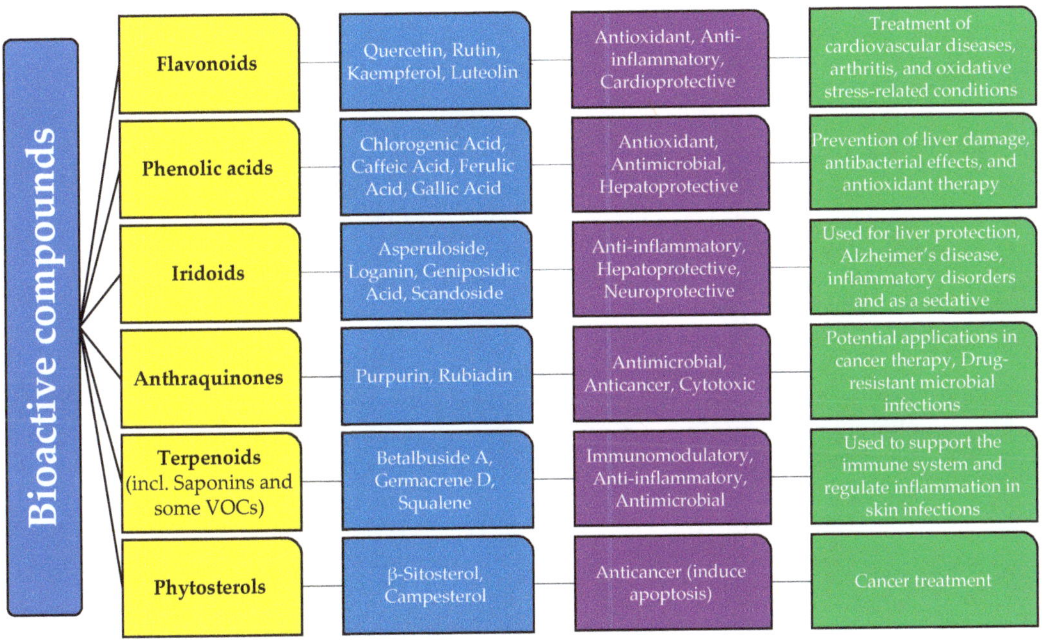

Figure 1. Relationship between bioactive compounds, biological activities, and medicinal uses of *Galium* species (Rubiaceae)/*Galium verum* L. according to the scientific research.

4. Relevance of the Topic and Current Research Trends

The data presented in this review have been carefully selected and organized to provide a comprehensive overview of the phytochemical constituents and biological effects of *G. verum* and the *Galium* genus as a whole, helping to obtain a clear understanding of the potential they offer. This literature review discusses a total of 83 scientific studies related to the composition and properties of *Galium* species (*Rubiaceae*). Notably, 60% of the published research focuses on *G. verum*, highlighting the strong interest in this species. The number of studies has increased significantly since 1978, with 30% of scientific studies being published after 2020 (Figure 2).

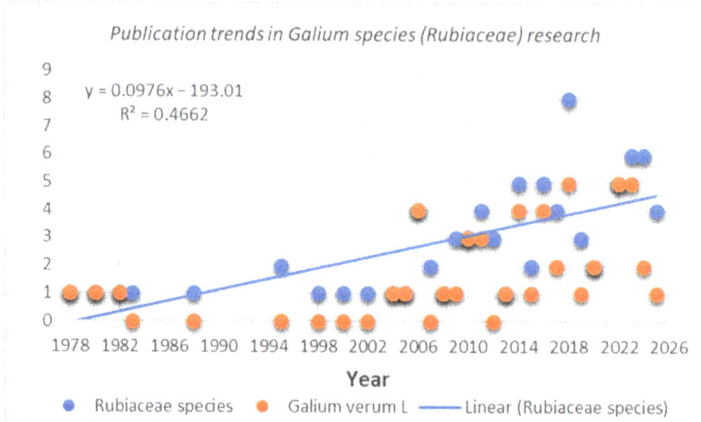

Figure 2. Publication trends in research connected with *Galium* species (Rubiaceae)/*Galium verum* L.

5. Conclusions

This review covers phytochemical studies of *Galium* species for the past 47 years (1978–2025). The reported bioactive compounds have been isolated mainly from *G.verum*, *G. aparine*, *G. mollugo]*, and *G. odoratum*. Based on the information collected, this review shows that plants of the genus *Galium*, including *G. verum*, are rich in diverse chemical compounds with strong biological activity. Most studies focus on the phenolic content of the plant extracts and their associated antioxidant activity. The increasing interest in biologically active compounds from *Galium* species reflects the growing recognition of their pharmacological potential. The topic remains highly relevant, as recent studies continue to explore their diverse phytochemical composition and therapeutic applications. Many of the bioactive compounds identified in *Galium* species, such as flavonoids, iridoids, phenolic acids, anthraquinones, and saponins, are also found in other members of the genus and the broader Rubiaceae family. These compounds have already been investigated for their medicinal properties and have demonstrated significant pharmacological effects, including antioxidant, anti-inflammatory, antimicrobial, hepatoprotective, and anticancer activities. Their established therapeutic applications further support the relevance of *Galium* species in modern medicine, highlighting the need for continued research to fully elucidate their mechanisms of action and clinical potential.

6. Future Directions

The scientific research on *Galium* species, particularly *G. verum*, supports their traditional medicinal applications. However, comprehensive studies on their full pharmacological potential remain limited. Future research should prioritize the clinical validation of isolated bioactive compounds to establish their efficacy and safety for therapeutic use. Additionally, further studies should explore the mechanisms of action, pharmacokinetics, and potential synergistic effects between different compounds. Expanding research to include large-scale in vivo and clinical trials will be essential in determining their role in modern medicine. Investigating new drug formulations, bioavailability improvements, and personalized medicine applications may also enhance their clinical relevance. Moreover, optimizing and standardizing extraction methods is crucial to ensuring the efficient isolation of bioactive compounds. Comparative studies on solvent selection, extraction efficiency, and compound stability should be conducted to determine the most effective techniques for preserving the pharmacological properties of *Galium* species. Additionally, future research should examine the influence of geographical and environmental factors on the phytochemical composition of *Galium* species, as variations in climate, soil composition, and altitude may significantly affect the concentration and diversity of bioactive compounds. Furthermore, further research to develop antioxidant-based therapies should be explored to enhance their potential in preventing and managing oxidative stress-related diseases.

Author Contributions: Conceptualization, M.K.P. and N.H.G.; resources, M.K.P.; writing—original draft preparation, M.K.P.; writing—review and editing, M.T.T.; supervision, M.H.T.; project administration, N.H.G.; funding acquisition, N.H.G. All authors have read and agreed to the published version of the manuscript.

Funding: This work is financially supported by the EU and the Bulgarian Ministry of Education and Science through project BG-RRP-2.004-0006-C02 "Development of scientific research and innovation at Trakia University in the service of health and sustainable well-being".

Institutional Review Board Statement: Not applicable.

Informed Consent Statement: Not applicable.

Data Availability Statement: Not applicable.

Conflicts of Interest: The authors declare no conflicts of interest.

References

1. Bungau, S.G.; Popa, V.-C. Between Religion and Science: Some Aspects Concerning Illness and Healing in Antiquity. *Transylv. Rev.* **2015**, *26*, 3–19. Available online: https://www.researchgate.net/publication/286442576_Between_Religion_and_Science_Some_Aspects_Concerning_Illness_and_Healing_in_Antiquity (accessed on 10 March 2025).
2. Davis, C.C.; Choisy, P. Medicinal plants meet modern biodiversity science. *Curr. Biol.* **2024**, *34*, R158–R173. [CrossRef] [PubMed]
3. Delprete, P.G.; Jardim, J.G. Systematics, taxonomy and floristics of Brazilian Rubiaceae: An overview about the current status and future challenges. *Rodriguésia* **2012**, *63*, 101–128. [CrossRef]
4. Esguerra, J.D.; Bernardo, J.M.; Gimao, K.M.; Peralta, M.E.; Tiu, C.J.; Hernandez, G.G.; Alejandro, G.J.; Tan, M.A. Mechanism-based antioxidant activity of Rubiaceae species collected from Ilocos Norte, Philippines. *Not. Sci. Biol.* **2024**, *16*, 2. [CrossRef]
5. Heitzman, M.E.; Neto, C.C.; Winiarz, E.; Vaisberg, A.J.; Hammond, G.B. Ethnobotany, phytochemistry and pharmacology of Uncaria. *Phytochemistry* **2025**, *66*, 5–29. [CrossRef]
6. Martins, D.; Nunez, C.V. Secondary Metabolites from Rubiaceae Species. *Molecules* **2015**, *20*, 13422–13495. [CrossRef]
7. Maldonado, C.; Barnes, C.J.; Cornett, C.; Holmfred, E.; Hansen, S.H.; Persson, C.; Antonelli, A.; Rønsted, N. Phylogeny predicts the quantity of antimalarial alkaloids within the iconic yellow *Cinchona* bark (Rubiaceae: *Cinchona calisaya*). *Front. Plant Sci.* **2017**, *8*, 391. [CrossRef] [PubMed]
8. Sanders, J.P.; Dawson, W.T. Efficacy of quinidine in malaria. *J. Am. Med. Assoc.* **1932**, *99*, 1773–1777. [CrossRef]
9. Mekonnen, B.; Cizungu, L.; Alegre, J.; Blondeel, H.; De Lombaerde, E.; Verbeeck, H.; Duchateau, L.; Schrevens, E.; Verheyen, K.; Boeckx, P.; et al. Smallholder farmers' knowledge on management of *Cinchona* in the Democratic Republic of the Congo. *Plant Ecol. Evol.* **2025**, *158*, 3–13. [CrossRef]
10. Robbrecht, E. Tropical Woody Rubiaceae. In *Opera Botanica Belgica*; National Botanic Garden of Belgium: Meies, Belgium, 1988; Volume 1, pp. 599–602. [CrossRef]
11. Bremer, B.; Andreasen, K.; Olsson, D. Subfamilial and tribal relationships in the Rubiaceae based on rbcL sequence data. *Ann. Mo. Bot. Gard.* **1995**, *82*, 383–397. [CrossRef]
12. Bremer, B. A review of molecular phylogenetic studies of Rubiaceae. *Ann. Mo. Bot. Gard.* **2009**, *96*, 4–26. [CrossRef]
13. Yang, L.E.; Meng, Y.; Peng, D.L.; Nie, Z.L.; Sun, H. Molecular Phylogeny of *Galium* L. of the Tribe Rubieae (Rubiaceae)—Emphasis on Chinese Species and Recognition of a New Genus *Pseudogalium*. *Mol. Phylogenet. Evol.* **2018**, *126*, 221–232. [CrossRef] [PubMed]
14. Turcov, D.; Barna, A.S.; Trifan, A.; Blaga, A.C.; Tanasa, A.M.; Suteu, D. Antioxidants from *Galium verum* as Ingredients for the Design of New Dermatocosmetic Products. *Plants* **2022**, *11*, 2454. [CrossRef]
15. Mavi, A.; Terzi, Z.; Özgen, U.; Yildirim, A.; Coşkun, M. Antioxidant properties of some medicinal plants: *Prangos ferulacea* (Apiaceae), *Sedum sempervivoides* (Crassulaceae), *Malva neglecta* (Malvaceae), *Cruciata taurica* (Rubiaceae), *Rosa pimpinellifolia* (Rosaceae), *Galium verum* subsp *verum* (Rubiaceae), *Urtica dioica* (urticaceae). *Biol. Pharm. Bull.* **2004**, *27*, 702–705. [CrossRef]
16. Tamas, M.; Stana, D.; Timis, S. Comparative phytochemical research of *Galium verum* L. and *G. mollugo]* L. *Not. Bot. Hort. Agrobot.* **2006**, *34*, 18–20.
17. Zhao, C.C.; Shao, J.H.; Li, X.; Kang, X.D.; Zhang, Y.W.; Meng, D.L.; Li, N. Flavonoids from *Galium verum* L. *J. Asian Nat. Prod. Res.* **2008**, *10*, 613–617. [CrossRef] [PubMed]

18. Zhao, C.C.; Shao, J.H.; Cao, D.; Zhang, Y.W.; Li, X. Chemical constituents of *Galium verum*. *China J. Chin. Mater. Medica.* **2009**, *34*, 2761–2764. Available online: https://pesquisa.bvsalud.org/portal/resource/pt/wpr-315368 (accessed on 16 November 2024).
19. Lakic, N.S.; Mimica-Dukic, N.M.; Isak, J.M.; Bozin, B.N. Antioxidant properties of *Galium verum* L. (Rubiaceae) extracts. *Centr. Eur. J. Biol.* **2010**, *5*, 331–337. [CrossRef]
20. Kim, D.K. Superoxide Quenching Activity of Phenolic Compounds from the Whole Plant of *Galium verum* var. asiaticum. *Nat. Prod. Sci.* **2011**, *17*, 261–266. Available online: https://koreascience.kr/article/JAKO201111436239799.page (accessed on 16 November 2024).
21. Zhao, R.; Chen, Z.; Jia, G.; Li, J.; Cai, Y.; Shao, X. Protective effects of diosmetin extracted from *Galium verum* L. on the thymus of U14-bearing mice. *Can. J. Physiol. Pharmacol.* **2011**, *89*, 665–673. [CrossRef]
22. Danila, A.O.; Gatea, F.; Radu, G.L. Polyphenol composition and antioxidant activity of selected medicinal herbs. *Chem. Nat. Comp.* **2011**, *47*, 22–26. [CrossRef]
23. Vlase, L.; Mocan, A.; Hanganu, D.; Benedec, D.; Gheldiu, A.; Crișan, G. Comparative study of polyphenolic content, antioxidant and antimicrobial activity of four *Galium* species (Rubiaceae). *Dig. J. Nanomater. Biostruct.* **2014**, *9*, 1085–1094. Available online: https://www.researchgate.net/publication/266208237 (accessed on 16 November 2024).
24. Moţ, A.C.; Coman, C.; Miron, C.; Damian, G.; Sarbu, C.; Silaghi-Dumitrescu, R. An assay for pro-oxidant reactivity based on phenoxyl radicals generated by laccase. *Food Chem.* **2014**, *143*, 214–222. [CrossRef] [PubMed]
25. Matei, A.O.; Gatea, F.; Radu, G.L. Analysis of phenolic compounds in some medicinal herbs by LC-MS. *J. Chromatogr. Sci.* **2015**, *53*, 1147–1154. [CrossRef]
26. Layali, I.; Ebrahimzadeh, M.A.; Joulaei, M. Antioxidant properties of *Galium verum*. *J. Life Sci. Pharm. Res.* **2016**, *6*, L31–L37. Available online: https://www.ijlpr.com/index.php/journal/article/view/380/264 (accessed on 16 November 2024).
27. Dong, J.M.; Ma, Y.L.; Zhang, Z.Y.; Li, R.; Zhu, Y.L.; Ma, L. Effects and related mechanism of flavone from *Galium verum* L. on peroxide induced oxidative injury in human umbilical vein endothelial cells. *Zhonghua Xin Xue Guan Bing Za Zhi* **2016**, *44*, 610–615. [CrossRef]
28. Ilyina, T.V.; Goryacha, O.V.; Kovaleva, A.M.; Koshovyi, O.M.; Shynkovenko, I.L. A comparative study of morphological features and flavonoid composition of *Galium* L. genus species. *Der. Pharm. Lett.* **2016**, *8*, 316–320. Available online: https://www.researchgate.net/publication/316888969_A_comparative_study_of_morphological_features_and_flavonoid_composition_of_galium_L_genus_species (accessed on 16 November 2024).
29. Cheng, C.; Zhang, H.; Li, Y.; Zhou, Y.; Lu, W.; Yao, L. The effect of Diosmin on the blood proteome in a rat model of venous thrombosis. *Int. J. Biol. Macromol.* **2017**, *104*, 778–787. [CrossRef]
30. Kuhtinskaja, M.; Vaher, M. Extraction and Analysis of Bioactive Compounds from Dipsacus Fullonum and *Galium Verum* for Lyme Borreliosis Treatment. *Biomed. J. Sci. Tech. Res.* **2018**, *11*, 8614–8616. [CrossRef]
31. Farcas, D.A.; Mot, C.A.; Zagrean-Tuza, C.; Toma, V.; Cimpoiu, C.; Hosu, A.; Parvu, M.; Roman, I.; Silaghi-Dumitrescu, R. Chemo-mapping and biochemical-modulatory and antioxidant/prooxidant effect of *Galium verum* extract during acute restraint and dark stress in female rats. *PLoS ONE* **2018**, *13*, e0200022. [CrossRef]
32. Shynkovenko, I.L.; Kashpur, N.V.; Ilyina, T.V.; Kovalyova, A.M.; Goryacha, O.V.; Koshovyi, O.M.; Kryvoruchko, O.V.; Komissarenko, A.M. The immunomodulatory activity of ethanolic extracts from *Galium verum* L. herb. *Ceska Slov. Farm.* **2018**, *67*, 101–106. [CrossRef]
33. Friščić, M.; Štibrić Baglama, M.; Milović, M.; Hazler Pilepić, K.; Maleš, Ž. Content of Bioactive Constituents and Antioxidant Potential of *Galium* L. Species. *Croat. Chem. Acta* **2018**, *91*, 411–417. [CrossRef]
34. Hanganu, D.; Burtescu, R.F.; Petrescu, S.; Pripon Furtuna, F.R.; Chișe, E.; Turcuș, V.; Benedec, D.; Oniga, I.; Olah, N.K. Galium Species—Polyphenolic Content And Their Antioxidant Potential, *Hop Med. Plants* **2019**, *26*, 85–94. [CrossRef]
35. Vuletic, M.; Jakovljevic, V.; Zivanovic, S.; Papic, M.; Papic, M.; Mladenovic, R.; Zivkovic, V.; Srejovic, I.; Jeremic, J.; Andjic, M.; et al. The Evaluation of Healing Properties of *Galium verum*-Based Oral Gel in Aphthous Stomatitis in Rats. *Molecules* **2022**, *27*, 4680. [CrossRef]
36. Ohindovschi, A.; Cojocaru-Toma, M. Identification of phenolic compounds from extract of Galium verum. Institute of Chemistry of the Academy of Sciences of Moldova. In *New Frontiers in Natural Product Chemistry*; Instrumentul Bibliometric National: Chișinău, Moldova, 2023; p. 28. [CrossRef]
37. Laanet, P.R.; Saar-Reismaa, P.; Jõul, P.; Bragina, O.; Vaher, M. Phytochemical Screening and Antioxidant Activity of Selected Estonian *Galium* Species. *Molecules* **2023**, *28*, 2867. [CrossRef]
38. Antoniak, K.; Studzińska-Sroka, E.; Szymański, M.; Dudek-Makuch, M.; Cielecka-Piontek, J.; Korybalska, K. Antiangiogenic, Anti-Inflammatory and Antioxidant Properties of *Bidens Tripartite* Herb, *Galium Verum* Herb and *Rumex Hydrolapathum* Root. *Molecules* **2023**, *28*, 4966. [CrossRef]
39. Rashed, A.; Mohamed, A.S.; Soliman, A. Ameliorative Effect of *Galium Verum* (Rubiaceae Family) Methanolic Extract on Folic Acid-Induced Acute Kidney Injury in Male Rats. *Iraqi J. Pharm. Sci.* **2023**, *32*, 14–24. [CrossRef]

40. Razzivina, V.; Vasiljeva, A.; Kronberga, A.; Skudrins, G.; Nakurte, I.; Zogota, M.; Mezaka, I.; Pugovics, O.; Grinberga, S.; Dambrova, M.; et al. Phenolic Content and Anti-Inflammatory Activity of Cultivated and Wild-Type *Galium odoratum* Extracts in Murine Bone Marrow-Derived Macrophages. *Antioxidants* **2024**, *13*, 1447. [CrossRef]
41. Wu, R.; Zhang, Z.; Qin, J.; Wu, Y.; Yang, F.; Li, J.; Yao, H.; Li, Y. Chemical constituents from *Galium aparine* and their chemotaxonomic significance. *Biochem. Syst. Ecol.* **2025**, *119*, 104943. [CrossRef]
42. Ilyina, T.; Kashpur, N.; Granica, S.; Bazylko, A.; Shinkovenko, I.; Kovalyova, A.; Goryacha, O.; Koshovyi, O. Phytochemical Profiles and In Vitro Immunomodulatory Activity of Ethanolic Extracts from *Galium aparine* L. *Plants* **2019**, *8*, 541. [CrossRef]
43. Corrigan, D.; Timoney, R.F.; Donnelly, D.M. Iridoids and alkanes in twelve species of *Galium* and Asperula. *Phytochemistry* **1978**, *17*, 1131–1133. [CrossRef]
44. Bojthe-Horvath, K.; Hetenyi, F.; Kocsis, A.; Szabo, M.; Varga-Balázs, M.; Mathe, I.J.; Tetenyi, P. Iridoid glycosides from *Galium verum* L. *Phytochemistry* **1980**, *21*, 2917–2919. [CrossRef]
45. Böjthe-Horváth, K.; Kocsis, A.; Párkány, L.; Simon, K. A new iridoid glycoside from *Galium verum* L. First X-ray analysis of a tricyclic iridoid glycoside. *Tetrahedron Lett.* **1982**, *23*, 965–966. [CrossRef]
46. Mitova, M.I.; Anchev, M.E.; Handjieva, N.V.; Popov, S.S. Iridoid patterns in *Galium* L. and some phylogenetic considerations. *Z. Nat. C* **2002**, *57*, 226–234. [CrossRef] [PubMed]
47. Demirezer, L.Ö.; Gürbüz, F.; Güvenalp, Z.; Ströch, K.; Zeeck, A. Iridoids, flavonoids and monoterpene glycosides from *Galium verum* subsp. *Verum*. *Turk. J. Chem.* **2006**, *30*, 525–534. Available online: https://journals.tubitak.gov.tr/chem/vol30/iss4/13 (accessed on 16 November 2024).
48. Lee, T.G.; Kim, D.K. Iridoid Compounds from the Whole Plant of *Galium verum* var. *asiaticum*. *Nat. Prod. Sci.* **2013**, *19*, 227–230. Available online: https://koreascience.or.kr/article/JAKO201330951777064.page (accessed on 16 November 2024).
49. Camero, C.M.; Germanò, M.P.; Rapisarda, A.; D'Angelo, V.; Amira, S.; Benchikh, F.; Braca, A.; De Leo, M. Anti-angiogenic activity of iridoids from *Galium tunetanum*. *Rev. Bras. Farmacogn.* **2018**, *28*, 374–377. [CrossRef]
50. Bradic, J.; Petkovic, A.; Tomovic, M. Phytochemical and Pharmacological Properties of Some Species of the *Genus galium* L. (*Galium verum* and *Mollugo*). *Serb. J. Exp. Clin. Res.* **2017**, *1*, 187–193. [CrossRef]
51. Heide, L.; Leistner, E. Enzyme activities in extracts of anthraquinone-containing cells of *Galium mollugo*. *Phytochemistry* **1983**, *22*, 659–662. [CrossRef]
52. Banthorpe, D.V.; White, J.J. Novel anthraquinones from undifferentiated cell cultures of *Galium verum*. *Phytochemistry* **1995**, *38*, 107–111. [CrossRef]
53. Zhao, C.C.; Shao, J.H.; Li, X.; Xu, J.; Wang, J.H. A new anthraquinone from *Galium verum* L. *Nat. Prod. Res.* **2006**, *20*, 981–984. [CrossRef] [PubMed]
54. Kanso, M.A.; Hijazi, M.A.; El-Lakany, A.; Aboul-Ela, M. Review on phytochemical constituents and pharmacological activities of genus *Galium*. *J. Appl. Pharm. Sci.* **2024**, *14*, 46–56. [CrossRef]
55. De Rosa, S.; Mitova, M.; Handjieva, N.; Popov, S.; Anchev, M. Rivalosides A and B, two 19-oxo triterpenoid saponins from *Galium* rivale. *J. Nat. Prod.* **2000**, *63*, 1012–1014. [CrossRef]
56. Ilyina, T.V.; Kovaleva, A.M.; Goryachaya, O.V.; Aleksandrov, A.N. Essential Oil from *Galium Verum* Flowers. *Chem. Nat. Compd.* **2009**, *45*, 587–588. [CrossRef]
57. Shynkovenko, I.L.; Ilyna, V.T.; Kovalyova, M.A.; Goryacha, V.O.; Golembiovska, I.O.; Koshovyi, M.O. Saponins of the extracts of *Galium aparine* and *Galium verum*. *Vîsnik Farm* **2018**, *4*, 16–23. [CrossRef]
58. Tava, A.; Biazzi, E.; Ronga, D.; Avato, P. Identification of the Volatile Components of *Galium verum* L. and *Cruciata leavipes* Opiz from the Western Italian Alps. *Molecules* **2020**, *25*, 2333. [CrossRef] [PubMed]
59. Ciotlaus, I.; Pojar-Fenesan, M.; Balea, A. Analysis of Volatile Organic Compounds from the Aerial Parts of Medicinal Plant, *Galium verum*. *Rev. Chim.* **2020**, *71*, 136–144. [CrossRef]
60. Tucakov, J. *Healing with Plants–Phytotherapy*; Culture: Beograd, Croatia, 1971; pp. 24–37.
61. Li, Q.-J.; Nan, M.-L.; He, Y.-F.; Wang, L.-P.; Zhao, Y.-W. Analysis of *Galium verum* L. SPE-CO^2 Extract by GC-MS. *Med. Plant* **2010**, *1*, 5–6. Available online: https://www.cabidigitallibrary.org/doi/pdf/10.5555/20113129801 (accessed on 16 November 2024).
62. Mocan, A.; Crişan, G.; Vlase, L.; Ivănescu, B.; Bădărău, A.S.; Arsene, A.L. Phytochemical investigations on four *Galium* species (Rubiaceae) from Romania. *Farmacia* **2016**, *64*, 95–99. Available online: https://farmaciajournal.com/arhiva/201601/art-15-Mocan_95-99.pdf (accessed on 16 November 2024).
63. Feijoo-Siota, L.; Rama, J.L.R.; Sánchez-Pérez, A.; Villa, T.G. Expression, activation and processing of a novel plant milk-clotting aspartic protease in *Pichia pastoris*. *J. Biotechnol.* **2018**, *268*, 28–39. [CrossRef]
64. Lee, S.-Y.; Park, S.-Y.; Park, H.-J. Immuno-Enhancing Effects of *Galium aparine* L. in Cyclophosphamide-Induced Immunosuppressed Animal Models. *Nutrients* **2024**, *16*, 597. [CrossRef] [PubMed]
65. Schmidt, M.; Polednik, C.; Roller, J.; Hagen, R. *Galium verum* aqueous extract strongly inhibits the motility of head and neck cancer cell lines and protects mucosal keratinocytes against toxic DNA damage. *Oncol. Rep.* **2014**, *32*, 1296–1302. [CrossRef] [PubMed]

66. Schmidt, M.; Scholz, C.; Gavril, G.; Otto, C.; Polednik, C.; Roller, J.; Hagen, R. Effect of *Galium verum* aqueous extract on growth, motility and gene expression in drug-sensitive and -resistant laryngeal carcinoma cell lines. *Int. J. Oncol.* **2014**, *44*, 745–760. [CrossRef]
67. Khalili, M.; Ebrahimzadeh, M.A.; Safdari, Y. Antihaemolytic activity of thirty herbal extracts in mouse red blood cells. *Arh. Za Hig. Rada I Toksikologiju* **2014**, *65*, 399–406. [CrossRef]
68. Goryacha, O.V.; Ilyina, T.V.; Kovalyova, A.M.; Koshovyi, O.M.; Krivoruchko, O.V.; Vladimirova, I.M.; Komisarenko, A.M. A hepatoprotective activity of *Galium verum* L. extracts against carbon tetrachloride-induced injuri in rats. *Der Pharma Chem.* **2017**, *7*, 80–83. Available online: http://www.derpharmachemica.com/archive.html (accessed on 16 November 2024).
69. Zagayko, A.L.; Briukhanova, T.O. A comparative study diuretic activity of *Galium verum* various extracts. *Ukr. Biopharm. J.* **2018**, *1*, 31–34. [CrossRef]
70. Milevic, A.; Simic, M.; Tomovic, M.; Rankovic, M.; Jakovljevic, V.; Bradic, J. The effects of methanol extract of *Galium verum* L. on cardiac redox state in hypertensive rats. *Braz. J. Pharm. Sci.* **2022**, *58*, e191062. [CrossRef]
71. Bradic, J.; Zivkovic, V.; Srejovic, I.; Jakovljevic, V.; Petkovic, A.; Turnic, T.N.; Jeremic, J.; Jeremic, N.; Mitrovic, S.; Sobot, T.; et al. Protective Effects of *Galium verum* L. Extract against Cardiac Ischemia/Reperfusion Injury in Spontaneously Hypertensive Rats. *Oxid. Med. Cell. Longev.* **2019**, *2019*, 4235405. [CrossRef]
72. Bradic, J.; Andjic, M.; Novakovic, J.; Kocovic, A.; Tomovic, M.; Petrovic, A.; Nikolic, M.; Mitrovic, S.; Jakovljevic, V.; Pecarski, D. Lady's Bedstraw as a Powerful Antioxidant for Attenuation of Doxorubicin-Induced Cardiotoxicity. *Antioxidants* **2023**, *12*, 1277. [CrossRef]
73. Beirami, A.D.; Akhtari, N.; Noroozi, R.; Hatamabadi, D.; Hasan, S.M.; Ayatollahi, S.A.; Ayatollahi, N.A.; Kobarfard, F. Bringing back *Galium aparine* L. from forgotten corners of traditional wound treatment procedures: An antimicrobial, antioxidant, and in-vitro wound healing assay along with HPTLC fingerprinting study. *BMC Complement. Med. Ther.* **2024**, *24*, 279. [CrossRef]
74. Aslantürk, S.; Çelik, T.A.; Karabey, B.; Karabey, F. Apoptotic Activities of Ethyl Acetate and Methanol Extracts of *Galium aparine* L. , *J. Pharm. Res. Int.* **2017**, *15*, 1–16. Available online: https://journaljpri.com/index.php/JPRI/article/view/203/406 (accessed on 16 November 2024).
75. Pashapour, S.; Heshmati, M.; Mousavi, Z.; Esmaeili, S. The Apoptotic Effect of Methanolic Extract of *Galium verum* on HT29 Cell Line. *J. Biol. Stud.* **2022**, *4*, 210–220. [CrossRef]
76. Pashapour, S.; Heshmati, M.; Mousavi, Z.; Esmaeili, S. Effect of whole methanolic extract of *Galium verum* on AGO cell line. *Toxicol. Commun.* **2022**, *4*, 10. [CrossRef]
77. Marković, M.S.; Pljevljakušić, D.S.; Pančić, A.S.; Rakonjac, L.B.; Nikolić, B.M.; Stankov, J.V.P. Ethnobotanical use of plants from the genus *Galium* in the Pirot District. *Pirot. Zb.* **2023**, *48*, 191–202. [CrossRef]
78. Peng, Y.; Demidchik, V.; Li, Y.; Shen, Z. Comparison of terpenoids in Nauclea officinalis and Paederia scandens and their anti-inflammatory effects on RAW264. 7 macrophages. *Fitoterapia* **2025**, *182*, 106411. [CrossRef]
79. Jarić, S.; Popović, Z.; Mačukanović-Jocić, M.; Djurdjević, L.; Mijatović, M.; Karadžić, B.; Mitrović, M.; Pavlović, P. An Ethnobotanical Study on the Usage of Wild Medicinal Herbs from Kopaonik Mountain (Central Serbia). *J. Ethnopharmacol.* **2007**, *111*, 160–175. [CrossRef]
80. Menković, N.; Šavikin, K.; Tasić, S.; Zdunić, G.; Stešević, D.; Milosavljević, S.; Vincek, D. Ethnobotanical study on traditional uses of wild medicinal plants in Prokletije Mountains (Montenegro). *J. Ethnopharmacol.* **2011**, *133*, 97–107. [CrossRef]
81. Mitic, V.D.; Stankov-Jovanovic, V.P.; Ilic, M.D.; Vasiljevic, P.J.; Zabar, A.L.; Stojanovic, G.S. The antioxidant, hemolytic and cholinesterase inhibition properties of *Galium verum* L. and *Tragopogon pratensis* subsp. *pratensis*. *Bulg. Chem. Commun.* **2014**, *46*, 269–276. Available online: http://bcc.bas.bg/BCC_Volumes/Volume_46_Number_2_2014/BCC-46-2-269-276-Mitic.pdf (accessed on 16 November 2024).
82. Popović, Z.; Smiljanić, M.; Matić, R.; Kostić, M.; Nikić, P.; Bojović, S. Phytotherapeutical plants from the Deliblato Sands (Serbia): Traditional pharmacopoeia and implications for conservation. *Indian J. Tradit. Knowl.* **2012**, *11*, 385–400. Available online: https://nopr.niscpr.res.in/handle/123456789/14378 (accessed on 16 November 2024).
83. Ilyina, T.V.; Goryacha, O.V.; Toryanik, E.L.; Kulish, I.A.; Kovaleva, A.M. Antimicrobial Activity of the Genus *Galium*, L. *Pharmacogn. Commun.* **2016**, *6*, 42–47. [CrossRef]
84. Semenescu, A.-D.; Moacă, E.-A.; Iftode, A.; Dehelean, C.-A.; Tchiakpe-Antal, D.-S.; Vlase, L.; Rotunjanu, S.; Muntean, D.; Chiriac, S.D.; Chioibaş, R. Recent Updates Regarding the Antiproliferative Activity of *Galium verum* Extracts on A375 Human Malignant Melanoma Cell Line. *Life* **2024**, *14*, 112. [CrossRef]
85. Asenov, I.; Gusev, C.H.; Kitanov, G.; Nikolov, S.T.; Petkov, T. *Gathering of Medicinal Plants*; Biler: Sofia, Bulgaria, 1998. (In Bulgarian)
86. Morariu-Briciu, D.M.; Bolintineanu, S.L.; Rata, A.; Semenescu, A.D.; Anton, A.; Jijie, R.; Kis, A.; Hrubaru, I.; Heghes, A. Assessment of the biosafety profile of *Galium verum* in vitro on myoblasts and in ovo on chorioallantoic membrane. *World J. Cardiol.* **2025**, *17*, 102310. [CrossRef] [PubMed]

87. Markov, V. The ancient Thracian megalithic sanctuary 'Markov Kamak' at Tsarev Peak in Rila Mountain: Semantic and functional analysis. In *Geoarchaeology and Archaeomineralogy*; Publishing House 'St. Ivan Rilski': Sofia, Bulgaria, 2008; pp. 177–179. Available online: http://satrae.swu.bg/media/5058/markovb.pdf (accessed on 16 November 2024).
88. Mocan, A.; Diuzheva, A.; Bădărău, S.; Moldovan, C.; Andruch, V.; Carradori, S.; Campestre, C.; Tartaglia, A.; De Simone, M.; Vodnar, D.; et al. Liquid Phase and Microwave-Assisted Extractions for Multicomponent Phenolic Pattern Determination of Five Romanian *Galium* Species Coupled with Bioassays. *Molecules* **2019**, *24*, 1226. [CrossRef]
89. Güvenalp, Z.; Kilic, N.; Kazaz, C.; Kaya, Y.; Demirezer, L. Chemical constituents of *Galium tortumense*. *Turk. J. Chem.* **2006**, *30*, 515–523. Available online: https://journals.tubitak.gov.tr/chem/vol30/iss4/12 (accessed on 16 November 2024).
90. Tzakou, O.; Mylonas, P.; Vagias, C.; Petrakis, P.V. Iridoid glucosides with insecticidal activity from *Galium melanantherum*. *Z. Naturforsch. C* **2007**, *62*, 597–602. [CrossRef]
91. Semenescu, A.D.; Moacă, E.A.; Iftode, A.; Dehelean, C.A.; Tchiakpe-Antal, D.S.; Vlase, L.; Vlase, A.M.; Muntean, D.; Chioibaş, R. Phytochemical and Nutraceutical Screening of Ethanol and Ethyl Acetate Phases of Romanian *Galium verum* Herba (*Rubiaceae*). *Molecules* **2023**, *28*, 7804. [CrossRef] [PubMed]
92. Saeed, S.A.; Javed, S. Exploring the economic value of underutilized plant species in Ayubia national park. *Pak. J. Botany* **2007**, *39*, 1435–1442. Available online: https://www.researchgate.net/publication/256298201_Exploring_the_Economic_Value_of_Underutilized_Plant_Species_in_Ayubia_National_Park (accessed on 16 November 2024).
93. Matejić, J.S.; Stefanović, N.; Ivković, M.; Živanović, N.; Marin, P.D.; Džamić, A.M. Traditional uses of autochthonous medicinal and ritual plants and other remedies for health in Eastern and South-Eastern Serbia. *J. Ethnopharmacol.* **2020**, *261*, 113186. [CrossRef]
94. Dias, M.C.; Pinto, D.C.G.A.; Silva, A.M.S. Plant Flavonoids: Chemical Characteristics and Biological Activity. *Molecules* **2021**, *26*, 5377. [CrossRef]
95. Nijveldt, R.J.; van Nood, E.; van Hoorn, D.E.C.; Boelens, P.G.; van Norren, K.; van Leeuwen, P.A.M. Flavonoids: A review of probable mechanisms of action and potential applications. *Am. J. Clin. Nutr.* **2001**, *74*, 418–425. [CrossRef]
96. Kessler, M.; Ubeaud, G.; Jung, L. Anti- and pro-oxidant activity of rutin and quercetin derivatives. *J. Pharm. Pharmacol.* **2003**, *55*, 131–142. [CrossRef]
97. Abdel-Daim, M.M.; Abo-El-Sooud, K.; Aleya, L.; Bungău, S.G.; Najda, A.; Saluja, R. Alleviation of Drugs and Chemicals Toxicity: Biomedical Value of Antioxidants. *Oxidative Med. Cell. Longev.* **2018**, *2018*, 6276438. [CrossRef]
98. Abdel-Daim, M.M.; Zakhary, N.I.; Aleya, L.; Bungău, S.G.; Bohara, R.A.; Siddiqi, N.J. Aging, Metabolic, and Degenerative Disorders: Biomedical Value of Antioxidants. *Oxidative Med. Cell. Longev.* **2018**, *2018*, 2098123. [CrossRef] [PubMed]
99. Dai, J.; Mumper, R.J. Plant Phenolics: Extraction, Analysis and Their Antioxidant and Anticancer Properties. *Molecules* **2010**, *15*, 7313–7352. [CrossRef] [PubMed]
100. Arts, I.C.W.; Hollman, P.C.H. Polyphenols and disease risk in epidemiologic studies. *Am. J. Clin. Nutr.* **2005**, *81*, 317S–325S. [CrossRef] [PubMed]
101. Higdon, J.V.; Frei, B. Tea Catechins and Polyphenols: Health Effects, Metabolism, and Antioxidant Functions. *Crit. Rev. Food Sci. Nutr.* **2003**, *43*, 89–143. [CrossRef]
102. Yang, C.S.; Landau, J.M.; Huang, M.T.; Newmark, H.L. Inhibition of carcinogenesis by dietary polyphenolic compounds. *Annu. Rev. Nutr.* **2001**, *21*, 381–406. [CrossRef]
103. Rasmussen, S.E.; Frederiksen, H.; Krogholm, K.S.; Poulsen, L. Dietary Proanthocyanidins: Occurrence, Dietary Intake, Bioavailability, and Protection against Cardiovascular Disease. *Mol. Nutr. Food Res.* **2005**, *49*, 159–174. [CrossRef]
104. Hertog, M.G.L.; Feskens, E.J.M.; Hollman, P.C.H.; Katan, M.B.; Kromhout, D. Dietary flavonoids and cancer risk in the Zutphen elderly study. *Nutr. Cancer* **1994**, *22*, 175–184. [CrossRef]
105. Cole, G.M.; Lim, G.P.; Yang, F.; Teter, B.; Begum, A.; Ma, Q.; Harris-White, M.E.; Frautschy, S.A. Prevention of Alzheimer's disease: Omega-3 fatty acid and phenolic antioxidant interventions. *Neurobiol. Aging* **2005**, *26*, 133–136. [CrossRef]
106. Ebrahimzadeh, M.A.; Nabavi, S.M.; Nabavi, S.F.; Bahramian, F.; Bekhradnia, A.R. Antioxidant and free radical scavenging activity of *H. officinalis*, L. Var. *angustifolius*, *V. odorata*, *B. hyrcana* and *C. speciosum*. *Pak. J. Pharm. Sci.* **2010**, *23*, 29–34. Available online: https://pubmed.ncbi.nlm.nih.gov/20067863/ (accessed on 16 November 2024). [PubMed]
107. Ebrahimzadeh, M.A.; Hosseinimehr, S.J.; Hamidinia, A.; Jafari, M. Antioxidant and free radical scavenging activity of *Feijoa sallowiana* fruits peel and leaves. *Pharmacologyonline* **2008**, *1*, 7–14. Available online: https://www.researchgate.net/publication/286282080_Antioxidant_and_free_radical_scavenging_activity_of_Feijoa_sallowiana_fruits_peel_and_leaves (accessed on 16 November 2024).
108. Naguib, Y.M.A. A fluorometric method for measurement of oxygen radical scavenging activity of water soluble antioxidants. *Anal. Biochem.* **2000**, *284*, 93–98. [CrossRef] [PubMed]
109. Wang, C.; Gong, X.; Bo, A.; Zhang, L.; Zhang, M.; Zang, E.; Zhang, C.; Li, M. Iridoids: Research Advances in Their Phytochemistry, Biological Activities, and Pharmacokinetics. *Molecules* **2020**, *25*, 287. [CrossRef]

110. Ghisalberti, E.L. Biological and pharmacological activity of naturally occurring iridoids and secoiridoids. *Phytomedicine* **1998**, *5*, 147–163. [CrossRef]
111. Viljoen, A.; Mncwangi, N.; Vermaak, I. Anti-inflammatory iridoids of botanical origin. *Curr. Med. Chem.* **2012**, *19*, 2104–2127. [CrossRef]
112. Dinda, B. *Pharmacology and Application of Naturally Occuring Iridoids*; Springer International Publishing: Berlin/Heidelberg, Germany, 2019; ISBN 9783030055752. [CrossRef]
113. Harborne, J.B. *Phytochemicals Methods*; Chapman and Hall Ltd.: London, UK, 1973; pp. 119–120. Available online: https://books.google.bg/books?id=2yvqeRtE8CwC&lpg=PR7&ots=xBdoT8VqT8&lr&hl=bg&pg=PR10#v=onepage&q&f=false (accessed on 16 November 2024).
114. Li, Y.; Jiang, J.G. Health functions and structure-activity relationships of natural anthraquinones from plants. *Food Funct.* **2018**, *9*, 6063–6080. [CrossRef]
115. Qun, T.; Zhou, T.; Hao, J.; Wang, C.; Zhang, K.; Xu, J.; Wang, X.; Zhou, W. Antibacterial activities of anthraquinones: Structure–activity relationships and action mechanisms. *RSC Med. Chem.* **2023**, *14*, 1446–1471. [CrossRef] [PubMed]
116. Biswas, T.; Dwivedi, U.N. Plant Triterpenoid Saponins: Biosynthesis, in Vitro Production, and Pharmacological Relevance. *Protoplasma* **2019**, *256*, 1463–1486. [CrossRef]
117. Woyengo, T.A.; Ramprasath, V.R.; Jones, P.J.H. Anticancer effects of phytosterols. *Eur. J. Clin. Nutr.* **2009**, *63*, 813–820. [CrossRef]
118. Shahzad, N.; Khan, W.; Shadab, M.D.; Ali, A.; Saluja, S.S.; Sharma, S.; Al-Allaf, F.A.; Abduljaleel, Z.; Ibrahim, I.A.A.; Abdel-Wahab, A.F.; et al. Phytosterols as a natural anticancer agent: Current status and future perspective. *Biomed. Pharm.* **2017**, *88*, 786–794. [CrossRef] [PubMed]
119. Berkhin, E.B. Methods of studying the action of new chemical compounds on kidney function. *Pharm. Chem. J.* **1977**, *11*, 3–11. [CrossRef]
120. Zahra, M.; Abrahamse, H.; George, B.P. Flavonoids: Antioxidant Powerhouses and Their Role in Nanomedicine. *Antioxidants* **2024**, *13*, 922. [CrossRef]
121. Watroly, M.N.; Sekar, M.; Fuloria, S.; Gan, S.H.; Jeyabalan, S.; Wu, Y.S.; Subramaniyan, V.; Sathasivam, K.V.; Ravi, S.; Mat Rani, N.N.I.; et al. Chemistry, Biosynthesis, Physicochemical and Biological Properties of Rubiadin: A Promising Natural Anthraquinone for New Drug Discovery and Development. *Drug Des. Dev. Ther.* **2021**, *15*, 4527–4549. [CrossRef] [PubMed]
122. Zhao, J.Q.; Hao, Y.Y.; Gong, T.T.; Wei, Y.F.; Zheng, G.; Du, Z.D.; Zou, B.J.; Yan, S.; Liu, F.H.; Gao, S.; et al. Phytosterol intake and overall survival in newly diagnosed ovarian cancer patients: An ambispective cohort study. *Front. Nutr.* **2022**, *9*, 974367. [CrossRef]

molecules

MDPI

Article

Whey Protein Enzymatic Breakdown: Synthesis, Analysis, and Discovery of New Biologically Active Peptides in Papain-Derived Hydrolysates

Michał Czelej [1,2], Katarzyna Garbacz [1,2], Tomasz Czernecki [2], Kamila Rachwał [2,*], Jacek Wawrzykowski [3,*] and Adam Waśko [2]

1 Biolive Innovation Sp. z.o.o., Dobrzańskiego 3, 20-262 Lublin, Poland; katarzyna.garbacz@up.lublin.pl (K.G.)
2 Department of Biotechnology, Microbiology and Human Nutrition, Faculty of Food Science and Biotechnology, University of Life Sciences in Lublin, Skromna 8, 20-704 Lublin, Poland; tomasz.czernecki@up.lublin.pl (T.C.); adam.wasko@up.lublin.pl (A.W.)
3 Department of Biochemistry, Faculty of Veterinary Medicine, University of Life Sciences in Lublin, Akademicka 12, 20-033 Lublin, Poland
* Correspondence: kamila.rachwal@up.lublin.pl (K.R.); wawrzykowski@up.lublin.pl (J.W.)

Abstract: Bioactive peptides derived from milk proteins offer promising potential that can be unlocked through hydrolysis. Enzymatic hydrolysis is particularly noteworthy because of its mild conditions and its efficacy in producing peptides with various biological activities. This study focused on creating whey protein hydrolysates using three enzymes: pepsin, trypsin, and papain. The degree of hydrolysis and the antioxidant properties of the resulting peptides were evaluated, and papain demonstrated the highest degree of hydrolysis, leading to its selection for further investigation. LC-MS was employed to identify peptide sequences from the papain-derived hydrolysate, resulting in the identification of 107 distinct peptide sequences These peptides were predicted to exhibit a range of potential biological activities, including antihypertensive, antidiabetic, antioxidant, antimicrobial, and immunomodulatory effects, as well as roles in regulating glucose homeostasis, maintaining cardiovascular health, and supporting overall metabolic function. In vitro tests revealed the significant antioxidant and antibacterial properties of the hydrolysate, confirming the potential of papain-derived peptides for use in functional food and pharmaceutical applications. The novelty of this study lies in the identification of novel peptides with promising biological activities. Additional in vitro and in vivo studies are required to fully elucidate the health benefits of these peptides.

Keywords: enzymatic hydrolysis; whey protein; biological activity of peptides; LC-MS identification of peptides

1. Introduction

Whey, a protein-rich fraction obtained during the acid or enzymatic processing of dairy products in cheese or casein production, is frequently considered a by-product, constituting approximately 85–90% of the milk volume. However, because of its high nutritional value and health-promoting properties, whey can be used for the production of dietary supplements and nutraceuticals [1,2]. This co-product contains various soluble milk components, including proteins, lipids, lactose, polyphenols, minerals, and vitamins [3]. Among the most prevalent proteins in whey are β-lactoglobulin, α-lactalbumin, bovine serum albumin, and immunoglobulins, with lactoferrin, lactoperoxidase, and proteose peptone present in lower quantities. Whey proteins also include glycomacropeptides released during plasmin-mediated hydrolysis, which are exclusively present in sweet whey [4].

Whey proteins are widely acknowledged for their unique composition and functional properties that render them valuable in the food industry. These proteins exhibit high solubility and are susceptible to heat denaturation owing to their globular conformation because of their highly diluted ingredients and perishability [2]. Consequently, various processing methods have been developed to enhance the usability of whey, with one of the most promising being hydrolysis, which produces peptides with potential biological activities [5].

Hydrolysis is crucial for unlocking the bioactive potential of whey proteins. It can be performed through chemical or enzymatic means as well as through fermentation or physical processes. Despite its cost-effectiveness and simplicity, chemical hydrolysis presents several drawbacks, including the potential for toxic residues and diminished nutritional value due to harsh processing conditions [6]. In contrast, enzymatic hydrolysis offers more favourable conditions, allowing the controlled release of peptides with specific biological activities [3,7]. The principal enzymes utilised include gastrointestinal enzymes (pepsin, pancreatin, trypsin, chymotrypsin), plant-derived enzymes (e.g., papain, bromelain, actinidin), and proteolytic microorganisms or microbial proteases (e.g., proteases from lactic acid bacteria and flavourzyme from *Aspergillus oryzae*) [6,8]. Despite the known benefits of enzymatic hydrolysis, the specific bioactive potential of papain-derived whey protein peptides, particularly in terms of their antioxidant and antimicrobial activities, remains underexplored. Additionally, the fermentation process utilises the proteolytic activity of microorganisms, whereas methods such as microwaves or ultrasound can also facilitate peptide production [9].

Different enzymatic digestion processes yield different quantities and types of peptides in the same food matrix. The selection of a particular enzyme to catalyse protein hydrolysis is guided by the evaluation of its selectivity and available literature data, indicating its applicability. Enzymatic hydrolysis of whey proteins employs various proteases, each influencing the composition and bioactivity of the resulting peptides. For example, Alcalase, a serine protease, efficiently generates antioxidant and ACE-inhibitory peptides, while trypsin and chymotrypsin, often used together, enhance the release of bioactive sequences [10–12]. Pepsin hydrolysis improves antioxidant and antihypertensive properties, whereas plant-derived enzymes such as papain, bromelain, and ficin contribute to antihypertensive peptide production [12,13]. Microbial proteases (Protease S and M) yield hydrolysates with a high degree of hydrolysis and significant bioactive properties [14,15]. The functional properties of peptides derived from whey proteins are influenced by their amino acid composition. For instance, peptides with aromatic and nonpolar residues tend to exhibit enhanced antioxidant activity, while cationic and aromatic sequences are associated with ACE inhibition. Additionally, other peptides may demonstrate antimicrobial, immunomodulatory, antidiabetic, or opioid-like activities [3,12,16].

In this study, the most commonly used gastrointestinal enzymes, pepsin and trypsin, were used for hydrolysis. Additionally, they were selected based on literature data suggesting that they are capable of generating peptides with dipeptidyl peptidase IV (DPPIV) and angiotensin-converting enzyme (ACE) inhibitory [17,18], bactericidal [19], antihypertensive, antioxidant [20], and cytoprotective [21] properties. In recent years, research has been conducted to obtain bioactive whey protein peptides using enzymes of plant origin. Previously, it was reported that plant-derived proteases (cardosins A and B, papain, bromelain, and ficin) could be utilised to obtain peptides with ACE inhibitory activity [13,22].

The enzymatic hydrolysis of whey proteins enhances their nutritional and functional properties, rendering them suitable for a diverse range of applications in the food and health industries. This process generates bioactive peptides with improved digestibility, solubility, and physiological activities, further increasing their potential benefits. Hydrolysis augments the nutritional value of whey proteins by cleaving them into smaller peptides and amino acids, which are more readily digested and absorbed. This process substantially reduces the antigenic properties of whey proteins, making them suitable for use in hypoallergenic food products [16]. Regarding effects on functional characteristics, enzymatic hydrolysis of whey proteins improves solubility across a wide pH range, promotes viscosity through water binding, and facilitates cohesion, adhesion, and elasticity [23]. Enzymatic hydrolysis can also enhance the foaming and emulsifying properties of whey proteins, rendering them suitable for use in sports nutrition and as stabilisers in acidic beverages [24].

Enzymatic hydrolysis is utilised to generate peptides with a diverse range of bioactive properties, which have applications in the development of specialised foods and beverages for sports nutrition and preventive nutrition for individuals with allergies to bovine milk proteins [25]. The selection of enzymes and hydrolysis conditions plays a crucial role in determining the specific benefits and applications of the resulting hydrolysates. It determines the degree of protein hydrolysis (DH), which influences the functional properties of the hydrolysates. Higher DH is also frequently correlated with increased bioactivity [11]. Consequently, different enzymes employed in hydrolysis can produce distinct peptide profiles with varying bioactivity [13,26].

Bioactive peptides released from whey proteins during hydrolysis exhibit a broad spectrum of health-promoting properties, including antimicrobial, antidiabetic, antioxidant, and immunomodulatory effects. These properties have generated significant interest in food and nutraceutical industries, particularly in the development of functional foods and supplements. Several commercially available products incorporate bioactive whey peptides for specific therapeutic purposes, such as antihypertensive, anti-inflammatory, and sleep-inducing effects [6]. Additionally, whey peptides may possess anticancer, cytoprotective, mineral-chelating, osteoanabolic, hypocholesterolemic, opioid, and antithrombotic properties. However, the market for functional foods enriched with whey-derived bioactive peptides is relatively underdeveloped, highlighting the need for further research in this area. The discovery of novel peptide sequences with specific biological properties may influence the development of innovative products enriched with health functions such as antioxidant activity, anticancer properties, or improvement of the gut microbiota.

The use of bioactive peptides in functional foods and supplements represents a highly pertinent and expanding field of research. Given the potential of whey as a rich source of such peptides, there is significant demand for efficient peptide production and characterisation methods. Owing to their health-promoting properties, these peptides hold considerable promise as ingredients in fortified foods, offering enhanced nutritional benefits. However, there is a paucity of reports in the literature regarding the activity of peptides generated from whey proteins using papain, and studies have not identified the specific sequences of peptides obtained using this method. This study aimed to evaluate and compare the hydrolysis efficiency and bioactive potential of whey peptides generated using pepsin, papain, and trypsin. Particular emphasis was placed on the identification of novel peptide sequences in papain hydrolysate and the assessment of their potential biological activity. This study employed a comprehensive approach that integrated experimental analysis of biological activities (antioxidant and antimicrobial), LC-MS analysis of the peptide composition obtained during papain hydrolysis, and in silico prediction of their activities. Owing to the acquisition and identification of new peptides, these findings may contribute to the development of novel food products, nutraceuticals, or therapeutic agents, supporting the growing interest in bioactive peptides for health promotion. This study aimed to evaluate the efficiency of papain in hydrolysing whey proteins, identifying novel bioactive peptides, and assessing their potential antioxidant and antimicrobial activities.

2. Results and Discussion

2.1. Degree of Hydrolysis (DH) of Whey Proteins by Various Enzymes

Enzyme activity plays a crucial role in protein hydrolysis; therefore, in the initial phase of the study, enzymatic hydrolysis of whey proteins was conducted using three distinct enzymes under identical reaction conditions (selected following preliminary optimisation). Various commercial proteases, including whey proteins, have been successfully evaluated for the production of bioactive hydrolysates from milk. In this study, reactions catalysed by trypsin, pepsin, and papain were selected for analysis. For each variant, the degree of hydrolysis was determined at different time intervals. Figure 1 illustrates the effects of enzyme specificity and reaction time on the degree of hydrolysis (DH). Among the three enzymes employed in this study, whey proteins hydrolysed with papain after a 3 h reaction exhibited significantly higher DH values than whey hydrolysed with trypsin and pepsin. The hydrolysis rates for trypsin, pepsin, and papain were 15 ± 1.6%, 22 ± 2.8%, and 33 ± 3.7%, respectively (Figure 1). Consequently, the highest efficiency of the enzymatic reaction, assessed by the ratio of released peptides to total protein content, was observed when papain hydrolysis was employed (DH 33 ± 3.7% after 3 h). It is also noteworthy that a reaction duration of merely half an hour facilitated a high degree of whey protein hydrolysis.

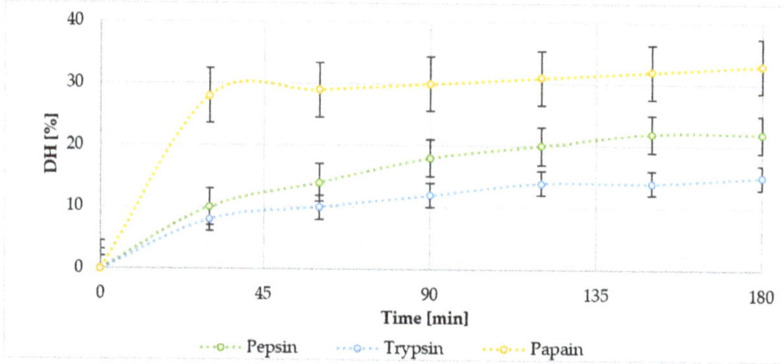

Figure 1. Degree of hydrolysis (%) of whey proteins by pepsin, trypsin, and papain at different time points.

Papain is an enzyme known for its advantages, including faster rates and the ability to operate under mild conditions. This unique property helps preserve the bioactivity of the released peptides, which is often compromised by harsher enzymatic or chemical hydrolysis processes, while also enabling a reduction in production costs and improving yield and productivity [13]. In addition, papain has a narrow pH range (5–7), but its activity is advantageous over a broad temperature range, including higher temperatures (<90 °C) [27].

Studies on whey hydrolysis have demonstrated different levels of hydrolysis for the different enzymes utilised. This is because the efficiency of enzymatic hydrolysis of whey proteins depends on factors such as the type of enzyme and substrate, their ratio, hydrolysis conditions, and mixing conditions [28]. For example, in a study conducted by Wang et al. [19], whey protein hydrolysis was performed using three different enzymes. A significantly lower degree of hydrolysis was observed in variants with 3 h hydrolysis with papain (DH 9.3 ± 0.3%), whereas superior results were obtained for samples hydrolysed with alkalase (6 h, DH 32.2 ± 2.5%) and trypsin (4 h, DH 25.2 ± 1.7%). However, the reaction times and temperatures applied were different. Additionally, Kaur et al. [27]

observed lower levels of whey protein hydrolysis using papain (DH of 17.69%), while results very similar to those obtained in this work (DH of 32.28%) were demonstrated by Du et al. [29] in their study.

2.2. Antioxidant Properties of Peptides Obtained via Enzymatic Hydrolysis of Whey Proteins

In the subsequent phase, the antioxidant properties of whey hydrolysates obtained via enzymatic hydrolysis using pepsin, trypsin, and papain were determined (Table 1). Given the increasing prevalence of civilisation diseases, interest in the antioxidant properties of food products has recently intensified. Antioxidant properties pertain to the capacity of certain molecules to neutralise excessive amounts of free oxygen radicals in the body, which are responsible for cellular damage and associated with the occurrence of diseases. Two methods were employed to determine antioxidant activity: the reduction of metal ions to lower-oxidation ions by the antioxidant under investigation (FRAP) and the ability to scavenge stable free radicals (ABTS+ and DPPH). The analyses conducted in this study showed the significant antioxidant potential of all hydrolysates obtained (Table 1).

Table 1. Antioxidant potential of peptides obtained via enzymatic hydrolysis of whey proteins.

Enzyme Treatment	ABTS (eq Trolox μmol/g)	FRAP (eq Trolox μmol/g)	DPPH (eq Trolox μmol/g)
Pepsin	297.44 ± 24.11 [a]	16.22 ± 2.03 [a]	4.87 ± 0.22 [c]
Trypsin	361.96 ± 31.02 [b]	19.68 ± 1.5 [b]	1.75 ± 0.03 [a]
Papain	527.36 ± 25.13 [c]	17.56 ± 2.16 [ab]	3.56 ± 0.17 [b]

The values followed by different letters in superscripts mark significant differences ($p < 0.05$) for each test obtained by ANOVA analysis and Tukey HSD test.

Assessment of ABTS+ cation radical scavenging activity is the predominant method used to quantify the antioxidant activity of food ingredients. Among the hydrolysates obtained in the 3 h reaction with various enzymes, the highest activity was observed for whey proteins digested with papain (527.36 ± 25.13 (eq Trolox μmol/g)), followed by trypsin and pepsin (361.96 ± 31.02 and 297.44 ± 24.11 (eq Trolox μmol/g), respectively).

Owing to its simplicity, short analysis time, and relatively high accuracy and reproducibility of results, an assay based on testing the reactivity of the DPPH (1,1-diphenyl-2-picrylhydrazyl) radical with the sample is one of the most widely utilised methods for measuring the scavenging potential of peptides. It is used to measure the total antioxidant potential of various food products. The results of the DPPH assay of whey hydrolysates extracted with different enzymes revealed the highest free radical scavenging potential of the formula obtained using trypsin (19.68 ± 1.5 (eq Trolox μmol/g)). This capacity using papain and pepsin was marginally lower (17.56 ± 2.16 and 16.22 ± 2.03 (eq Trolox μmol/g), respectively).

The FRAP method quantifies antioxidant capacity based on the influence of antioxidants present in the sample on the rate of reduction of the ferric iron (III)/ferricyanide complex to ferrous iron (II). In this study, the assay demonstrated the highest reducing potential in the whey hydrolysate prepared using pepsin catalysis (4.87 ± 0.22 (eq Trolox μmol/g)), whilst a marginally lower value was observed for the hydrolysate prepared using papain (3.56 ± 0.17 (eq Trolox μmol/g)). The hydrolysate obtained using trypsin exhibited the lowest antioxidant potential (1.75 ± 0.03 (eq Trolox μmol/g)).

The differences observed in the free-radical-reducing activity of whey hydrolysates prepared using different enzymes may be attributed to the specificity of the enzyme for a particular site in the peptide chain. This phenomenon is also associated with the degree of hydrolysis (DH) of the constituent proteins, which ultimately results in hydrolysates containing different amino acid compositions [30]. DH and the enzymes utilised to catalyse hydrolysis play a crucial role in determining the reducing power of protein hydrolysates. The observed differences in antioxidant activity among the tested protein hydrolysates can be associated with the specific amino acid profiles of the peptides [31]. The amino acid sequence also exerts a significant influence on the potency of the antioxidant activity of peptides owing to variations in the activity of individual amino acids related to differences in the side chain structure. This activity is attributed to readily oxidised groups: the indole group in tryptophan, imidazole group in histidine, thiol in cysteine, phenolic hydroxyl group in tyrosine, and thioether in methionine [32]. Ohashi et al. [33] demonstrated that tyrosine-containing tripeptides exhibited higher antioxidant activity against the hydrophilic radical ABTS than histidine-containing tripeptides, suggesting an essential role for tryptophan and tyrosine residues in the determination of radical scavenging activity. The tripeptides examined showed weak scavenging activity against the hydrophobic DPPH radical, and their antioxidant activity against linoleic acid peroxidation demonstrated a high correlation with ABTS assays and a low correlation with FRAP and DPPH assays [33]. This explains the differences in the antioxidant potential assay results observed in this study.

2.3. Antibacterial Activity of Whey Peptides

At this stage of the investigation, only whey hydrolysate produced using papain was analysed. This hydrolysate was selected based on its superior degree of hydrolysis and potent antioxidant activity (Table 1) [34,35].

The effects of whey peptides on the growth of eight bacterial isolates obtained from spoilt food were investigated. Growth inhibition zones were used as a measure of the antimicrobial activity of whey hydrolysates. Growth inhibition zones surrounding the wells containing whey-derived peptides were observed for four bacterial strains tested (*Bacillus* sp., *Bacillus megaterium*, *Staphylococcus capitis*, and *Rhizobium radiobacter*) (Table 2). The highest antibacterial activity was observed against Bacillus sp. with an inhibition zone of 11 mm. No growth inhibition was detected in *B. cereus*, *B. pumilus*, *E. aurantiacum*, or *B. diminut*. These results indicate a selective inhibitory effect of the peptides contained in whey hydrolysates on the growth of certain bacterial strains. The observed effect can be attributed to the capacity of bacteria, including *Bacillus* spp., to secrete extracellular proteases capable of inactivating antibacterial peptides [36].

Table 2. Antimicrobial activity of whey peptides hydrolysed with the use of papain.

Bacterial Species	G(+)/G(−)	Growth Inhibition Zone (mm)
Bacillus sp.	G(+)	11
Bacillus cereus	G(+)	0
Bacillus megaterium	G(+)	8
Bacillus pumilus	G(+)	0
Staphylococcus capitis	G(+)	10
Exiguobacterium aurantiacum	G(+)	0
Brevundimonas diminuta	G(−)	0
Rhizobium radiobacter	G(+)	9

Numerous previous studies have demonstrated that enzymatic hydrolysis of whey proteins results in the release of antimicrobial peptides, which are encrypted in whey proteins. The positive effect of papain enzymatic hydrolysis on antimicrobial activity has previously been demonstrated for papain hydrolysates of buffalo and camel milk whey proteins [37–39].

Peptides derived from β-lactoglobulin degradation, including the AASDISLLDAQS-APLR peptide identified in this study, were responsible for the observed antimicrobial activity of the hydrolysate. This effect may also be attributable to the presence of other sequences with antimicrobial activity in the obtained peptides derived from the hydrolysis of β-lactoglobulin, namely VAGTWY, VLVLDTDYK, and IPAVFK, which were previously identified by Pellegrini et al. [40]. The presence of antimicrobial peptides in the hydrolysate suggests that the addition of these peptides to food products may exert an inhibitory effect on the growth of certain undesirable bacteria present in food.

2.4. Identification of Peptides Derived from Whey and Their Predicted Biological Activity

Following the hydrolysis methodology involving papain and the aforementioned conditions, 107 peptides were extracted and identified. LC-MS analysis revealed peptides of varying lengths ranging from 7 to 27 amino acids. A comprehensive list of all identified peptide sequences, including information on the proteins from which they were derived and the biological activities of the peptides, as determined from data available in databases and predicted from the sequences, is presented in Table S1.

The molecular weights of peptides obtained from the hydrolysis of whey proteins are contingent on the enzymatic reaction conditions employed, particularly the enzyme type utilised. The bioactivity of the resultant hydrolysate was determined based on its final composition and amino acid sequence. In this study, multiple predicted biological activities were attributed to each peptide. It is not uncommon for a single peptide to exhibit multiple functions because of the interconnectedness of metabolic pathways that govern specific functions. Furthermore, certain peptides may function as signalling molecules, thereby exerting systemic effects.

Based on peptide sequences obtained using LC-MS, the biological activities of several peptides were identified using a database search (BIOPEP-UWM database). These include zinc-binding peptides, such as VEELKPTPEGDLEIL and ELKPTPEGDLEIL, derived from β-lactoglobulin digestion. Previous studies have demonstrated that peptides interact with zinc ions to form chemically stable and soluble chelates. These chelates are involved in elemental transport and can prevent zinc from interacting with various compounds in the gastrointestinal tract, such as phytic acid. Zinc peptide chelates can be utilised as a novel route for supplementing the human body with zinc, as the zinc present in such a chelate can enter the body via the peptide absorption mode [41]. Such zinc-binding peptides may have valuable nutritional applications as dietary zinc carriers to enhance the bioavailability and bioaccessibility of this element. Furthermore, peptides possessing zinc ligands are pharmacologically relevant as zinc-dependent enzyme inhibitors and are potentially efficacious in controlling inflammatory diseases [42].

The APFPEVF peptide derived from α-S1-casein digestion was identified. It has been recognised for its potential application in the prevention and treatment of pathological conditions associated with alpha-glucosidase [43,44]. The databases also provided information on the activity of peptides obtained during the hydrolysis of whey using β-casein, namely VYPFPGPIH, LVYPFPGPIH, and YPFPGPIPNS. The VYPFPGPIH peptide has been reported to inhibit prolyl endopeptidase (PEP) activity, which has been associated with neurodegenerative disorders.

PEP inhibitors are considered capable of reversing memory loss induced by amnesic compounds [45]. LVYPFPGPIH has been identified as an ACE inhibitor that exhibits antihypertensive effects, whereas YPFPGPIPNS is known as β-casomorphin-11, which is an opioid receptor agonist. Bioactive peptides from this family are capable of binding to and activating opioid receptors located in various regions of the body (including the immune system, gastrointestinal tract, and potentially the central nervous system) and may differentially affect processes such as immunosuppression, gastrointestinal nutrient absorption, opioid signalling, hyperglycaemia, and oxidative stress [46,47].

Analysis of the predicted activity of other peptides indicated that they may exert a variety of beneficial physiological effects, including reducing blood pressure, preventing cardiovascular disease, exhibiting hypolipidaemic effects, maintaining glucose homeostasis, regulating stomach mucosal membrane activity, influencing the nervous system, and functioning as antidiabetic, anticancer, anti-inflammatory, immunomodulatory, antimicrobial, antioxidant, and osteoanabolic agents.

Previous studies have demonstrated that the milk proteome comprises peptides that are inactive in the native protein, but upon release, constitute biologically active peptides capable of interacting with relevant receptors and regulating physiological functions in the body. These peptides have diverse biological activities. Peptides released from whey proteins have demonstrated antihypertensive (ACE inhibitors), antioxidant, anticancer, cognitive, and memory-enhancing effects [13].

Antioxidant and antimicrobial activities are considered to be the primary common characteristics of biologically active peptides. In the present study, 16 peptides potentially responsible for the observed antimicrobial activity of the hydrolysates were identified. In contrast, 58 peptides derived from whey digestion were potentially associated with in vitro antioxidant activity. Antioxidant activity is also associated with cancer prevention. Among the identified peptides, 12 exhibited potential anticancer activity. Peptides with annotated activities, such as the protein associated with Myc (PAM) inhibitor, DPP-III inhibitor, and regulator of phosphoglycerate kinase activity, may also be postulated to exert anticancer effects. Peptides with immunomodulatory and anti-inflammatory properties (including the aminopeptidase inhibitor Xaa-Pro and DPP-III inhibitor) may possess more generalised systemic functions, partially related to cancer prevention and immunity.

One of the most prevalent biological activities of peptides is the inhibition of angiotensin-converting enzyme (ACE), which in silico analyses attributed to all the peptides obtained in this study. This effect involves inhibition of the angiotensin-converting enzyme, which converts angiotensin I (AT I) into angiotensin II (AT II), consequently reducing the blood levels of ATII, which in excess constricts the vessels, resulting in an increase in blood pressure. Previous research has reported that several milk- and whey-derived peptides exhibit high in vitro ACE inhibitory activity (IPP peptides, LIVTQ, IIAE, LVYPFP) [48]. Among the peptides identified in this investigation, APFPEVF was previously predicted to possess ACE inhibitory activity [49].

In addition to hypotensive peptides, blood-pressure-lowering and anti-atherosclerotic effects are also attributed to peptides with calmodulin-dependent cyclic nucleotide phosphodiesterase (CaMPDE) inhibitor, DPP-III inhibitor, and renin inhibitor activity, as well as partially to peptides stimulating vasoactive substance release. Peptides with hypolipidaemic effects are also partially associated with the prevention of cardiovascular disease. This effect was attributed to peptides with HMG-CoA reductase inhibitor activity. In our investigation, in silico analyses indicated that one of the identified peptides (RELKDLKGYGGVS) may exhibit such activity. By inhibiting the HMGR activity, these peptides reduce the rate of cholesterol biosynthesis [50,51].

In contrast to the aforementioned activities, among the predicted activities of the peptides shown in the in silico analyses, anti-diabetic, antiviral, anti-sclerotic, and gut mucosa-regulating activities are considered particularly noteworthy [52]. Several categories of peptide activity are associated with antidiabetic potential and the maintenance of glucose homeostasis. Of the anticipated activities attributed to the peptides identified in this study, peptides with potential DPP-IV inhibitor and alpha-glucosidase inhibitor activities, as well as those stimulating glucagon-like peptide 1 release and regulating phosphoglycerate kinase, may exhibit such effects. Regarding peptides with antiviral activity, the study identified 17 peptides that were found to have aminopeptidase Xaa-Pro inhibitory activity, which may provide an antiretroviral effect. The group of peptides with predicted effects on the nervous system is equally significant. These include peptides with potential neuropeptide, opioid, antiamnestic, and β-casomorphin-5 butyrylcholinesterase inhibitor activities.

3. Materials and Methods

3.1. Materials

Commercial bovine whey protein isolate (84% protein content) was procured from BioTechUSA Ltd. (Budapest, Hungary). The amino acid composition of the products is presented in Table 3.

Table 3. Amino acid content of WPI used in the study (mg per 100 g WPI).

Essential Amino Acids (mg)		Conditionally Essential Amino Acids (mg)		Nonessential Amino Acids (mg)	
Histidine	1500	Arginine	2008	Alanine	3836
Isoleucine	4712	Cysteine	2552	Aspartic acid	8564
Leucine	8680	Glutamine and glutamic acid	17,208	Glycine	1428
Methionine	1880	Proline	4424	Serine	3804
Phenylalanine	2556	Tyrosine	2384		
Threonine	5176				
Tryptophan	1368				
Valine	4564				

3.2. Preparation of Whey Hydrolysates

Enzymatic hydrolysis was used to obtain peptides from the whey proteins. Three distinct enzymes were utilised for hydrolysis: pepsin (from porcine gastric mucosa, ≥400 units/mg protein, P7125, Sigma-Aldrich, Saint Louis, MO, USA), papain (from papaya latex crude powder, 1.5–10 units/mg solid, P3375, Sigma-Aldrich, Saint Louis, MO, USA), and trypsin (from bovine pancreas, lyophilised powder, ≥10,000 BAEE units/mg protein, T1426, Sigma-Aldrich, Saint Louis, MO, USA), with the objective of selecting the enzyme that yielded the optimal degree of hydrolysis and facilitated the production of peptides with the highest antioxidant activity. The protein isolate was dissolved in Milli-Q water and preheated, and the pH of the solution was subsequently adjusted to the optimum value for the action of the individual enzymes, namely 3.0, 6.0, and 8.0 for pepsin, papain, and trypsin, respectively. Enzymatic hydrolysis was conducted for 3 h with constant agitation at an enzyme/substrate ratio of 1:10 (w/w), at 37 °C for pepsin and trypsin, and 70 °C for papain. The reaction was terminated by heating the mixture at 100 °C for 15 min. Subsequently, the hydrolysate was cooled to 37 °C and centrifuged at 3000× g for 30 min. The resultant supernatant was lyophilised and stored at 4 °C for further analysis (and the degree of hydrolysis and antioxidant activity were determined for each variant).

3.3. Determination of Degree of Hydrolysis

The degree of hydrolysis was determined by quantifying the soluble peptides present in the mixture at predetermined time intervals from the initiation of the hydrolysis process (0, 0.5, 1, 2, and 3 h). For this purpose, 500 μL of the hydrolysate was extracted at specified time points and immediately combined with 10% trichloroacetic acid in a 1:1 (v/v) ratio. The samples were subsequently incubated for 15 min at room temperature, followed by centrifugation (5500× g for 10 min). To ascertain the concentration of soluble peptides in the supernatant, a spectrophotometric method was employed to measure absorbance at 280 nm. The degree of hydrolysis was calculated as the percentage of soluble peptides relative to the total protein content in the mixture.

$$DH\,[\%] = \frac{protein\ content\ after\ hydrolysis}{\text{total protein content in sample}} \cdot 100\%$$

3.4. Determination of Antioxidant Potential

Antioxidant activity of the peptides was determined as previously described by Czelej et al. [53] using 2,20-azino-bis(3-ethylbenzthiazoline-6-sulfonic acid (ABTS•+), 1,1-diphenyl-2-picrylhydrazyl (DPPH), and Ferric Reducing Antioxidant Power (FRAP) assays. Samples were prepared by combining 10 mg of hydrolysate with 1 mL of deionised water (5 min, 15 Hz, Retsch Mixer MM400; Haan, Germany). The samples were centrifuged for 3 min (15 °C, 33 000× g, Hettich 32R centrifuge, Tuttlingen, Germany), and the supernatant was used for subsequent analysis. The samples were prepared in triplicates.

The Ferric Reducing Antioxidant Power of the whey peptides was assessed using a 10 mmol/L solution of 2,4,6-Tris(2-pyridyl)-s-triazine (TPTZ) diluted in 40 mmol/L HCl combined with 20 mmol/L FeCl3 · $6H_2O$ and acetate buffer (300 mmol/L, pH 3.6) at a 1:1:10 (*v*:*v*:*v*) ratio. Then, 50 µL of the samples containing the peptide solution was combined with 150 µL of FRAP reagent, homogenised, and incubated for 5 min at 25 °C. Subsequently, the absorbance was measured at 593 nm (using a Marcel s330 spectrophotometer, Zielonka, Poland) against a blank sample (containing water instead of the peptide sample). The reducing antioxidant power was assessed by reference to a standard curve established using Trolox standards.

Free radical scavenging activity was evaluated using the stable radical DPPH assay. Aliquots (50 µL) of the peptide solution were combined with 150 µL of methanolic DPPH solution. Samples were incubated in the dark at 25 °C for 60 min with agitation. The absorbance of each sample was measured spectrophotometrically at 517 nm against a blank sample. The antioxidant activity of the peptides was evaluated by comparison with a standard curve plotted against the Trolox standards.

Radical Cation Decolourisation Activity was assayed using (ABTS•+). The ABTS•+ working solution was prepared by combining an equal volume of 7 mM ABTS and 2.4 mM potassium persulfate in deionised water and allowed to stand for 16 h prior to the measurements. The resulting working solution was diluted with phosphate-buffered saline (PBS) until the absorbance reached 0.7 at λ = 734 nm. Then, 50 µL of the working solution was added to 1 mL of the peptide mixture sample, and the absorbance of the samples was measured at 734 nm relative to the blank.

3.5. Antibacterial Activity

The antimicrobial activity of the whey peptides was evaluated using a well diffusion assay. This study encompassed eight bacterial strains previously isolated from decomposed fruits and vegetables (*Bacillus* sp., *Bacillus cereus*, *Bacillus megaterium*, *Bacillus pumilus*, *Staphylococcus capitis*, *Exiguobacterium aurantiacum*, *Brevundimonas diminuta*, and *Rhizobium radiobacter*) [53]. Bacterial strains were cultured in Mueller–Hinton broth (Biomaxima, Lublin, Poland) at 37 °C for 24 h. Subsequently, 100 µL of the bacterial culture was applied to Petri dishes containing Mueller–Hinton agar and was distributed uniformly across the surface. For this, 8 mm diameter wells were excised in the medium. Then, 70 µL of the test peptide at a concentration of 50 mg/mL was introduced into the wells. The plates were incubated for 24 h at 37 °C, and the bacterial growth inhibition zones surrounding the wells were measured.

3.6. Identification and Characterisation of Bioactive Peptides by LC-MS

For peptide identification, 3 mg of each sample after papain hydrolysis was reconstituted in 400 μL of 100 mM ammonium bicarbonate buffer. The peptides were filtered through a Vivacon 30 kDa molecular weight cutoff filter (Sartorius Stedim Biotech, Goettingen, Germany). The samples were analysed using an LC-MS system comprising an Evosep One HPLC System (Evosep Biosystems, Odense, Denmark) coupled with an Orbitrap Exploris 480 mass spectrometer (Thermo Scientific, Sunnyvale, CA, USA). The peptide solution (100 μL) was loaded onto Evotips Pure C18 disposable trap columns according to the manufacturer's instructions. The peptides were fractionated for 88 min with a predefined Evosep gradient at a flow rate of 220 nL/min on an analytical column (Dr Maisch C18 AQ, 1.9 μm beads, 150 μm ID, 15 cm long, Evosep Biosystems, Odense, Denmark). The data-dependent acquisition parameters were as follows: top 40 precursors selected for MS2 analysis, collisional induced fragmentation NCE 30%, spray voltage 2.1 kV, funnel RF level 40, and heated capillary temperature 275 °C. Full MS scans covered the mass range of 300–1600 m/z with a resolution of 60,000, a maximum injection time set to Auto, and a normalised AGC target of 300%. MS2 scans were acquired with a resolution of 15,000, auto maximum injection time, and Standard AGC target. The ion isolation window was set to 1.6 m/z, dynamic exclusion was set to 20 s, and the minimum intensity threshold was 5×10^3.

Raw data were pre-processed with Mascot Distiller (version 2.8, Matrixscience, London, UK) and peptides/proteins were identified with Mascot suite (version 2.8, Matrixscience) after offline mass recalibration with MScan (version 3.0, http://proteom.ibb.waw.pl/mscan; accessed on 14 February 2023). The search parameters were as follows: enzyme—none, variable modifications—oxidation (M), max missed cleavages—2, fragment ion tolerance—0.01 Da, parent ion tolerance set individually after recalibration within range 7–11 ppm. The database always includes popular contaminants (common Repository of Adventitious Proteins (cRAP), 115 sequences, 86,853,323,495 residues). Species-specific database: Bos taurus (47,245 sequences) from Uniprot.

3.7. In Silico Analysis of LC-MS-Identified Peptides

The biological activities of the obtained peptides were analysed based on their amino acid sequences using the BIOPEP-UWM database [54]. Identified peptide sequences were verified for known bioactivities by comparing them against the database's collection of biologically active peptides. With regard to peptides without a direct match, potential activity was predicted based on their structural and compositional similarities to known bioactive sequences. This approach allowed for a comprehensive assessment of the functional potential of the identified whey-protein-derived peptides.

3.8. Statistical Analysis

Statistical analyses were performed using Python 3.10 (SciPy package and statsmodels). One-way ANOVA followed by Tukey's post hoc test were applied to compare samples treated with different enzymes for each antioxidant parameter (ABTS, FRAP, DPPH). Results are presented as mean ± standard deviation, and p values < 0.05 were considered statistically significant.

4. Conclusions

In contemporary research, food-derived proteins are increasingly recognised not only for their nutritional value but also as a significant source for identifying bioactive peptide sequences. In this study, the matrix selected was whey, which contains proteins that offer substantial potential for the extraction of bioactive peptides. This study focused on whey, a matrix with considerable potential for extracting bioactive peptides. This article elucidates the hydrolysis of whey proteins and the identification of peptides released during enzymatic reactions, along with their biological activities. These findings demonstrate that high efficiency in the enzymatic hydrolysis process can be achieved by utilising papain at a relatively elevated reaction temperature of 70 °C. Consequently, 107 distinct peptide sequences were obtained and identified using LC-MS.

By employing optimised enzymatic hydrolysis conditions, the majority of the identified peptide sequences represented novel peptides that have not been previously described or recorded in databases. In silico analyses correlated these sequences with a broad spectrum of predicted biological activity. Furthermore, in vitro assays confirmed the antioxidant activity of the whey hydrolysates and their selective antimicrobial properties.

The research presented in this work provides extensive data on novel peptides derived from whey proteins and their potential biological activities. These findings suggest that the hydrolysates obtained could be utilised in the development of functional foods and beverages, dietary supplements, or nutraceuticals. This research establishes a foundation for further investigations to validate the predicted activities observed in in silico and in vitro experiments. Additionally, there is a need to assess their bioavailability and properties in vivo to achieve a comprehensive understanding of their health effects. Future studies should also explore the feasibility of leveraging these peptides for pharmaceutical applications, as well as in functional foods, dietary supplements, and nutraceuticals, where their bioactive properties could offer significant health benefits.

Supplementary Materials: The following supporting information can be downloaded at: https://www.mdpi.com/article/10.3390/molecules30071451/s1, Table S1: The identified peptide sequences derived via papain-catalysed hydrolysis of whey proteins, information on proteins from which they are derived and predicted biological activities of the peptides.

Author Contributions: Conceptualisation, M.C., J.W. and A.W.; methodology, M.C. and T.C.; software, K.G., K.R. and T.C.; validation, M.C., J.W., K.G. and A.W.; investigation, M.C. and K.R.; writing—original draft preparation, M.C.; writing—review and editing, M.C., J.W. and A.W.; visualisation, K.G. and K.R.; supervision, A.W. All authors have read and agreed to the published version of the manuscript.

Funding: This research was funded within the framework of the Polish Ministry of Science and Higher Education Program Implementation PhD (DWD/487/2020).

Institutional Review Board Statement: Not applicable.

Informed Consent Statement: Not applicable.

Data Availability Statement: Data are contained within the article and Supplementary Materials.

Conflicts of Interest: Michał Czelej and Katarzyna Garbacz are employed by the company Biolive Innovation Sp., simultaneously conducting implementation PhDs, therefore the research included in this publication is co-financed by the Polish Ministry of Science and Higher Education. The remaining authors declare that the research was conducted in the absence of any commercial or financial relationships that could be construed as a potential conflict of interest.

References

1. Yu, Y.-J.; Amorim, M.; Marques, C.; Calhau, C.; Pintado, M. Effects of whey peptide extract on the growth of probiotics and gut microbiota. *J. Funct. Foods* **2016**, *21*, 507–516. [CrossRef]
2. Brandelli, A.; Daroit, D.J.; Corrêa, A.P.F. Whey as a source of peptides with remarkable biological activities. *Food Res. Int.* **2015**, *73*, 149–161. [CrossRef]
3. Zhao, C.; Ashaolu, T.J. Bioactivity and safety of whey peptides. *LWT—Food Sci. Technol.* **2020**, *134*, 109935. [CrossRef]
4. Madureira, A.R.; Pereira, C.I.; Gomes, A.M.P.; Pintado, M.E.; Xavier Malcata, F. Bovine whey proteins—Overview on their main biological properties. *Food Res. Int.* **2007**, *40*, 1197–1211. [CrossRef]

5. Madadlou, A.; Abbaspourrad, A. Bioactive whey peptide particles: An emerging class of nutraceutical carriers. *Crit. Rev. Food Sci. Nutr.* **2018**, *58*, 1468–1477. [CrossRef]
6. Olvera-Rosales, L.B.; Cruz-Guerrero, A.E.; García-Garibay, J.M.; Gómez-Ruíz, L.C.; Contreras-López, E.; Guzmán-Rodríguez, F.; González-Olivares, L.G. Bioactive peptides of whey: Obtaining, activity, mechanism of action, and further applications. *Crit. Rev. Food Sci. Nutr.* **2023**, *63*, 10351–10381. [CrossRef]
7. Sila, A.; Bougatef, A. Antioxidant peptides from marine by-products: Isolation, identification and application in food systems. A review. *J. Funct. Foods* **2016**, *21*, 10–26. [CrossRef]
8. Li, J.; Hartinger, C.; Zhu, F. Physicochemical properties of infant formula model emulsions stabilised by different whey protein hydrolysates and characteristics of interfacial peptides. *Food Hydrocoll.* **2023**, *145*, 109035. [CrossRef]
9. Saadi, S.; Saari, N.; Anwar, F.; Hamid, A.A.; Ghazali, H.M. Recent advances in food biopeptides: Production, biological functionalities and therapeutic applications. *Biotechnol. Adv.* **2015**, *33*, 80–116. [CrossRef]
10. López, E.C.; Eberhardt, A.; Marino, F.; Mammarella, E.J.; Sihufe, G.A.; Manzo, R.M. Physicochemical characterisation of ACE-inhibitory and antioxidant peptides from Alcalase® whey protein hydrolysates using fractionation strategies. *Int. J. Dairy Technol.* **2022**, *75*, 538–552. [CrossRef]
11. Halavach, T.M.; Kurchenko, V.P.; Tarun, E.I.; Yantsevich, A.V.; Shchur, V.V.; Tsygankow, V.G.; Lodygin, A.D.; Evdokimov, I.A.; Poklar Ulrih, N. Effect of hydrolysis degree with Alcalase on antioxidant and antigenic properties of whey and colostrum protein hydrolysates. *J. Agric. Food Res.* **2024**, *15*, 100975. [CrossRef]
12. Gammoh, S.; Alu'datt, M.H.; Alhamad, M.N.; Alrosan, M.; Al-husein, B.; AL-U'datt, D.G.; Al-kandari, S.; Rababah, T.; Ammari, Z.; Albiss, B.A.; et al. Enzymatic bioactive peptides from sonicated whey proteins of camel milk: Impacts of nanopeptides on structural properties, antioxidant activity and inhibitory activity of alpha-amylase and ACE. *Int. J. Dairy Technol.* **2022**, *75*, 791–802. [CrossRef]
13. Peslerbes, M.; Fellenberg, A.; Jardin, J.; Deglaire, A.; Ibáñez, R.A. Manufacture of whey protein hydrolysates using plant enzymes: Effect of processing conditions and simulated gastrointestinal digestion on angiotensin-I-converting enzyme (ACE) inhibitory activity. *Foods* **2022**, *11*, 2429. [CrossRef] [PubMed]
14. Kankanamge, R.; Jeewanthi, C.; Paik, H.-D.; Kim, M.-H.; Lee, N.-K.; Kim, S.-Y.; Yoon, Y.C. Characteristics of whey protein hydrolysates from cheese whey, favors on various food application. *Chem. Ind. Chem. Eng. Q.* **2014**, *20*, 503–509. [CrossRef]
15. Kankanamge, R.; Jeewanthi, C.; Kim, M.-H.; Lee, N.-K.; Yoon, Y.C.; Paik, H.-D. Peptide analysis and the bioactivity of whey protein hydrolysates from cheese whey with several enzymes. *Korean J. Food Sci. Anim. Resour.* **2017**, *37*, 62–70. [CrossRef]
16. Halavach, T.M.; Kurchenko, V.P.; Zhygankov, V.G.; Evdokimov, I.A. Determination of physicochemical, immunochemical and antioxidant properties, toxicological and hygienic assessment of whey protein concentrate and its hydrolysate. *Foods Raw Mater.* **2015**, *3*, 105–114. [CrossRef]
17. Jia, C.L.; Hussain, N.; Joy Ujiroghene, O.; Pang, X.Y.; Zhang, S.W.; Lu, J.; Liu, L.; Lv, J.P. Generation and characterization of dipeptidyl peptidase-IV inhibitory peptides from trypsin-hydrolyzed α-lactalbumin-rich whey proteins. *Food Chem.* **2020**, *318*, 126333. [CrossRef]
18. Chatterjee, A.; Kanawjia, S.K.; Khetra, Y.; Saini, P. Discordance between in silico & in vitro analyses of ACE inhibitory & antioxidative peptides from mixed milk tryptic whey protein hydrolysate. *J. Food Sci. Technol.* **2015**, *52*, 5621–5630. [CrossRef]
19. Wang, R.; He, S.; Xuan, Y.; Cheng, C. Preparation and characterization of whey protein hydrolisates-Zn complexes. *J. Food Meas. Charact.* **2020**, *14*, 254–261. [CrossRef]
20. Giromini, C.; Lovegrove, J.A.; Givens, D.I.; Rebucci, R.; Pinotti, L.; Maffioli, E.; Tedeschi, G.; Sundaram, T.S.; Baldi, A. In vitro-digested milk proteins: Evaluation of angiotensin-1-converting enzyme inhibitory and antioxidant activities, peptidomic profile, and mucin gene expression in HT29-mtx cells. *J. Dairy Sci.* **2019**, *102*, 10760–10771. [CrossRef]
21. Ballatore, M.B.; del Rosario Bettiol, M.; Braber, N.L.V.; Aminahuel, C.A.; Rossi, Y.E.; Petroselli, G.; Erra-Balsells, R.; Cavaglieri, L.R.; Montenegro, M.A. Antioxidant and cytoprotective effect of peptides produced by hydrolysis of whey protein concentrate with trypsin. *Food Chem.* **2020**, *319*, 126472. [CrossRef] [PubMed]
22. Estévez, N.; Fuciños, P.; Fuciños, C.; Jauregi, P.; Tovar, C.A.; Rúa, M.L. Hydrolysis of whey protein as a useful approach to obtain bioactive peptides and a β-lg fraction with different biotechnological applications. *Food Hydrocoll.* **2020**, *109*, 106095. [CrossRef]
23. Jeewanthi, R.K.C.; Lee, N.-K.; Paik, H.-D. Improved functional characteristics of whey protein hydrolysates in food industry. *Korean J. Food Sci. Anim. Resour.* **2015**, *35*, 350–359. [CrossRef] [PubMed]
24. West, C.; Gallagher, D. Whey protein—A source of digestible nutrients but palatability issues remain. *Food Sci. Technol.* **2007**, *21*, 28–30. [CrossRef]
25. Melnikova, E.I.; Bogdanova, E.V.; Koshevarova, I.B. Nutritional evaluation of whey protein hydrolysate: Chemical composition, peptide profile, and osmolarity. *Food Sci. Technol.* **2022**, *42*, e110721. [CrossRef]
26. Zapata Bustamante, S.; Gil González, J.; Sforza, S.; Tedeschi, T. Bioactivity and peptide profile of whey protein hydrolysates obtained from Colombian double-cream cheese production and their products after gastrointestinal digestion. *Food Sci. Technol.* **2021**, *145*, 111334. [CrossRef]

27. Kaur, S.; Vasiljevic, T.; Huppertz, T. Milk Protein Hydrolysis by Actinidin—Kinetic and Thermodynamic Characterisation and Comparison to Bromelain and Papain. *Foods* **2023**, *12*, 4248. [CrossRef]
28. Kordala, N.; Bednarska, M.; Adamczak, M. Health-promoting properties of bioactive peptides (BAP) in dairy products—Biotechnological and medical aspects. *Med. Og. Nauk. Zdr.* **2021**, *27*, 107–116.[CrossRef]
29. Du, X.; Jing, H.; Wang, L.; Huang, X.; Wang, X.; Wang, H. Characterization of structure, physicochemical properties, and hypoglycemic activity of goat milk whey protein hydrolysate processed with different proteases. *LWT—Food Sci. Technol.* **2022**, *159*, 113257. [CrossRef]
30. Kumar, D.; Chatli, M.K.; Singh, S.; Mehta, N.; Kumar, P. Antioxidant and antimicrobial activity of camel milk casein hydrolysates and its fractions. *Small Rumin. Res.* **2016**, *139*, 20–25. [CrossRef]
31. Wu, H.C.; Chen, H.M.; Shiau, C.Y. Free amino acids and peptides as related to antioxidant properties in protein hydrolysates of mackerel (*Scomber austriasicus*). *Food Res. Int.* **2003**, *36*, 949–957. [CrossRef]
32. Matsui, R.; Honda, R.; Kanome, M.; Hagiwara, A.; Matsuda, Y.; Togitani, T.; Ikemoto, N.; Terashima, M. Designing antioxidant peptides based on the antioxidant properties of the amino acid side-chains. *Food Chem.* **2018**, *245*, 750–755. [CrossRef] [PubMed]
33. Ohashi, Y.; Onuma, R.; Naganuma, T.; Ogawa, T.; Naude, R.; Nokihara, K.; Muramoto, K. Antioxidant properties of tripeptides revealed by a comparison of six different assays. *Food Sci. Technol. Res.* **2015**, *21*, 695–704. [CrossRef]
34. Martysiak-Żurowska, D.; Wenta, W. A comparison of ABTS and DPPH methods for assessing the total antioxidant capacity of human milk. Acta scientiarum polonorum. *Acta Sci. Pol. Technol. Aliment.* **2012**, *11*, 83–89.
35. Chen, J.; Lindmark-Månsson, H.; Gorton, L.; Åkesson, B. Antioxidant capacity of bovine milk as assayed by spectrophotometric and amperometric methods. *Int. Dairy. J.* **2003**, *13*, 927–935. [CrossRef]
36. Thwaite, J.E.; Hibbs, S.; Titball, R.W.; Atkins, T.P. Proteolytic Degradation of Human Antimicrobial Peptide LL-37 by Bacillus anthracis May Contribute to Virulence. *Antimicrob. Agents* **2006**, *50*, 2316–2322. [CrossRef]
37. Abdel-Hamid, M.; Goda, H.A.; De Gobba, C.; Jenssen, H.; Osman, A. Antibacterial activity of papain hydrolyzed camel whey and its fractions. *Int. Dairy J.* **2016**, *61*, 91–98. [CrossRef]
38. Salami, M.; Moosavi-Movahedi, A.A.; Ehsani, M.R.; Yousefi, R.; Haertlé, T.; Chobert, J.M.; Razavi, S.H.; Henrich, R.; Balalaie, S.; Ebadi, S.A.; et al. Improvement of the antimicrobial and antioxidant activities of camel and bovine whey proteins by limited proteolysis. *J. Agric. Food Chem.* **2010**, *58*, 3297–3302. [CrossRef]
39. Meignanalakshmi, S.; Vinoth Kumar, S. Antibacterial activity of papain hydrolysates of buffalo milk whey milk whey protein against mastitis pathogens. *Int. J. Pharma Bio Sci.* **2013**, *4*, 1133–1138.
40. Pellegrini, A.; Dettling, C.; Thomas, U.; Hunziker, P. Isolation and characterization of four bactericidal domains in the bovine β-lactoglobulin. *BBA—Gen. Subj.* **2001**, *1526*, 131–140. [CrossRef]
41. Fu, T.; Zhang, S.; Sheng, Y.; Feng, Y.; Jiang, Y.; Zhang, Y.; Yu, M.; Wang, C. Isolation and characterization of zinc-binding peptides from mung bean protein hydrolysates. *Eur. Food Res. Technol.* **2020**, *246*, 113–124. [CrossRef]
42. Udechukwu, M.C.; Dang, C.; Udenigwe, C.C. Identification of zinc-binding peptides in ADAM17-inhibiting whey protein hydrolysates using IMAC-Zn^{2+} coupled with shotgun peptidomics. *Food Prod. Process Nutr.* **2021**, *3*, 5. [CrossRef]
43. Maugard, T.; Bordenave-Juchereau, S.; Piot, J.M.; Ben-Henda, Y.; Sirvent, P.; Peltier, S. Compositions for Preventing and/or Treating Pathological Conditions Associated with Alpha-Glucosidase. US 2018/0104303 A1, 19 April 2018.
44. Peltier, S.; Sirvent, P.; Maugard, T. Compositions and Methods for Treating Diabetes, Fatty Liver, Cardiopathies, Insulin Resistance, Carbohydrate and Fat Me-tabolism. US 9962420B2, 8 May 2018.
45. Hsieh, C.-H.; Wang, T.-Y.; Hung, C.-C.; Hsieh, Y.-L.; Hsu, K.-C. Isolation of prolyl endopeptidase inhibitory peptides from a sodium caseinate hydrolysate. *Food Funct.* **2016**, *7*, 565–573. [CrossRef] [PubMed]
46. Meisel, H.; Frister, H. Chemical characterization of bioactive peptides from in vivo digests of casein. *J. Dairy Res.* **1989**, *56*, 343–349. [CrossRef]
47. de Vasconcelos, M.L.; Oliveira, L.M.F.S.; Hill, J.P.; Vidal, A.M.C. Difficulties in Establishing the Adverse Effects of β-Casomorphin-7 Released from β-Casein Variants—A Review. *Foods* **2023**, *12*, 3151. [CrossRef]
48. Chamata, Y.; Watson, K.A.; Jauregi, P. Whey-Derived Peptides Interactions with ACE by Molecular Docking as a Potential Predictive Tool of Natural ACE Inhibitors. *Int. J. Mol. Sci.* **2020**, *21*, 864. [CrossRef]
49. FitzGerald, R.J.; Cermeño, M.; Khalesi, M.; Kleekayai, T.; Amigo-Benavent, M. Application of in silico approaches for the generation of milk protein-derived bioactive peptides. *J. Funct. Foods* **2020**, *64*, 103636. [CrossRef]
50. Bansal, A.B.; Cassagnol, M. HMG-CoA Reductase Inhibitors. In *StatPearls*; StatPearls Publishing: Treasure Island, FL, USA, 2024. Available online: https://www.ncbi.nlm.nih.gov/books/NBK542212/ (accessed on 25 January 2024).
51. Pak, V.V.; Koo, M.; Kwon, D.Y.; Yun, L. Design of a highly potent inhibitory peptide acting as a competitive inhibitor of HMG-CoA reductase. *Amino Acids* **2012**, *43*, 2015–2025. [CrossRef]
52. Maestri, E.; Pavlicevic, M.; Montorsi, M.; Marmiroli, N. Meta-Analysis for Correlating Structure of Bioactive Peptides in Foods of Animal Origin with Regard to Effect and Stability. *Compr. Rev. Food Sci. Food Saf.* **2019**, *18*, 3–30. [CrossRef]

53. Czelej, M.; Czernecki, T.; Garbacz, K.; Wawrzykowski, J.; Jamioł, M.; Michalak, K.; Walczak, N.; Wilk, A.; Waśko, A. Egg Yolk as a New Source of Peptides with Antioxidant and Antimicrobial Properties. *Foods* **2023**, *12*, 3394. [CrossRef]
54. Minkiewicz, P.; Iwaniak, A.; Darewicz, M. BIOPEP-UWM Database of Bioactive Peptides: Current Opportunities. *Int. J. Mol. Sci.* **2019**, *20*, 5978. [CrossRef]

molecules

Article

Effect of Frying Temperature on Lipid Binding, Fatty Acid Composition, and Nutritional Quality of Fish Crackers Prepared from Carp (*Ciprinus carpio* L.) and Tapioca Starch (*Manihot esculentus*)

Grzegorz Tokarczyk [1], Grzegorz Bienkiewicz [2], Patrycja Biernacka [1,*], Sylwia Przybylska [1], Wojciech Sawicki [3] and Małgorzata Tabaszewska [4,5]

1 Department of Fish, Plant and Gastronomy Technology, West Pomeranian University of Technology in Szczecin, Papieża Pawła VI 3, 71-459 Szczecin, Poland; grzegorz.tokarczyk@zut.edu.pl (G.T.); sylwia.przybylska@zut.edu.pl (S.P.)

2 Department of Commodity Science, Quality Assessment, Process Engineering and Human Nutrition, West Pomeranian University of Technology in Szczecin, Papieża Pawła VI 3, 71-459 Szczecin, Poland; grzegorz.bienkiewicz@zut.edu.pl

3 Department of Applied Microbiology and Physiology of Human Nutrition, West Pomeranian University of Technology in Szczecin, Papieża Pawła VI 3, 71-459 Szczecin, Poland; wojciech.sawicki@zut.edu.pl

4 Department of Plant Products Technology and Nutrition Hygiene, University of Agriculture in Krakow, Balicka 122, 30-149 Krakow, Poland; malgorzata.tabaszewska@urk.edu.pl

5 Department of Human Nutrition and Metabolomics, Pomeranian Medical University in Szczecin, Broniewskiego Street 24, 71-460 Szczecin, Poland

* Correspondence: patrycja.biernacka@zut.edu.pl

Abstract: Background: The growing consumption of snack foods such as chips driving demand for healthier, more nutritious alternatives. This study investigated the effect of frying temperature on oil absorption, oil binding capacity, and fatty acid composition of fish-based snacks made from a 1:1 ratio of tapioca starch and carp meat obtained after the separation of the remains of its industrial filleting. **Methods:** The snacks were deep-fried at 160 °C, 170 °C, and 180 °C, and analyzed for expansion, oil absorption, oil binding capacity, fatty acid profiles, and nutritional indices. Oxidation levels and free fatty acids were also measured, ensuring compliance with legal limits. **Results:** Deep-frying at 180 °C resulted in significantly higher snack expansion (95.20%) than the 50% expansion observed at 160 °C and 170 °C. However, snacks deep-fried at 180 °C absorbed the most oil (29.07%) and exhibited the lowest oil binding capacity (8.84%), whereas deep-frying at 160 °C and 170 °C led to oil binding capacities of 15.83% and 18.58%, respectively. Fatty acid profiles also showed temperature-dependent changes, with increased oil absorption reducing omega-3 to omega-6 ratios. Importantly, deep-frying for 45 s at all temperatures did not lead to excessive oxidation or free fatty acid levels beyond regulatory thresholds. Nutritional indices of the deep-fried product were comparable to those of vegetable oils, while before deep-frying, they resembled those of seafood products like shellfish and seaweed. **Conclusions:** While higher frying temperatures improve the texture and expansion of fish-based snacks, they also increase oil absorption and reduce oil binding. Based on these findings, deep-frying at 180 °C was suggested as the optimal condition to balance product texture, oil absorption, and nutritional quality, making the snacks a healthier alternative to conventional deep-fried products.

Keywords: fish crackers; *Ciprinus carpio*; tapioca starch; fatty acid; nutritional quality

1. Introduction

In the food industry, snacks like potato chips, breadsticks, crisps, and crackers are omnipresent, and their popularity continues to grow. In 2023, the retail value of the European savory snacks market amounted to around €40 billion, representing nearly 3.5% of the European food and beverages market. The consumption of savory snacks across Europe varies from country to country but on average around 4 kg were purchased per year per capita [1]. One notable traditional fish-based snack is crackers, which are known by various names across Asia—for example, they are referred to as wafers or crackers in India and "Keropok" in Malaysia [2].

While popular among all age groups, starch-based snacks typically lack high-quality protein and essential minerals. Incorporating fish in appropriate quantities, characterized by high-quality protein and a favorable amino acid profile, significantly enhances the nutritional value of these snacks. The carp (*Cyprinus carpio* L.) is an economically important farmed fish in central Europe and is a good species for this purpose [3]. Carp, in particular, is a valuable source of protein (approximately 16–18 g per 100 g of raw fillet) [4] and essential fatty acids, including omega-3 (EPA and DHA) and omega-6, which play a crucial role in cardiovascular health [5]. Additionally, it provides important micronutrients such as phosphorus, selenium, and vitamins A and D. However, the anatomical structure of carp, which includes a high number of small bones, makes it challenging to process and less favored in traditional fillet-based products [6]. The study was conducted using carp meat obtained after the separation of the remains of industrial filleting. This approach enhances resource efficiency, reduces waste, and retains high-quality protein, essential fatty acids (omega-3 and omega-6), and key micronutrients, making it a sustainable and nutritionally valuable ingredient for fish-based snacks [7]. It was known that the type of flour or starch used to make crackers influences their quality. Various types of starch/flour have been studied [8] for the production of crackers, such as tapioca, rice, or sago starches. From these studies, there was a consensus that sago and tapioca provided better cracker expansion than other starches. Tapioca is considered a base food for humans in many countries and is the main ingredient, alongside comminuted fish flesh, used to make fish crackers [6,9].

Another important problem is the high content of fat, which is largely absorbed in the expansion process during deep-frying, increasing the calorific value of the product [10]. The fat content of deep-fried snacks is usually high, up to 50% [11]. During deep-frying, oil at high temperatures (160–190 °C) undergoes various physical and chemical transformations, such as hydrogenation, oxidation, and polymerization. These changes influence the nutritional value and safety of the deep-fried products [12,13].

In the case of products such as keropok (fish crackers), oil plays a crucial role during deep-frying, not only by aiding in expansion and enhancing texture and sensory qualities but also by interacting with starch. These interactions result in the formation of starch–lipid and starch–lipid–protein complexes, which influence the structural and nutritional properties of the product. Studies indicate that these complexes, particularly those formed with exogenous lipids introduced during deep-frying, can alter starch's molecular structure into a more compact V-type arrangement, limiting enzymatic digestion and bioavailability [14]. Zhang and Hamaker [15] elucidated the role of starch–lipid complex formation (in binary systems), and starch–lipid–protein complex formation (in ternary systems), suggesting changes related to structural integrity and reduced digestibility. Oil absorption during deep-frying is different from interactions in gelatinization processes. Deep-frying is a high-temperature process in which the oil penetrates inside the product, removing water from it [16]. Oil absorption is affected by initial water content, product shape, surface porosity, frying method, and temperature [17,18]. Deep-frying remains an efficient, convenient, and economical processing method that produces microbiologically safe food with desirable sensory properties, such as color, aroma, and taste [19]. However, high oil absorption during deep-frying has nutritional implications, increasing the total fat content of the product. While the inclusion of fats in the diet is essential for providing energy and supporting physiological functions, the excessive consumption of fats, particularly as part of a high-fat diet—where dietary fat provides more than 35% of daily caloric intake—has been linked to the development of chronic diseases such as obesity, cardiovascular disease, and certain types of cancer [20,21]. It is important to note that these effects are associated with overall dietary patterns rather than the consumption of individual foods in isolation. Therefore, strategies to control oil absorption during deep-frying could help to improve the nutritional profile of deep-fried products without compromising their sensory quality.

The objective of this study was to investigate the effect of frying temperature on the binding of lipids and the fatty acid profile of fish snacks made from carp (*Cyprinus carpio* L.) and tapioca starch (*Manihot esculenta*). Specifically, this research focused on exploring the mechanisms of oil absorption and changes in the fatty acid profile, including the preservation of essential fatty acids such as omega-3 and omega-6. It also aimed to assess the impact of lipid transformations occurring during deep-frying on the oxidative stability of the product, a factor directly related to food safety. Furthermore, this study sought to provide insights into minimizing undesirable fat content while maintaining the nutritional integrity and sensory qualities of the product. The research developed and evaluated a novel fish-based snack utilizing carp and tapioca starch, addressing consumer demand for healthier snack options while preserving desirable sensory and nutritional properties.

2. Results and Discussion

2.1. Physical and Chemical Quality Assessment

To assess the quality of crackers (Figure 1) prepared from tapioca starch and carp meat obtained after the separation of the remains of its industrial filleting in a 1:1 ratio, the basic physical parameters of deep-fried fish snacks were analyzed in triplicate.

Two key parameters—linear expansion and bulk density (Table 1)—are evaluated, which are directly related to the organoleptic qualities of the snacks, such as their size, texture, and crispiness [9,22]. The results show that deep-frying at higher temperatures, particularly 180 °C, led to a markedly greater linear expansion, nearly doubling the size of the crackers, to lower frying temperatures of 160 °C and 170 °C (54% increase). This expansion is accompanied by a lighter, airier texture. Bulk density is inversely related to frying temperature, with snacks deep-fried at 180 °C exhibiting significantly lower bulk density than those deep-fried at lower temperatures. A reduction in bulk density is typically associated with improved crispiness and mouthfeel, as the product becomes less compact and more porous. This phenomenon can be attributed to the increased evaporation of water at higher temperatures, which accelerates the gelatinization of starch and the formation of a crispy structure, enhancing the textural qualities of the product [23]. The reduction in water content with increasing frying temperature further supports these findings. As the frying temperature increases, the moisture content in the crackers decreases significantly, from 8.58% at lower temperatures to an average of 3.8% at 180 °C. This aligns with previous studies, such as those by Jothi et al. [24], who reported similar trends in vacuum-fried potato chips. The accelerated evaporation of water at higher temperatures is a key factor in achieving the desired texture and expansion in deep-fried products, as it led to the formation of a porous structure with lower moisture content. Additionally, the ash content decreased with the increase in frying temperature, from 2.37 ± 0.07% for crackers deep-fried at 160 °C to 0.91 ± 0.03% for crackers deep-fried at 180 °C. Significant differences in the amount of ash are observed along with increasing the volume and decreasing the bulk density of the snacks [22]. The reduction in ash content observed in the deep-fried crackers is likely due to the migration of mineral components from the meat to the frying oil during the process. This could be explained by the fact that certain minerals, such as calcium and phosphorus (often referred to as lime from bones), may be present in small amounts in the meat used in snack production. Since the meat is recovered from fillet residues, it is possible that minute fragments of bone, which contain these minerals, are present in the product. During deep-frying, the high temperatures could cause these mineral residues to melt and dissolve into the oil [25,26].

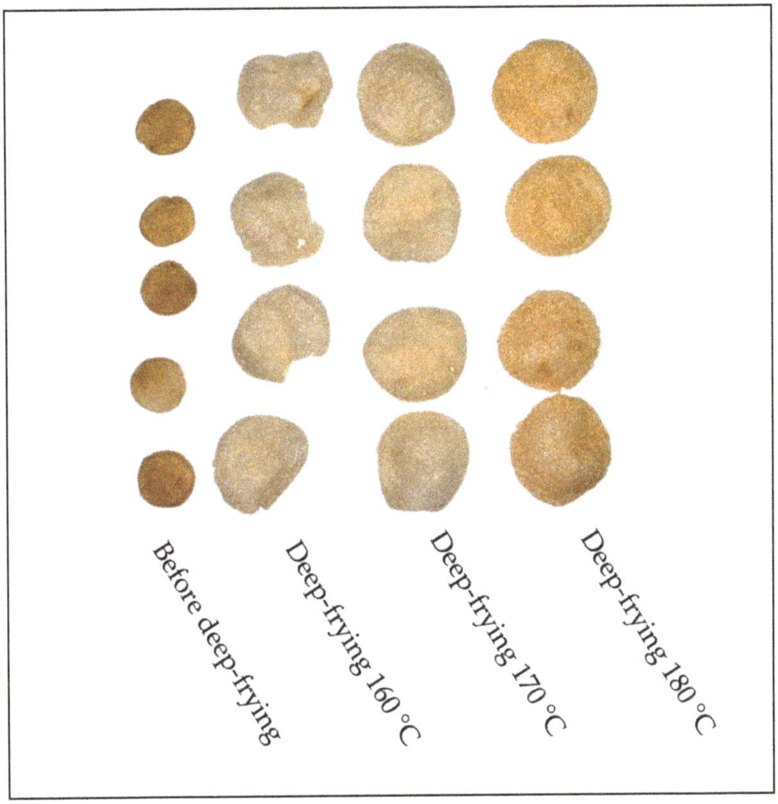

Figure 1. Photographs of crackers prepared from carp and tapioca before and after deep-frying at 160 °C, 170 °C, and 180 °C.

Table 1. Changes in the content of water, ash, and the value of physical parameters during deep-frying fish crackers.

	Frying Temperature [°C]			
Parameters	**160**	**170**	**180**	**Before Deep-Frying**
Water [%]	3.86 ± 0.08 [a]	3.84 ± 0.02 [a]	3.78 ± 0.03 [a]	8.58 ± 0.15
Ash [%]	2.37 ± 0.07 [a]	1.26 ± 0.07 [b]	0.91 ± 0.03 [c]	3.84 ± 0.08
Bulk density [g/cm^3]	0.65 ± 0.12 [a]	0.26 ± 0.24 [a]	0.21 ± 0.18 [b]	1.00 ± 0.04
Linear expansion [%]	54.8 ± 2.5 [a]	52.8 ± 1.6 [a]	95.2 ± 2.1 [b]	

The mean ± SD (standard deviation) within rows with different small letters differs significantly ($p < 0.05$) between frying temperature (n = 3); n—number of samples.

2.2. Influence of Frying Temperature on Lipid Content and Oil Absorption Dynamics

Table 2 summarizes the results of fat content, and the amount of oil absorbed during deep-frying.

Table 2. The influence of frying temperature on changes in the content of fat fractions in the analyzed snacks.

Fat Fraction	Frying Temperature [°C]				
	160	170	180	Before Deep-Frying	Fish
Oil absorption [%] (n = 36)	26.7 ± 2.4 [a]	24.6 ± 2.1 [a]	29.1 ± 1.5 [b]		
Fat content [%] (n = 3)	22.5 ± 0.1 [a]	20.0 ± 1.3 [b]	26.5 ± 1.1 [c]	1.2 ± 0.3	4.5 ± 0.3
Bonded fat [%] (n = 36)	15.8 ± 1.6 [a]	18.6 ± 1.7 [a]	8.8 ± 1.3 [b]		

The mean ± SD (standard deviation) within rows with different small letters differs significantly ($p < 0.05$) between frying temperature; n—number of samples.

The interaction of lipids with starch and protein is observed already at the stage of cracker production. The fat content in the samples before deep-frying is less than 1.5%, while the fat content in the carp meat was 4.5%. With 50% fish addition, the expected fat content in the cracker before deep-frying is approximately 2.3%, indicating that around 44% of the fat is strongly bound in the starch–lipid–protein system, resisting extraction with a solvent mixture. This binding likely resulted from intensive mixing in the presence of water, facilitating lipid interactions. The formation of inclusion complexes between lipids and starch, particularly with fatty acids like lauric acid, is well documented [27–29]. In three-component systems (starch-lipid-protein), interactions become more complex, involving ionic and hydrophobic bonds with proteins [15,28].

Table 2 shows the effect of frying temperature on oil absorption and binding. Oil absorption increased with frying temperature, with statistically significant differences observed between 170 °C and 180 °C. This is closely related to cracker expansion (Table 1). At 160 °C and 170 °C, 15.8% to 18.6% of the oil was strongly bound, but increasing the temperature to 180 °C reduced binding to 8.8%, despite higher oil absorption. This suggests that higher temperatures weaken strong interactions between oil, starch, and protein. The small standard deviations observed in the results reflect the controlled experimental conditions and large sample sizes; however, they may not fully capture the inherent variability of deep-frying processes, which can be influenced by factors such as oil temperature fluctuations, and moisture content. The relationship between oil absorption and fat binding during deep-frying is complex and influenced by several factors, including temperature, microstructure, and time. At higher frying temperatures, such as 180 °C, the rapid evaporation of water from the fish crackers and the increased porosity of the snack's surface result in higher oil absorption. However, this rapid process also leads to a reduction in the degree of fat binding, as the higher temperature results in a faster expulsion of moisture from the snack, leaving less time for the oil to strongly interact with the starch and protein matrix. In contrast, at lower frying temperatures, the oil has more time to bond with the starch and protein structures, leading to a higher degree of fat binding despite lower overall oil absorption [30].

The microstructure of the crackers also plays a crucial role in these interactions. The innovative crackers with filleted carp meat had a more porous surface compared to traditional keropoks, which likely contributed to increased oil uptake. Studies have shown that oil absorption is a microstructural phenomenon, with porosity and interactions with other components playing key roles [31–35]. However, the rapid structural changes occurring at higher temperatures (such as 180 °C) may cause a decrease in the amount of oil that can be tightly bound to the food matrix. This reduced binding capacity at higher temperatures may explain the lower degree of oil retention at 180 °C compared to lower temperatures, despite the higher overall oil uptake. These interactions between temperature, oil absorption, and fat binding underline the importance of controlling deep-frying parameters to optimize both the sensory and nutritional qualities of the product.

2.3. Effect of Frying Temperature on Fatty Acid Content

Similarly to the fat content and oil absorption, the fatty acid composition of fish, oil used for deep-frying, and lipids extracted from fish crackers before and after deep-frying are analyzed at three temperatures. The analysis is performed in triplicate. The total amount of fatty acids in fish is 606.82 mg/g of extracted lipid, while in snacks before deep-frying, it was only 60.76 mg/g, indicating strong interactions between fish lipids and tapioca starch during mixing and gelatinization. After deep-frying, the total amount of extracted fatty acids increases from 779 mg/g at 160 °C to 888 mg/g at 180 °C, reflecting higher oil absorption at elevated temperatures. However, the degree of fatty acid binding decreases with increasing frying temperature (Tables 2 and 3).

Table 3. Effect of frying temperature on fatty acid composition (mg fatty acid on 1 g fat) extracted from fish crackers.

			Frying Temperature [°C]			
Fatty Acid	Fish	Before Deep-Frying	160	170	180	Oil
C10:0	0.21 ± 0.04	-	0.11 ± 0.02 a	0.14 ± 0.05 a	0.09 ± 0.03 a	0.10 ± 0.02
C12:0	0.79 ± 0.03	-	0.14 ± 0.06 a	0.12 ± 0.04 a	0.16 ± 0.03 a	0.07 ± 0.01
C14:0	4.27 ± 0.14	-	0.25 ± 0.05 a	0.34 ± 0.11 a	0.33 ± 0.06 a	0.38 ± 0.01
C16:0	80.05 ± 2.24	14.85 ± 0.94	40.02 ± 2.08 a	42.34 ± 2.18 a	51.73 ± 3.01 b	47.8 ± 0.91
C16:1	12.94 ± 1.07	1.57 ± 0.09	1.58 ± 0.11 a	1.73 ± 0.14 a	2.27 ± 0.04 b	1.56 ± 0.03
C17:0	3.61 ± 0.09	-	0.22 ± 0.03 a	0.26 ± 0.04 a	0.31 ± 0.05 a	0.12 ± 0.01
C18:0	238.74 ± 8.33	5.12 ± 0.14	16.22 ± 0.08 a	17.97 ± 0.84 a	21.25 ± 1.09 b	20.22 ± 0.54
C18:1 ω-9	220.04 ± 7.09	27.63 ± 1.09	492.87 ± 9.09 a	510.8 ± 8.88 a	525.89 ± 9.54 a	576.67 ± 4.84
C18:2 ω-6	13.29 ± 0.32	9.16 ± 1.14	153.44 ± 3.07 a	164.85 ± 2.94 b	189.15 ± 4.08 c	195.13 ± 3.15
C18:3 ω-3	1.52 ± 0.11	1.23 ± 0.07	55.05 ± 3.94 a	60.46 ± 4.08 a	73.85 ± 1.07 b	83.8 ± 1.09
C20:1 ω-9	2.61 ± 0.15	1.39 ± 0.07	8.67 ± 0.64 a	9.72 ± 0.64 a	9.63 ± 0.66 a	10.89 ± 0.55
C20:2 ω-6	3.68 ± 0.21	-	5.26 ± 0.12 a	5.86 ± 0.71 a	7.54 ± 1.08 a	7.35 ± 0.14
C20:4 ω-3	4.98 ± 0.43	1.63 ± 0.05	2.4 ± 0.10 a	2.65 ± 0.15 a	3.64 ± 0.35 b	-
C20:5 ω-3	1.98 ± 0.14	-	0.36 ± 0.02 a	0.45 ± 0.08 b	0.46 ± 0.06 b	-
C22:4 ω-6	1.03 ± 0.06	-	0.28 ± 0.01 a	0.26 ± 0.03 a	0.31 ± 0.04 b	-
C24:1 ω-9	1.72 ± 0.08	-	0.15 ± 0.02 a	0.22 ± 0.11 b	0.37 ± 0.14 c	-
C22:5 ω-3	1.67 ± 0.09	-	0.86 ± 0.03 a	0.63 ± 0.04 b	0.39 ± 0.07 c	-
C22:6 ω-3	13.69 ± 0.94	1.18 ± 0.09	1.26 ± 0.09 a	1.30 ± 0.14 a	1.58 ± 0.24 b	-
SFA	327.67 ± 7.06	19.97 ± 0.12	56.96 ± 0.12 a	61.17 ± 0.14 b	73.87 ± 0.24 c	68.69 ± 0.03
MUFA	237.31 ± 3.19	30.59 ± 1.14	503.27 ± 6.94 a	522.47 ± 6.85 a	538.16 ± 7.08 b	589.12 ± 3.05
PUFA	41.84 ± 0.67	13.2 ± 0.08	218.91 ± 0.09 a	236.46 ± 0.11 b	276.92 ± 0.11 c	286.28 ± 0.64
Total FA	606.82 ± 3.38	63.76 ± 0.67	779.14 ± 4.03 a	820.10 ± 3.19 b	888.95 ± 3.54 c	944.09 ± 1.82

The mean ± SD (standard deviation) within rows with different small letters differs significantly ($p < 0.05$) between frying temperature; (n = 3); n—number of samples.

Assuming the total amount of fatty acids in the oil is 100% compared to the total amount of these acids extracted from deep-fried snacks, it is found that the percentage of binding of the total amount of fatty acids depends on the frying temperature (in Table 3) and is similar to that in the case of total fat (Table 2). Comparing the effect of frying temperature on the amount of individual fatty acid fractions, it is found that the least fatty acids were recovered after deep-frying at 160 °C. Comparing the effect of deep-frying temperature on the amount of individual fatty acid fractions, it is found that the least fatty acids were recovered after deep-frying at 160 °C, i.e., saturated fatty acids (SFA) 83%, monounsaturated fatty acids (MUFA) 85%, and polyunsaturated fatty acids (PUFA) 76%, respectively, compared to the oil itself. However, at a temperature of 180 °C, the content of individual groups of fatty acids is, respectively as follows: SFA, 107.5%; MUFA, 91%; PUFA, 98%. The over 100% increase in the SFA fraction was caused by the release of fatty acids from the fish meat, present in the 50% share in fish snacks. These findings align with studies by Wang et al. [36], who demonstrated that water content influences starch–fatty acid complex formation during deep-frying. For samples with 8% water content (similar to the fish snacks in this study), they reported oil complexation degrees of 14.78% for corn starch and 9.21% for rice starch, consistent with the results presented here. Fatty acids could enter the amylose helix, forming more stable amylose–fatty acid complexes [37,38]. However, most of these types of complexes were formed at the stage of mixing the starch solution with lipid and in the process of its gelatinization. These results underscore the importance of optimizing frying conditions to balance sensory attributes with nutritional quality.

2.4. Effect of Frying Temperature on Lipid Quality

Deep-frying has a significant impact on the quality of the oil and the quality of the product that absorbs the oil during deep-frying. The degradation of oil may affect fat binding and absorption during deep-frying [33]. The described experiment characterized the oxidation level and degree of hydrolysis of fat lipid extracted from fish snacks prepared from filleted carp meat and tapioca starch (Table 4). The analysis is performed in triplicate. Uniquely, the comminuted fish meat–tapioca composition of the snacks presents a distinctive interaction between fish lipids and starch, which may affect how lipids are absorbed and degraded compared to typical starch-based products such as potato chips. This makes fish-based snacks a novel matrix for studying the lipid degradation process during deep-frying.

Table 4. Effect of frying temperature on fat quality extracted from crackers.

	Frying Temperature [°C]				
Parameters	**160**	**170**	**180**	**Before Deep-Frying**	**Oil**
PV [meq O_2/kg fat]	5.8 ± 0.3 a	3.7 ± 0.2 b	3.4 ± 0.4 b	8.6 ± 1.3	3.1 ± 0.5 b
AsV	1.7 ± 0.1 a	4.2 ± 0.1 b	3.1 ± 0.2 c	4.9 ± 1.4	1.8 ± 0.1 d
TOTOX	13.7 ± 0.6 a	11.8 ± 0.4 b	10.8 ± 1.0 b	22.3 ± 2.3	18.0 ± 1.0 c
AV [mg KOH/g fat]	2.0 ± 0.0 a	2.2 ± 0.3 a	1.9 ± 0.1 a		1.2 ± 0.1 b

PV—peroxide value; AsV—anisidine value; AV—acid value; the mean ± SD (standard deviation) within rows with different small letters differs significantly ($p < 0.05$) between frying temperature; (n = 3); n—number of samples.

The quality of the oil used in this study is maintained at a high level throughout the entire deep-frying process, with a TOTOX index of 18.02 and an acid value of 1.2 mg KOH. These values were notably lower than the permissible limits for oil, as set by the Polish Ministry of Health [39], indicating that the oil remained in a good condition even after repeated use. This suggests that the protein–starch matrix of the fish snacks may protect the oil from excessive degradation, possibly by limiting oxidation. In contrast, oil quality typically deteriorates rapidly in traditional starch-based snacks, often exceeding legal oxidation limits [40]. The result suggests that fish-based snacks may offer a healthier alternative to traditional snacks due to lower degradation of the oil. Increasing the frying temperature above 160 °C reduced the number of primary oxidation products, likely due to their thermal decomposition and complex formation with the starch matrix, consistent with other studies [40,41]. The total oxidation level expressed as TOTOX differed statistically significantly between the oil after deep-frying and the lipid extracted from fish snacks, primarily due to higher levels of secondary oxidation products in the extracted lipids. The acid value (AV) increased during deep-frying, but frying temperature had no significant effect on lipid hydrolysis, likely due to the short frying time. This may indicate that the amylose–protein–lipid complexes in the fish snacks form a hydrolysis-resistant matrix, protecting the oil from breakdown [42,43]. However, a statistically significant difference is observed in the degree of hydrolysis between the oil after deep-frying and the lipids extracted from the product. The lipid extracted from the snacks showed a greater degree of hydrolysis.

2.5. The Influence of Frying Temperature on Nutritional Quality Indices of Lipids

Fatty acids, which are often found in dietary fats, can have either beneficial or detrimental effects on disease prevention and therapy. Nutritional indices for fatty acids are very important parameters when assessing the quality of the lipid fraction of food [44]. Table 5 compares the values of these indices for raw fish and finished products before and after deep-frying. The analysis is performed in triplicate. One of the most important indices characterizing the appropriate balance of fatty acids in the diet is the ω-3 to ω-6 PUFA ratio. Dietary recommendations indicate that the optimal ratio in the entire diet is a ratio of 1 to 4. However, ω-6 acids dominate in the Central European diet [45,46]. Therefore, it is important to enrich the diet with products with the highest ω-3 to ω-6 ratio [47]. Such products include fish and dishes prepared from them. Table 5 shows the changes in the value of this index in the deep-frying process. Its threefold decrease is observed compared to raw fish, which is caused by the very high absorption of oil in the final product. However, there was no influence of deep-frying temperature on changes in the value of this index.

Table 5. Effect of frying temperature on nutritional indices of fish snacks.

			Frying Temperature [°C]			
Indices	**Fish**	**Before Deep-Frying**	**160**	**170**	**180**	**Oil**
ω-3/ω-6	1.32 ± 0.11	0.44 ± 0.03	0.37 ± 0.03 a	0.38 ± 0.042 a	0.40 ± 0.04 a	0.41 ± 0.11
PUFA/SFA	0.13 ± 0.04	0.66 ± 0.02	3.84 ± 0.22 a	3.87 ± 0.24 a	3.75 ± 0.14 a	4.17 ± 0.09
ω-3 PUFA	23.84 ± 0.84	4.04 ± 0.06	59.57 ± 1.24 a	65.04 ± 1.66 b	79.46 ± 1.19 c	83.80 ± 1.15
Σ LC ω-3 PUFA	22.32 ± 0.46	2.81 ± 0.11	4.88 ± 0.44 a	5.03 ± 0.34 a	6.07 ± 0.33 b	0.00 ± 0.00
ω-6 PUFA	18.00 ± 0.94	9.16 ± 0.08	158.98 ± 3.35 a	170.97 ± 3.76 b	197.00 ± 4.12 c	202.48 ± 6.09
DHA/EPA	6.91 ± 0.06	-	3.50 ± 0.02 a	2.89 ± 0.06 a	3.43 ± 0.04 a	-
IA	0.35 ± 0.03	0.34 ± 0.03	0.06 ± 0.02 a	0.06 ± 0.01 a	0.07 ± 0.01 a	0.06 ± 0.01
TI	1.52 ± 0.09	0.57 ± 0.05	0.10 ± 0.02 a	0.10 ± 0.03 a	0.11 ± 0.03 a	0.09 ± 0.01
HPI	2.79 ± 0.03	2.06 ± 0.02	12.45 ± 0.01 b	12.21 ± 0.03 b	10.31 ± 0.03 a	12.21 ± 0.06
HH	3.05 ± 0.01	2.75 ± 0.03	17.54 ± 0.02 a	17.37 ± 0.02 a	15.27 ± 0.04 b	17.76 ± 0.01
FLQ	2.58 ± 0.02	1.85 ± 0.04	0.21 ± 0.04 a	0.21 ± 0.03 a	0.23 ± 0.02 a	-

ω-3—omega 3; ω-6—omega 6; PUFA—polyunsaturated fatty acids; SFA—saturated fatty acids; Σ LC—sum of long-chain fatty acids; DHA—docosahexaenoic acid; EPA—eicosapentaenoic acid; IA—index of atherogenicity; TI—index of thrombogenicity; HPI—health-promoting index; HH—hypocholesterolemic/hypercholesterolemic ratio; FLQ—quality of fish lipids; the mean ± SD (standard deviation) within rows with different small letters differs significantly ($p < 0.05$) between frying temperature; (n = 3); n—number of samples.

Another parameter supplementing this indicator is the amount of long-chain n-3 fatty acids (LC ω-3 PUFA). The DHA/EPA ratio is an important index for evaluating the nutritional quality of fish and fish-based products, as both docosahexaenoic acid (DHA) and eicosapentaenoic acid (EPA) were long-chain omega-3 fatty acids with significant health benefits, particularly in reducing inflammation and supporting cardiovascular health [48]. The ratio of DHA to EPA in the raw fish used in this study is 6.91, indicating a relatively balanced presence of these two essential fatty acids in the comminuted meat carp. Compared to other publications, this is a relatively high result [49,50]. If the differences in the

DHA/EPA ratio across the frying temperatures are statistically insignificant, it suggests that frying temperature (within the tested range of 160 °C to 180 °C) does not have a meaningful impact on the relative preservation of DHA and EPA in fish snacks. Further indices characterizing the nutritional value of fat are the index of atherogenicity (IA), which characterizes the atherogenic potential of FAs (fatty acids), and the index of thrombogenicity (IT), which characterizes the thrombogenic potential of FAs, indicating the tendency to form clots in blood vessels. It is shown that the product before deep-frying has parameters similar to those of shellfish [51] or some seaweed [52]. However, the deep-frying process and high oil absorption significantly worsen these indicators. It particularly reduces IT, which takes values typical of rapeseed oils [53]. Both the hypocholesterolemic/hypercholesterolemic (HH) ratio and the health-promoting index (HPI) show significant increases after deep-frying compared to the raw comminuted fish meat. The HH ratio increases from 3.05 to 17.54 (160 °C), 17.37 (170 °C), and 15.27 (180 °C) after deep-frying, while the HPI increases from 2.79 to 12.45 (160 °C), 12.21 (170 °C), and 10.31 (180 °C). These changes are largely due to the absorption of oil, which is rich in monounsaturated fatty acids (MUFA), contributing to the higher values of these nutritional indices. While these data may suggest an improvement in lipid quality, particularly in cholesterol metabolism, this does not necessarily mean that the deep-fried product is healthier than the raw fish. The increase in MUFA, while generally considered beneficial for cardiovascular health [54], replaces some of the more nutritionally critical omega-3 polyunsaturated fatty acids found in fish, such as EPA and DHA. These omega-3 PUFAs are known for their potent anti-inflammatory and cardioprotective effects, and their relative reduction in the deep-fried product means a loss of the specific health benefits associated with consuming fish [55]. Therefore, although the HH and HPI indices are improved, this does not fully capture the degradation in the quality of PUFA, which is essential for the health benefits that fish naturally provide. Furthermore, the process of deep-frying increases the total fat content of the product, resulting in a higher calorific density. Increased oil absorption contributes to the increase in calorific intake, which could have negative metabolic consequences if consumed regularly. Therefore, despite the seemingly improved fatty acid profile suggested by the HH and HPI values, the overall nutritional balance of the deep-fried snack may be less optimal compared to the raw fish. In the case of FLQ, this index is used to evaluate the quality of lipids in terms of their content of long-chain polyunsaturated fatty acids (LC-PUFA), particularly the proportion of omega-3 fatty acids like DHA and EPA in total fat content. For comminuted fish meat, the FLQ is 2.58, indicating the naturally high omega-3 content. After deep-frying, the FLQ decreases. This decrease indicates a significant loss of omega-3 fatty acids due to the deep-frying process. The absorption of oil with no omega-3 reduces the content of these valuable fatty acids in the final product. Studies on deep-fried fish products have similarly shown a loss of omega-3s due to the replacement of fish oil with frying oil, especially when using high temperatures or extended frying times [56].

2.6. Effect of Frying Temperature on Sensory Assessment

The results of the sensory evaluation, which is conducted using a 5-point rating scale, show a distinct trend of improved overall sensory quality as the deep-frying temperature rises (Table 6). The sensory analysis is performed by a research panel composed of 10 qualified persons. For instance, snacks deep-fried at 180 °C received the highest scores for color (4.9), taste (4.8), and texture (4.9), reflecting a preference for the crispness and golden-brown color typically associated with higher frying temperatures.

Table 6. Effect of frying temperature on sensory evaluation of fish snacks.

	Frying Temperature [°C]		
	160	170	180
Color [1–5 pkt]	4.7 ± 0.1 a	4.7 ± 0.0 a	4.9 ± 0.0 b
Taste [1–5 pkt]	4.2 ± 0.1 a	4.6 ± 0.1 b	4.9 ± 0.1 c
Aroma [1–5 pkt]	3.9 ± 0.0 a	4.9 ± 0.1 c	4.6 ± 0.1 b
Texture [1–5 pkt]	3.8 ± 0.1 a	4.0 ± 0.1 b	4.9 ± 0.0 c

The mean ± SD (standard deviation) within rows with different small letters differs significantly ($p < 0.05$) between frying temperature (n = 10); n—number of samples.

However, the aroma score is significantly lower at 180 °C (4.6 ± 0.1) compared to 170 °C (4.9 ± 0.1), suggesting that higher temperatures might lead to slight aroma degradation, potentially due to excessive oil oxidation or volatile compound loss. This trend aligns with the findings reported in the literature. For example, Durmaz and Yuksel (2021) demonstrated that higher deep-frying temperatures enhanced the color and texture of wheat-based chips due to increased Maillard reaction activity and structural crispness [2]. The moderate decline in aroma at 180 °C, despite improvements in other attributes, might be attributed to the thermal degradation of volatile flavor compounds, as noted in studies on sweet potato crisps and fish frying processes [57].

3. Materials and Methods

3.1. Materials

Tapioca starch (*Manihot esculentus*) was purchased from Eiamheng Modified Starch Co, Ltd. (EH brand, Thailand). Manageable remains of industrial filleting of farmed carp (*Cyprinus carpio*), such as backbones, collarbones, or parts of fins, were obtained fresh from the fish processing plant in Poland and transported in ice to the laboratory. Fine food salt was purchased from Mariager Salt Specialties A/S (Mariager, Denmark) and sugar was purchased from Krajowa Spółka Cukrowa S.A. (Toruń, Poland).

3.2. Sample Preparation

The fish remains were washed with chilled potable tap water and then were passed through the drum separator type NF 13DX having a diameter of holes of 4 mm (Bibun, Japan), and cleaned thoroughly in screw separator type SUM 420 having a diameter of holes of 2.5 mm (Bibun, Japan). That was how clean comminuted fish meat was received. The comminuted fish meat was mixed with starch in a ratio of 1:1, 2% salt, 1% sugar, and 30% water (% by weight based on the total weight of starch and wet fish meat). The ingredients were mixed mechanically (approx. 30 s) using a cutter mixer (Empero, Türkiye) until a smooth paste was obtained. The semi-solid paste was then stuffed into cellulose sausage casings (diameter of 4 cm and 30 cm length) using an electric sausage stuffer 282,083 (Hendi, Poland). The stuffed casings were steamed for 90 min using a convection steam oven iCombi PRO 101E (Rational, Germany). After steaming the steamed pastes were cooled in cold water to minimize shrinkage and chilled for 24 h in a refrigerator at 5 ± 1 °C. The gelatinized semi-product was cut manually into slices about 2 mm thick and dried in Profi Line food dehydrator (Hendi, Poland) at 50 °C for 12 h until moisture content was around 10 ± 2%. The dry slice of fish snack was deep-fried in rapeseed oil (Kruszwica, Poland) at 160 °C, 170 °C, and 180 °C for 10 s using electric fryer Kitchen Line 205,839 (Hendi, Poland). The deep-fried crackers were evaluated for different quality analyses. For each analysis, 3 replicates of 12 chips were prepared for each frying temperature analyzed. Physical determinations included measurements obtained from 36 chips (n = 36).

For chemical determinations, 3 parallel replicates were performed from 36 crushed chips (n = 3).

3.3. *Proximate Analysis*

The water content was determined by drying the sample in an oven at 105 °C until a constant weight was achieved. The crude protein content was determined using the Kjeldahl method, and a conversion factor of 6.25 was applied to convert total nitrogen into crude protein. Ash content was determined by ashing the samples in an oven at 550 °C for 8–12 h [58–60].

3.4. *Determination of Linear Expansion (%)*

Linear expansion was obtained after deep-frying the dried crackers in rapeseed oil at 160 °C, 170 °C, and 180 °C. The dried cracker was ruled with three lines across using a fine oil marker pen. Each line was measured before and after deep-frying. Measurements were performed on twenty samples from each temperature. The percentage linear expansion was calculated according to the method used by Nurul [61], as follows:

$$\text{Linear expansion}[\%] = \frac{\text{Length after puffing} - \text{Length before puffing}}{\text{Length before puffing}} \times 100 \quad (1)$$

3.5. *Determination of Bulk Density (g/cm^3)*

To assess the bulk density of fish snacks at first the volume (v) of the crackers was determined in triplicate in each measurement series using sesame seed displacement according to Sahin and Sumnu [62]. Then, the weight (m) of snacks was determined using an electronic scale RADWAG WTC 2000 (Radwag, Poland). Bulk density (ρ) was calculated as follows:

$$\rho\left[\text{g/cm}^3\right] = \frac{\text{m}}{\text{v}} \quad (2)$$

3.6. *Determination of Oil Absorption (%)*

The percentage of absorbed oil was calculated according to the method used by Nurul [61] as follows:

$$\text{Oil absorption}[\%] = \frac{\text{Weight of cracker after deep} - \text{frying [g]} - \text{weight of cracker before deep} - \text{frying [g]}}{\text{Weight of cracker before deep} - \text{frying [g]}} \times 100 \quad (3)$$

The fish crackers were weighed before and after deep-frying in rapeseed oil, using an electronic scale RADWAG WTC 2000 (Radwag, Poland). Measurements were made on twenty samples from each temperature tested and then the average was taken.

3.7. *Determination of the Degree of Bounded Oil (%)*

The degree of bound oil was calculated by the difference in the content of oil absorbed, determined according to point 3.6, compared to the amount of oil determined via extraction using the Bligh and Dyer method [63], according to point 3.8, as follows:

$$\text{Bounded oil [\%]} = \text{Absorbed oil (\%)} - \text{Bligh and Dyer oil (\%)} \quad (4)$$

3.8. *Determination of Lipid Content*

Lipids were extracted using the Bligh and Dyer [63] method. Single-phase lipid solubilization with a chloroform–methanol mixture (1:1) was used. Quantification results were expressed as grams of lipid per 100 g of products.

3.9. Determination of Lipids Quality Parameters

The peroxide value (PV) was determined in the lipids extracted using the Bligh and Dyer method [63], according to EN-ISO 3960:2017 [64], based on the iodometric determination of iodine liberated by the peroxides with a starch indicator and a sodium thiosulfate standard solution. Results were expressed as milliequivalents of active oxygen per kilogram of lipids (meqO_2/kg of lipids).

Anisidine value (AsV) was determined in the lipid extract according to the EN-ISO 6885:2007 [65] method, based on the reaction between α- and β-unsaturated aldehydes and p-anisidine reagent. AsV was expressed as 100 times the absorbance measured at 350 nm (Thermo Scientific, Genesys 20, Waltham, MA, USA) in a 1 cm path length cuvette from a solution containing 10 mg of lipid in 1 mL of reaction medium.

Total oxidation (TOTOX) products were calculated as follows:

$$\text{TOTOX} = 2\text{PV} + \text{AsV} \tag{5}$$

The acid value (AV) was determined by the titration of 0.1 N KOH in methanol, according to EN ISO 660:2020 [66]. The results were presented in milligrams of KOH per gram of fat.

3.10. Fatty Acids Composition

To obtain the fatty acid methyl esters (FAMEs), the extracted lipids underwent alkaline hydrolysis using 0.5 N sodium methylate (CH_3ONa) [22]. Subsequently, the FAMEs were separated using a gas chromatography apparatus coupled with a mass spectrometer (Agilent Technologies 7890A, Santa Clara, CA, USA) and equipped with a split/splitless-type injector. The separation conditions for the FAMEs were as follows: a was ysed SPTM 2560 column (100 m length, 0.25 mm inner diameter, and 0.20 μm film thickness, catalog no. 24056); helium was used as the carrier gas with a constant flow rate of 1.2 mL/min; the split ratio was 1:50; the injector and detector temperatures were set at 220 °C; and the programmed furnace temperature was started at 140 °C for 5 min, and then ramped up to 240 °C at a rate of 4 °C/min. The total analysis time was 45 min.

The qualitative interpretation of chromatograms was based on comparing the retention times and mass spectra of the specific FAMEs in the sample with those of analogous FAME standards provided by Sigma Company, Tokyo, Japan (Lipid Standard). C19:0 (Merck, Poland) was used as the internal standard for quantification purposes.

3.11. Nutritional Quality Indices of Lipids

Indices were calculated using fatty acid profiles. The n-3/n-6 index was obtained by dividing the omega-3 by the omega-6 fatty acids. The DHA/EPA index indicates the ratio between docosahexaenoic acid (DHA) and eicosapentaenoic acid (EPA). The PUFA/SFA index represents the ratio of polyunsaturated fatty acids (PUFA) to saturated fatty acids (SFA).

The index of thrombogenicity (TI) [67] was calculated as follows:

$$\text{TI} = \frac{\text{C14}:0 + \text{C16}:0 + \text{C18}:0}{(0.5 \times \sum \text{MUFA}) + (0.5 \times \sum \text{n} - 6\text{PUFA}) + (3 \times \sum \text{n} - 3\text{PUFA}) + \left(\frac{\text{n}-3}{\text{n}-6}\right)} \tag{6}$$

This index of atherogenicity (IA) [67] was calculated as follows:

$$\text{IA} = \frac{\text{C12}:0 + (4 \times \text{C14}:0) + \text{C16}:0}{\sum \text{MUFA}} \tag{7}$$

The hypocholesterolemic/hypercholesterolemic ratio (HH) [68] more accurately reflects the effects of fatty acids on cardiovascular health compared to the PUFA/SFA ratio and was calculated as follows:

$$HH = \frac{C18:1n-9 + C18:2n-6 + C18:3n-3 + C20:4n-6 + C20:5n-3 + C22:5n-3 + C22:6n-3}{C14:0 + C16:0} \quad (8)$$

The health-promoting index (HPI) [44] was calculated as follows:

$$HPI = \frac{\sum MUFA}{C12:0 + 4 \times C14:0 + C16:0} \quad (9)$$

The quality of fish lipids (FLQ) [69] was calculated as follows:

$$FLQ = \frac{100 \times (C22:6n-3 + C20:5n-3)}{\sum Total\ FA} \quad (10)$$

3.12. Sensory Assessment

A panel of ten trained people (n = 10) with no prior history of taste or aroma impairments evaluated good sensory qualities using the hedonic approach. Samples were presented at random and coded with three-digit codes to avoid bias. A 5-point rating system assessed color, taste, aroma, and texture, with 1 denoting "undesirable" and 5 denoting "very desirable". The results of the profile analysis were shown as polar plots. By PN-ISO 5496:1997 and PN-ISO 3972:2016-07, each panelist underwent evaluation and training in sensory sensitivity [70,71].

3.13. Statistical Analysis

All experiments were conducted in three replications. The results were expressed as mean ± standard deviation (SD). Statistical analyses of the results were performed using the Statistica 13.1 program, with a significance level of $p < 0.05$, using the post hoc test of Tukey's significant difference [72].

4. Conclusions

Snack food is gaining an increasingly wider group of supporters, and its sales are still growing. Generally, these types of products are not considered "healthy", so it is important to enrich these products with easily digestible proteins and high-quality lipids. In addition, it is important to understand the mechanisms of interaction of food ingredients during processing, as they have a significant impact on the calorific value, nutritional value, and sensory characteristics of this type of snack food.

This study showed the influence of the frying temperature of fish cracker products (crackers made of tapioca starch with 50% of farmed carp meat) on physical parameters (degree of expansion) and biochemical parameters (fat content and its interactions), which can serve as a model for similar snacks based on fish and starch. It was found that the frying temperature of 180 °C resulted in almost twice the expansion of the snack than the temperature of 160 °C and its density is much lower, and these parameters have a direct impact on the sensory values of snacks. Moreover, at a higher deep-frying temperature of 180 °C, the product absorbs more oil, but it interacts with starch significantly less than at lower frying temperatures. Higher frying temperature (above 170 °C), for a relatively short time, up to 1 min, does not increase the oxidation level and even have a beneficial effect on reducing the amount of peroxides through their thermal decomposition. The sensory evaluation confirmed that a higher frying temperatures enhanced the overall desirability of the product, particularly in terms of texture and color, which aligns with consumer expectations for deep-fried snacks. The product presented in this work is also characterized by very valuable nutritional indices for assessing fatty acids (IA, IT, HH, HPI, FLQ) for this type of product; however, the deep-frying process causing high oil absorption significantly reduces these indices. Future works suggest the further exploration of methods to reduce oil absorption in deep-fried snacks, while maintaining favorable sensory and nutritional properties, especially through alternative deep-frying techniques or pre-treatments.

Author Contributions: Conceptualization, G.T.; Methodology, G.T., G.B., P.B., S.P., W.S. and M.T.; Formal analysis, G.T., P.B. and G.B.; Resources, G.T.; Data curation, S.P.; Writing—original draft, G.T., W.S., P.B. and M.T.; Writing—review & editing, G.T., G.B. and S.P.; Visualization, S.P., W.S. and M.T.; Supervision, G.T. and G.B.; Project administration, G.T. and G.B. All authors have read and agreed to the published version of the manuscript.

Funding: This research was funded by the European Union from the financial resources of the European Maritime and Fisheries Fund Operational Program "Fisheries and the Sea 2014–2020". Action 2.1 Innovation under Priority 2—Supporting environmentally sustainable, resource-efficient, innovative, competitive and knowledge-based aquaculture. Research work number: 518-9110-518.08.85.08958—10.124—7.1.11.01.1.1; Research project number: 00004-6521.1-OR1600005/17/20.

Institutional Review Board Statement: This study complied with PN-ISO 3972:2016-07 and PN-ISO 5496:1997 criteria and comprised sensory analyses conducted by a trained panel. It is not necessary to have permission to perform sensory panel research. All participants were given an information sheet outlining the purpose of their involvement, and their informed consent was obtained. This document described the study's methods, possible hazards, and participants' rights.

Informed Consent Statement: Not applicable.

Data Availability Statement: The original contributions presented in this study are included in the article. Further inquiries can be directed to the corresponding author.

Conflicts of Interest: The authors declare no conflict of interest.

References

1. European Snacks Association. Available online: https://www.esasnacks.eu/ (accessed on 9 December 2024).
2. Durmaz, A.; Yuksel, F. Deep Fried Wheat Chips Added with Potato Peel Flour—Effect on Quality Parameters. *Qual. Assur. Saf. Crops Foods* **2021**, *13*, 115–124. [CrossRef]
3. Rynek Karpia w Polsce—Trade.Gov.Pl. Available online: https://www.trade.gov.pl/aktualnosci/rynek-karpia-w-polsce/ (accessed on 11 December 2024).
4. Kaliniak-Dziura, A.; Skałecki, P.; Florek, M.; Kędzierska-Matysek, M.; Sobczak, P. Chemical Composition and Elements Concentration of Fillet, Spine and Bones of Common Carp (*Cyprinus carpio*) in Relation to Nutrient Requirements for Minerals. *Animals* **2024**, *14*, 1311. [CrossRef] [PubMed]
5. Ahmed, A. Evaluation of the Nutritional Quality of Farmed Common Carp (*Cyprinus carpio* L.) Based on Fatty and Amino Acids Profile. *Acta Aquat. Turc.* **2022**, *18*, 159–167. [CrossRef]
6. Skalecki, P.; Florek, M.; Litwińczuk, A.; Staszowska, A.; Kaliniak, A. Wartość Użytkowa i Skład Chemiczny Mięsa Karpi (*Cyprinus carpio* L.) i Pstrągów Tęczowych (Oncorhynchus Mykiss Walb.) Pozyskanych z Gospodarstw Regionu Lubelskiego. *Rocz. Nauk. Pol. Tow. Zootech.* **2013**, *9*, 57–62.
7. Bacelar, R.G.A.; Moura, N.d.O.; Sousa, M.d.S.; Filho, J.H.S.; Rodrigues, K.D.S.; de Melo, E.S.; Muratori, M.C.S. Mechanically Separated Meat Prepared with Edible Tilapia Filleting Waste from a Public Fish Market. *Acta Sci.* **2023**, *45*, e60993. [CrossRef]
8. Roder, N.; Ellis, P.; Butterworth, P. Starch Molecular and Nutritional Properties: A Review. *Adv. Mol. Med.* **2005**, *1*, 5–14.
9. Chudasama, B.; Zofair, S.; Bhola, D.; Dave, T. Development and Characterization of Fish Crackers Prepared from the Bull's Eye (Priacanthus Hamrur, Forsskal, 1775) Fish Meat and Different Starches. *J. Entomol. Zool. Stud.* **2019**, *7*, 401–406.
10. Asokapandian, S.; Swamy, G.J.; Hajjul, H. Deep Fat Frying of Foods: A Critical Review on Process and Product Parameters. *Crit. Rev. Food Sci. Nutr.* **2020**, *60*, 3400–3413. [CrossRef]
11. Arslan, M.; Xiaobo, Z.; Shi, J.; Rakha, A.; Hu, X.; Zareef, M.; Zhai, X.; Basheer, S. Oil Uptake by Potato Chips or French Fries: A Review. *Eur. J. Lipid Sci. Technol.* **2018**, *120*, 1800058. [CrossRef]
12. Aladedunye, F.; Przybylski, R.; Matthaus, B. Performance of Antioxidative Compounds under Frying Conditions: A Review. *Crit. Rev. Food Sci. Nutr.* **2017**, *57*, 1539–1561. [CrossRef]
13. Li, X.; Cheng, X.; Wu, G.; Huang, J.; Zhang, H.; Jin, Q.; Wang, X. Individual and Combined Effects of Frying Load and Deteriorated Polar Compounds on the Foaming of Edible Oil. *Food Res. Int.* **2020**, *134*, 109206. [CrossRef] [PubMed]

14. Krishnan, V.; Mondal, D.; Thomas, B.; Singh, A.; Praveen, S. Starch-Lipid Interaction Alters the Molecular Structure and Ultimate Starch Bioavailability: A Comprehensive Review. *Int. J. Biol. Macromol.* **2021**, *182*, 626–638. [CrossRef] [PubMed]
15. Zhang, G.; Hamaker, B.R. Starch-Free Fatty Acid Complexation in the Presence of Whey Protein. *Carbohydr. Polym.* **2004**, *55*, 419–424. [CrossRef]
16. Mellema, M. Mechanism and Reduction of Fat Uptake in Deep-Fat Fried Foods. *Trends Food Sci. Technol.* **2003**, *14*, 364–373. [CrossRef]
17. Parimala, K.R.; Sudha, M.L. Effect of Hydrocolloids on the Rheological, Microscopic, Mass Transfer Characteristics during Frying and Quality Characteristics of Puri. *Food Hydrocoll.* **2012**, *27*, 191–200. [CrossRef]
18. Jiamjariyatam, R. Use of Riceberry Bran to Reduce Oil Absorption in Puffed Cracker. *Int. Food Res. J.* **2019**, *26*, 441–450.
19. Kurek, M.; Ščetar, M.; Galić, K. Edible Coatings Minimize Fat Uptake in Deep Fat Fried Products: A Review. *Food Hydrocoll.* **2017**, *71*, 225–235. [CrossRef]
20. Lawrence, G.D. Perspective: The Saturated Fat-Unsaturated Oil Dilemma: Relations of Dietary Fatty Acids and Serum Cholesterol, Atherosclerosis, Inflammation, Cancer, and All-Cause Mortality. *Adv. Nutr.* **2021**, *12*, 647–656. [CrossRef]
21. Tong, Y.; Gao, H.; Qi, Q.; Liu, X.; Li, J.; Gao, J.; Li, P.; Wang, Y.; Du, L.; Wang, C. High Fat Diet, Gut Microbiome and Gastrointestinal Cancer. *Theranostics* **2021**, *11*, 5889. [CrossRef]
22. Association of Official Analytical Chemists. Fatty Acids in Encapsulated Fish Oils. In *AOAC Official Methods of Analyses of Association of Analytical Chemist*, 18th ed.; Method 991.39; AOAC International: Rockville, MD, USA, 2007.
23. Dehghannya, J.; Ngadi, M. Recent Advances in Microstructure Characterization of Fried Foods: Different Frying Techniques and Process Modeling. *Trends Food Sci. Technol.* **2021**, *116*, 786–801. [CrossRef]
24. Jothi, J.S.; Le, T.N.D.; Kawai, K. Effects of Trehalose and Corn Starch on the Mechanical Glass Transition Temperature and Texture Properties of Deep-Fried Food with Varying Water and Oil Contents. *J. Food Eng.* **2020**, *267*, 109731. [CrossRef]
25. Karp Nacinany: Nacinanie Karpia Do Smażenia—Beszamel.Pl. Available online: https://beszamel.se.pl/przepisy/dania-glowne-rybne/karp-nacinany-nacinanie-karpia-do-smazenia-re-SRii-wGAp-yJ6p.html (accessed on 11 December 2024).
26. Li, X.; Yu, L.; Xie, Y.; Li, C.; Fang, Z.; Hu, B.; Wang, C.; Chen, S.; Wu, W.; Li, X.; et al. Effect of Different Cooking Methods on the Nutrient, and Subsequent Bioaccessibility and Biological Activities in Boletus Auripes. *Food Chem.* **2023**, *405*, 134358. [CrossRef] [PubMed]
27. Parada, J.; Santos, J.L. Interactions between Starch, Lipids, and Proteins in Foods: Microstructure Control for Glycemic Response Modulation. *Crit. Rev. Food Sci. Nutr.* **2016**, *56*, 2362–2369. [CrossRef] [PubMed]
28. Wang, S.; Chao, C.; Cai, J.; Niu, B.; Copeland, L.; Wang, S. Starch–Lipid and Starch–Lipid–Protein Complexes: A Comprehensive Review. *Compr. Rev. Food Sci. Food Saf.* **2020**, *19*, 1056–1079. [CrossRef]
29. Okumus, B.N.; Tacer-Caba, Z.; Kahraman, K.; Nilufer-Erdil, D. Resistant Starch Type V Formation in Brown Lentil (*Lens culinaris* Medikus) Starch with Different Lipids/Fatty Acids. *Food Chem.* **2018**, *240*, 550–558. [CrossRef]
30. Hu, X.; Li, Z.; Wang, F.; Mu, H.; Guo, L.; Xiao, J.; Liu, Y.; Li, X. Formation of Starch–Lipid Complexes during the Deep-Frying Process and Its Effects on Lipid Oxidation. *Foods* **2022**, *11*, 3083. [CrossRef]
31. Touffet, M.; Trystram, G.; Vitrac, O. Revisiting the Mechanisms of Oil Uptake during Deep-Frying. *Food Bioprod. Process.* **2020**, *123*, 14–30. [CrossRef]
32. Sandhu, J.S.; Takhar, P.S. Verification of Hybrid Mixture Theory Based Two-Scale Unsaturated Transport Processes Using Controlled Frying Experiments. *Food Bioprod. Process.* **2018**, *110*, 26–39. [CrossRef]
33. Yang, D.; Zhu, L.; Wu, G.; Li, X.; Li, P.; Zhang, H.; Liu, T. Whether the Degradation of Frying Oil Affects Oil Absorption: Tracking Fresh and Degraded Oil in Fried Potato Strips during Frying and Cooling and Microstructure Characterization. *Food Bioprod. Process.* **2022**, *133*, 87–99. [CrossRef]
34. Liu, Y.; Tian, J.; Zhang, T.; Fan, L. Effects of Frying Temperature and Pore Profile on the Oil Absorption Behavior of Fried Potato Chips. *Food Chem.* **2021**, *345*, 128832. [CrossRef]
35. Pratama, Y.; Ulfah, T.; Bintoro, V.P. Effect of Basil (*Ocimum americanum* L.) Proportion on Physical and Organoleptical Properties of Basil Cracker. *J. Appl. Food Technol.* **2018**, *5*, 1–5. [CrossRef]
36. Wang, H.; Wu, Y.; Wang, N.; Yang, L.; Zhou, Y. Effect of Water Content of High-Amylose Corn Starch and Glutinous Rice Starch Combined with Lipids on Formation of Starch–Lipid Complexes during Deep-Fat Frying. *Food Chem.* **2019**, *278*, 515–522. [CrossRef] [PubMed]
37. Chang, F.; He, X.; Fu, X.; Huang, Q.; Jane, J.L. Effects of Heat Treatment and Moisture Contents on Interactions between Lauric Acid and Starch Granules. *J. Agric. Food Chem.* **2014**, *62*, 7862–7868. [CrossRef] [PubMed]
38. Kawai, K.; Takato, S.; Sasaki, T.; Kajiwara, K. Complex Formation, Thermal Properties, and in-Vitro Digestibility of Gelatinized Potato Starch–Fatty Acid Mixtures. *Food Hydrocoll.* **2012**, *27*, 228–234. [CrossRef]

39. Rozporządzenie Ministra Zdrowia z Dnia 25 Września 2012 r. w Sprawie Określenia Maksymalnych Poziomów Substancji Zanieczyszczających, Które Mogą Znajdować Się w Tłuszczach Stosowanych Do Smażenia, Oraz Kryteriów Dla Metod Analitycznych Stosowanych Do Ich Oznaczania. Available online: https://isap.sejm.gov.pl/isap.nsf/DocDetails.xsp?id=WDU2012000 1096 (accessed on 9 September 2024).
40. Lolos, M.; Oreopoulou, V.; Tzia, C. Oxidative Stability of Potato Chips: Effect of Frying Oil Type, Temperature and Antioxidants. *J. Sci. Food Agric.* **1999**, *79*, 1524–1528. [CrossRef]
41. Iwegbue, C.M.A.; Osijaye, K.O.; Igbuku, U.A.; Egobueze, F.E.; Tesi, G.O.; Bassey, F.I.; Martincigh, B.S. Effect of the Number of Frying Cycles on the Composition, Concentrations and Risk of Polycyclic Aromatic Hydrocarbons (PAHs) in Vegetable Oils and Fried Fish. *J. Food Compos. Anal.* **2020**, *94*, 103633. [CrossRef]
42. Song, J.H.; Kim, S.; Kim, J.; Kim, M.J.; Lee, S.M.; Jang, M.I.; Lee, J.H. Oxidative Properties and Moisture Content in Repeatedly Used Oils for French Fries and Breaded Chickens during Frying. *Eur. J. Lipid Sci. Technol.* **2017**, *119*, 1600279. [CrossRef]
43. Cervantes-Ramírez, J.E.; Cabrera-Ramirez, A.H.; Morales-Sánchez, E.; Rodriguez-García, M.E.; Reyes-Vega, M.d.l.L.; Ramírez-Jiménez, A.K.; Contreras-Jiménez, B.L.; Gaytán-Martínez, M. Amylose-Lipid Complex Formation from Extruded Maize Starch Mixed with Fatty Acids. *Carbohydr. Polym.* **2020**, *246*, 116555. [CrossRef]
44. Chen, J.; Liu, H. Nutritional Indices for Assessing Fatty Acids: A Mini-Review. *Int. J. Mol. Sci.* **2020**, *21*, 5695. [CrossRef]
45. Li, F.; Duan, Y.; Li, Y.; Tang, Y.; Geng, M.; Oladele, O.A.; Kim, S.W.; Yin, Y. Effects of Dietary N-6:N-3 PUFA Ratio on Fatty Acid Composition, Free Amino Acid Profile and Gene Expression of Transporters in Finishing Pigs. *Br. J. Nutr.* **2015**, *113*, 739–748. [CrossRef]
46. Gonzalez-Becerra, K.; Barron-Cabrera, E.; Muñoz-Valle, J.F.; Torres-Castillo, N.; Rivera-Valdes, J.J.; Rodriguez-Echevarria, R.; Martinez-Lopez, E. A Balanced Dietary Ratio of N-6:N-3 Polyunsaturated Fatty Acids Exerts an Effect on Total Fatty Acid Profile in RBCs and Inflammatory Markers in Subjects with Obesity. *Healthcare* **2023**, *11*, 2333. [CrossRef]
47. Yang, Y.; Xia, Y.; Zhang, B.; Li, D.; Yan, J.; Yang, J.; Sun, J.; Cao, H.; Wang, Y.; Zhang, F. Effects of Different N-6/n-3 Polyunsaturated Fatty Acids Ratios on Lipid Metabolism in Patients with Hyperlipidemia: A Randomized Controlled Clinical Trial. *Front. Nutr.* **2023**, *10*, 1166702. [CrossRef] [PubMed]
48. Elagizi, A.; Lavie, C.J.; O'keefe, E.; Marshall, K.; O'keefe, J.H.; Milani, R.V. An Update on Omega-3 Polyunsaturated Fatty Acids and Cardiovascular Health. *Nutrients* **2021**, *13*, 204. [CrossRef] [PubMed]
49. Všetičková, L.; Suchý, P.; Straková, E.; Karmaoui, A. Factors Influencing the Lipid Content and Fatty Acids Composition of Freshwater Fish: A Review. *Artic. Asian J. Fish. Aquat. Res.* **2019**, *5*, 1–10. [CrossRef]
50. Kheiri, A.; Aliakbarlu, J.; Tahmasebi, R. Antioxidant Potential and Fatty Acid Profile of Fish Fillet: Effects of Season and Fish Species. *Vet. Res. Forum* **2022**, *13*, 91. [CrossRef]
51. Wu, Z.X.; Hu, X.P.; Zhou, D.Y.; Tan, Z.F.; Liu, Y.X.; Xie, H.K.; Rakariyatham, K.; Shahidi, F. Seasonal Variation of Proximate Composition and Lipid Nutritional Value of Two Species of Scallops (*Chlamys farreri* and *Patinopecten yessoensis*). *Eur. J. Lipid Sci. Technol.* **2019**, *121*, 1800493. [CrossRef]
52. Dellatorre, F.G.; Avaro, M.G.; Commendatore, M.G.; Arce, L.; Díaz de Vivar, M.E. The Macroalgal Ensemble of Golfo Nuevo (Patagonia, Argentina) as a Potential Source of Valuable Fatty Acids for Nutritional and Nutraceutical Purposes. *Algal. Res.* **2020**, *45*, 101726. [CrossRef]
53. Ratusz, K.; Symoniuk, E.; Wroniak, M.; Rudzińska, M. Bioactive Compounds, Nutritional Quality and Oxidative Stability of Cold-Pressed Camelina (*Camelina sativa* L.) Oils. *Appl. Sci.* **2018**, *8*, 2606. [CrossRef]
54. Bajramova, A.; Spégel, P. A Comparative Study of the Fatty Acid Profile of Common Fruits and Fruits Claimed to Confer Health Benefits. *J. Food Compos. Anal.* **2022**, *112*, 104657. [CrossRef]
55. Lupette, J.; Benning, C. Human Health Benefits of Very-Long-Chain Polyunsaturated Fatty Acids from Microalgae. *Biochimie* **2020**, *178*, 15–25. [CrossRef]
56. Vieira, E.C.S.; Mársico, E.T.; Conte-Junior, C.A.; Damiani, C.; Canto, A.C.V.d.C.S.; Monteiro, M.L.G.; Silva, F.A. da Effects of Different Frying Techniques on the Color, Fatty Acid Profile, and Lipid Oxidation of Arapaima Gigas. *J. Food Process Preserv.* **2018**, *42*, e13820. [CrossRef]
57. Nursyahirah, S.; Rozzamri, A. Effects of Frying on Fish, Fish Products and Frying Oil—A Review. *Food Res.* **2022**, *6*, 14–32. [CrossRef]
58. AOAC Dry Matter Method 945.12. In *Official Methods of Analysis of the AOAC*, 21st ed.; AOAC International: Washington, DC, USA, 2019.
59. AOAC Crude Ash Method 920.153. In *Official Methods of Analysis of the AOAC*, 21st ed.; AOAC International: Washington, DC, USA, 2019.
60. AOAC Crude Protein Method 945.18. In *Official Methods of Analysis of the AOAC*, 21st ed.; AOAC International: Washington, DC, USA, 2019.
61. Nurul, H.; Boni, I.; Noryati, I. The Effect of Different Ratios of Dory Fish to Tapioca Flour on the Linear Expansion, Oil Absorption, Colour and Hardness of Fish Crackers. *Int. Food Res. J.* **2009**, *16*, 159–165.

62. Sahin, S.; Sumnu, S.G. Rheological Properties of Foods. In *Physical Properties of Foods*; Springer: New York, NY, USA, 2006; pp. 39–105. [CrossRef]
63. Bligh, E.G.; Dyer, W.J. A Rapid Method of Total Lipid Extraction and Purification. *Can. J. Biochem. Physiol.* **1959**, *37*, 911–917. [CrossRef]
64. *PN EN ISO 3960:2017*; Animal and Vegetable Fats and Oils—Determination of Peroxide Value—Iodometric (Visual) Endpoint Determination. International Organization for Standardization: Geneva, Switzerland, 2017.
65. *EN ISO 6885:2016*; Animal and Vegetable Fats and Oils—Determination of Anisidine Value. International Organization for Standardization: Geneva, Switzerland, 2016.
66. *EN ISO 660:2020*; Animal and Vegetable Fats and Oils—Determination of Acid Value and Acidity. International Organization for Standardization: Geneva, Switzerland, 2020.
67. Ulbricht, T.L.V.; Southgate, D.A.T. Coronary Heart Disease: Seven Dietary Factors. *Lancet* **1991**, *338*, 985–992. [CrossRef]
68. Zhang, X.; Ning, X.; He, X.; Sun, X.; Yu, X.; Cheng, Y.; Yu, R.Q.; Wu, Y. Fatty Acid Composition Analyses of Commercially Important Fish Species from the Pearl River Estuary, China. *PLoS ONE* **2020**, *15*, e0228276. [CrossRef]
69. Chen, S.; Bobe, G.; Zimmerman, S.; Hammond, E.G.; Luhman, C.M.; Boylston, T.D.; Freeman, A.E.; Beitz, D.C. Physical and Sensory Properties of Dairy Products from Cows with Various Milk Fatty Acid Compositions. *J. Agric. Food Chem.* **2004**, *52*, 3422–3428. [CrossRef]
70. Analiza Sensoryczna—Metodologia—Wprowadzenie i Szkolenie Oceniających w Wykrywaniu i Rozpoznawaniu Zapachów PN-ISO 5496:1997/KATALOG GŁÓWNY Systemu Biblioteczno-Informacyjnego Uniwersytetu Jana Długosza w Częstochowie—BIBLIOTEKA GŁÓWNA—UJD. Available online: https://www.katalog.bu.ujd.edu.pl/cgi-bin/koha/opac-detail.pl?myhash=0%C3%973D4ABDCAA57B35DAB908F24503DF6620&mysearchid=6742&bib=239275 (accessed on 6 August 2024).
71. *PN-ISO 3972:2016-07*; Analiza Sensoryczna—Metodyka—Metody Badania Wrażliwości Sensorycznej. International Organization for Standardization: Geneva, Switzerland, 2016.
72. TIBCO Statistica Electronic Manual. Available online: https://www.scribd.com/document/321061529/STATISTICA-Electronic-Manual (accessed on 14 August 2024).

molecules

MDPI

Article

Impact of Cooking Techniques on the Dietary Fiber Profile in Selected Cruciferous Vegetables

Karolina Nowak [1], Sascha Rohn [2] and Michał Halagarda [3,*]

1 Department of Product Packaging, Krakow University of Economics, ul. Rakowicka 27, 31-510 Kraków, Poland
2 Institute of Food Technology and Food Chemistry, Technische Universität Berlin, Gustav-Meyer-Allee 25, 13355 Berlin, Germany
3 Department of Food Product Quality, Krakow University of Economics, ul. Sienkiewicza 5, 30-033 Kraków, Poland
* Correspondence: michal.halagarda@uek.krakow.pl

Abstract: Cruciferous vegetables of the plant order Brassicales are an attractive dietary component and a valuable source of fiber. However, the nutritional–physiological properties are different when comparing soluble and insoluble fibers. Another significant impact is the transformation of fibers by different influencing factors during food preparation. Cruciferous vegetables, especially, are dominantly processed to soften the matrix. As a result, during cooking, the polysaccharides are dissolved, swelled, or degraded to a certain extent, influencing the composition and the nutritional–physiological properties. The aim of the present study was to analyze the impact of different cooking procedures on changes in the dietary fiber content profile of three different plants: white cauliflower (*Brassica oleracea* L. var. *botrytis*), broccoli (*B. oleracea* L. var. *italica*), and Brussels sprouts (*B. oleracea* L. var. *gemmifera*). The sample material was subjected to direct ("in the water") and steam cooking. The dietary fiber content and the content of its fractions were determined using an enzymatic analysis method. The results of the research show that the cooking process had a significant influence on the content of dietary fiber fractions in cruciferous vegetables. The concentration of insoluble dietary fiber decreased, whereas the content of soluble dietary fiber increased. When considering the average influence of each process, both steam cooking and direct cooking had a similar impact on changes in the concentrations of dietary fiber fractions. It can therefore be concluded that, when considering dietary fiber content, both processes can be equally well chosen as a thermal treatment for cruciferous vegetables.

Keywords: Brassica vegetables; white cauliflower; broccoli; Brussels sprouts; dietary fiber

1. Introduction

Definitions of the term "dietary fiber" have been specified, among several others, by the Codex Alimentarius, the European Food Safety Authority (EFSA), Health Canada, and the U.S. Food and Drug Administration (FDA) [1]. The general definition says that dietary fiber (DF) is the edible part of plants that is not enzymatically digested and adsorbed by the human digestive tract after consumption [2]. DF reaches the colon, where it is either degraded further by the gut microbiome [3] or, after binding to water, simply excreted with the feces [4]. They have positive effects on the human organism by regulating stool weight and intestinal motility, binding to cholesterol or even residues and contaminants, and affecting the homeostasis of nutrients during digestion and absorption [4,5].

DFs belong primarily to the carbohydrate group, as they are dominantly polysaccharides with some modifications. Traditionally, there is a differentiation between two types of DF: water-soluble DF (SDF) and insoluble DF (IDF) [6]. The first type includes, for example, pectins, gums, and mucilages, while the second comprises cellulose, hemicellulose, and lignins [2]. These fractions affect the human organism differently. The viscosity of the chyme affects the form of the stool and the digestive processes, especially the pace of digestion and the absorption of nutrients. SDF increases the viscosity of the chyme, while IDF seems to have only a little effect [4,7]. SDF also facilitates bowel motility, because this fraction forms a gel-like consistency, enabling easier bowel movements [4].

DF in the human diet comes primarily from vegetables, fruits, and grains, as it is obviously a natural component of the cell walls of these plant materials. About 30–40% of the DF in the human diet comes from vegetables [2]. Kalmpourtzidou [8] showed that the consumption of vegetables is insufficient in most countries around the world. Brassica vegetables from the plant order *Brassicales* are an especially attractive dietary component due to their organoleptic characteristics such as taste, smell, and nutritional value, which originate from glucosinolates that are also regarded as very healthy [9]. However, they can be also good sources of DF, as the structure of their stalks and florets is quite rigid and difficult to degrade or digest [10], especially when consumed raw.

Very prominent Brassica vegetables are, among others, broccoli, cauliflower, and Brussels sprouts [9]. These have gained attention because of the proposed positive effect on cancer risk reduction [11]. According to Rodríguez et al. [12], their total DF content can reach up to 28–30% of the dry weight of the vegetables. In the cruciferous vegetables mentioned before, the concentration of total DF ranges between 1 and 4.1 g/100 g of fresh weight [13].

However, the effects of cooking need to be considered, as a certain transformation of DF can be expected. The vegetables are often prepared at home at a higher temperature (boiling, steaming, frying, baking, etc.) [14], which has a general impact on the composition of the vegetables. Some compounds are leached out into the cooking water, while others are transformed into smaller molecules with varying fates [15–18]. However, the exact mechanisms can be related to the cooking treatments but may also vary, depending on composition and matrix. Cooking methods such as boiling and steaming unlock distinct transformations in the dietary fiber matrix of cruciferous vegetables, potentially enhancing or diminishing their health-promoting properties. These transformations are hypothesized to vary significantly between species due to unique structural compositions [19], unveiling a nuanced interplay between thermal treatment and fiber bioavailability. Therefore, the aim of the present study was to analyze the impact of different cooking procedures on changes in the dietary fiber content profile of selected cruciferous vegetables. For comparing a potential dependency of species, the research material consisted of three different plants: white cauliflower (*Brassica oleracea* L. var. *botrytis*), broccoli (*B. oleracea* L. var. *italica*), and Brussels sprouts (*B. oleracea* L. var. *gemmifera*). The sample material was subjected to direct ("in the water") and steam cooking. The dietary fiber content and the content of its fractions were determined using an enzymatic analysis method.

2. Results and Discussion

The contents of total DF and its fractions, SDF and IDF, in raw, non-processed broccoli, Brussels sprouts, and white cauliflower (Table 1) generally corresponded to the data in the literature. The present values were slightly higher than those obtained by Hedges and Lister [20], Kalala et al. [21], or Lafarga et al. [22] and much higher than those reported by Melim et al. [23] for broccoli, Brussels sprouts, and cauliflower and by Kapusta-Duch et al. [24] for purple cauliflower. At the same time, the present values were slightly lower than those noted by Khanum et al. [25]. Conversely, Núñez-Gómez et al. [26] observed slightly lower DF and IDF contents but a slightly higher SDF concentration. Berndtsson [27] reported slightly higher or lower values depending on the year in which the tests were conducted. When expressed on a fresh matter basis, DF content in cooked broccoli (4.32 g/100 g) was slightly lower and in cauliflower (3.02 g/100 g) slightly higher in this study compared to the values reported by Ferjančič et al. [28] (4.41 g/100 g and 2.8 g/100 g, respectively). Based on the findings described by Wennberg et al. [19], it can be assumed that the discrepancies between the present study's results and those reported by other authors may be due to differences in the cultivars used. According to Berndtsson [27], differences may be also due to the timepoint during the season.

Table 1. Comparison of total dietary fiber content and its insoluble and soluble fractions in broccoli, Brussels sprouts, and white cauliflower with consideration of the effect of thermal processing (g/100 g on a dry matter basis).

Parameter	Vegetable		Type of Processing			Linear Mixed Models		
			Raw	Steam Cooking	Water Cooking	Steam Cooking vs. Raw	Water Cooking vs. Raw	Water Cooking vs. Steam Cooking
Total dietary fiber (DF)	Broccoli	$\bar{x} \pm$ SD	38.72 ± 0.26	36.81 ± 0.4	39.7 ± 0.17	$p < 0.001$ *	$p < 0.001$ *	$p < 0.001$ *
	Brussels sprouts	$\bar{x} \pm$ SD	39.21 ± 0.51	38.8 ± 0.33	38.39 ± 0.09	$p = 0.059$	$p = 0.001$ *	$p = 0.004$ *
	White cauliflower	$\bar{x} \pm$ SD	33.93 ± 2.49	34.81 ± 0.02	36.21 ± 0.27	$p = 0.291$	$p = 0.017$ *	$p < 0.001$ *
Insoluble dietary fiber (IDF)	Broccoli	$\bar{x} \pm$ SD	36.23 ± 0.17	26.38 ± 0.58	26.1 ± 0.09	$p < 0.001$ *	$p < 0.001$ *	$p = 0.162$
	Brussels sprouts	$\bar{x} \pm$ SD	35.22 ± 0.20	27.17 ± 0.14	28.09 ± 0.85	$p < 0.001$ *	$p < 0.001$ *	$p = 0.007$ *
	White cauliflower	$\bar{x} \pm$ SD	31.68 ± 2.17	24.52 ± 1.86	24.73 ± 1.34	$p < 0.001$ *	$p < 0.001$ *	$p = 0.786$
Soluble dietary fiber (SDF)	Broccoli	$\bar{x} \pm$ SD	2.49 ± 0.26	10.43 ± 0.99	13.61 ± 0.08	$p < 0.001$ *	$p < 0.001$ *	$p < 0.001$ *
	Brussels sprouts	$\bar{x} \pm$ SD	3.99 ± 0.32	11.63 ± 0.47	10.31 ± 0.94	$p < 0.001$ *	$p < 0.001$ *	$p = 0.003$ *
	White cauliflower	$\bar{x} \pm$ SD	2.21 ± 0.26	10.29 ± 1.84	11.48 ± 1.61	$p < 0.001$ *	$p < 0.001$ *	$p = 0.153$

* Statistically significant ($p < 0.05$); SD—standard deviation.

The research aimed to assess the influence of selected thermal processes on the total dietary fiber (DF) content in cruciferous vegetables, focusing on the impact of plant materials and cooking procedures, as detailed in Table 1. The results showed that, in the case of Brussels sprouts, the total DF content decreased as a result of simple cooking in water. In contrast, an increase in total DF concentration was noted for broccoli and cauliflower. Steam cooking resulted in a significant reduction in total DF in the case of broccoli only. With regard to IDF, a significant decrease was noted for all vegetables tested and both cooking procedures. A difference in processing influence was only significant in the case of Brussels sprouts, where steam cooking had a pronounced effect on IDF concentration. The content of SDF increased significantly in the case of all the tested vegetables. In the case of broccoli, steam cooking had a significantly weaker effect, whereas, in the case of Brussels sprouts, an inverse impact was noted.

When considering the average impact of thermal processes on the three selected vegetables, the type of processing did not have a significant influence on total DF (Table 2). Both steam cooking and water cooking significantly decreased the concentration of IDF (on average, from 34.38 g/100 g to 26.02 g/100 g and 26.3 g/100 g, respectively) and increased the content of SDF (on average, from 2.9 g/100 g to 10.78 g/100 g and 11.8 g/100 g, respectively) in the vegetables tested. According to Ozyurt and Ötle [29], high temperatures during these thermal processes can break down polysaccharides, leading to the release of oligosaccharides, which contributes to the observed increase in SDF. However, in this study, no significant differences between the two analyzed thermal processes were identified.

Table 2. The influence of the selected thermal processing techniques on total dietary fiber content and its insoluble and soluble fractions (g/100 g on a dry matter basis).

Parameter		Process			Linear Mixed Models		
		Raw	Steam Cooking	Water Cooking	Steam Cooking vs. Raw	Water Cooking vs. Raw	Water Cooking vs. Steam Cooking
Total dietary fiber (DF)	$\bar{x} \pm SD$	37.29 ± 2.85	36.81 ± 1.8	38.1 ± 1.59	$p = 0.825$	$p = 0.7$	$p = 0.447$
Insoluble dietary fiber (IDF)	$\bar{x} \pm SD$	34.38 ± 2.35	26.02 ± 1.5	26.3 ± 1.67	$p = 0.006$ *	$p = 0.009$ *	$p = 0.834$
Soluble dietary fiber (SDF)	$\bar{x} \pm SD$	2.9 ± 0.89	10.78 ± 1.16	11.8 ± 1.71	$p < 0.001$ *	$p = 0.001$ *	$p = 0.39$

* Statistically significant ($p < 0.05$); SD—standard deviation.

There is scarce information in the literature on the effect of heat treatment on the content of DF and its two fractions, IDF and SDF, in vegetables. In the present study, a slight but still statistically significant decrease in total DF content was noted as a result of water cooking and, in the case of Broccoli, as a result of steam cooking, too. Considering the average effect on all three tested vegetables, no significant influence on total DF was noted for either of the thermal processes. These results concur with the outcomes described by Nyman et al. [30], which showed that cooking did not significantly affect the DF content of Brussels sprouts. Kalala et al. [21] also found that steaming cauliflower, broccoli, and Brussels sprouts did not significantly affect total DF. However, in the present study, a significant increase in the SDF fraction was observed as a result of both processes. Similarly, Khanum et al. [25], for water-cooked cauliflower, and Kalala et al. [21], for steamed cauliflower, broccoli, and Brussels sprouts, noted a significant increase in SDF fractions. Compared to the results of the present study, the impact was much lower in the case of cauliflower as in the studies described by Kalala et al. [21] or Khanum et al. [25]. At the same time, those authors noted a simultaneous decrease in IDF, a finding that is generally consistent with the results of the present study.

As indicated in Table 1, the reduction in the case of steam-cooked cauliflower was insignificant in the present study. Similarly, Rehman et al. [31] also studied the influence of cooking on its IDF fraction. They showed that, when boiling cauliflower in water, there is a decrease in both neutral detergent fiber and acid detergent fiber. This means that during cooking, these polysaccharidic compounds partially break down. As a result, smaller oligosaccharides and small simple sugars are formed by hydrolysis, which is favored by the heat and the pH conditions during aqueous cooking. Consequently, DF concentrations in the vegetables decrease [31]. Also, according to Khanum et al. [25], the reduction in fiber content in vegetables after cooking may be related to the degradation of IDF. Cellulose is released and also partially degraded further [32]. Steam cooking involves indirect heat transfer through water vapor, which results in a more gentle cooking process and a slower impact on the cellular structures of the vegetables. This may help preserve the integrity of certain dietary fiber fractions, which is reflected in the higher share of IDF fractions in DF compared to water-cooked samples (Table 2). In contrast, Puupponen-Pimiä et al. [33] showed that, in the case of cauliflower, there was an increase in total DF, SDF, and IDF concentrations as a result of blanching combined with freezing. The statistical significance of these results was, however, not verified. Those authors suggested that these increases were due to the mechanical impact of ice crystals on cell wall structures, leading to an improved extraction. However, the mechanical transformation of the cell walls can also force hydrolysis, leading to a better extraction but also to a more probable degradation to smaller compounds.

With regard to nutritional–physiological aspects, nutritionists mostly prefer to maintain IDF in the food [34,35] as its rigidity in structure and complex chemical composition disables a fast breakdown and offers more probability for positively affecting gut passage [36]. Its mechanical stimulation increases fecal bulk, accelerates colonic transit, and alleviates symptoms of constipation, contributing to improved bowel function [37]. IDF is also considered a pre-requisite substrate for the gut microbiome, as it fosters microbial diversity and enhances the release of beneficial secondary metabolites of colonic fermentation, such as short-chain fatty acids (SCFA), particularly butyrate, which exhibit anti-inflammatory properties and support the integrity of the colonic mucosa [3]. These metabolites are vital for maintaining gut health and overall homeostasis, reducing inflammation, and potentially offering protective effects against colorectal diseases. The fermentation of dietary fiber by gut microbiota and the subsequent production of SCFA further underscore the health benefits of maintaining IDF in the diet [38,39]. The findings on fiber transformation during cooking processes highlight key considerations for dietary recommendations. The observed increase in SDF content, along with a decrease in IDF, suggests that cooking methods significantly influence the composition of dietary fiber in vegetables. While IDF is crucial for promoting gut motility and microbiome diversity, SDF provides unique benefits, including enhanced nutrient absorption, the modulation of blood glucose levels, and improved cholesterol metabolism [40]. Individuals should be encouraged to diversify their preparation methods for fiber-rich vegetables like broccoli, cauliflower, and Brussels sprouts. Raw or minimally cooked options minimize fiber degradation and help preserve IDF, supporting intestinal motility and microbiota health, while moderate cooking can increase SDF content, enhancing its effects on metabolic health. Tailoring cooking practices to specific health goals, such as supporting digestive health with higher IDF intake or managing blood sugar levels with increased SDF, could offer personalized nutritional strategies.

In order to illustrate the differences between the selected cruciferous vegetables and their thermal processing on DF and its fractions, as well as water content, PCA was employed (Figure 1). The first two main components received explained 100% of the total variance, with the first component explaining 62.87% and the second explaining 37.13%. As shown in Figure 1a, the first component is associated with a higher IDF/SDF ratio, while the second component corresponds to higher total DF content.

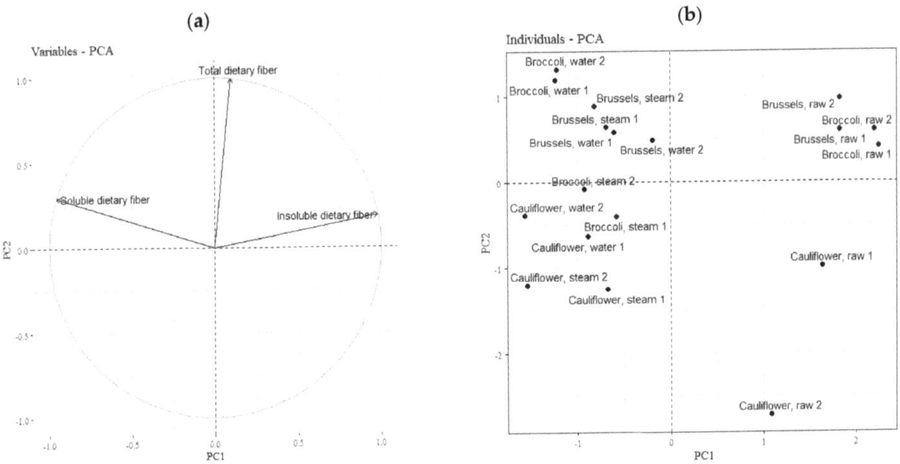

Figure 1. The results of the Principal Component Analysis (PCA). (**a**) The variables factor map; (**b**) The individuals factor map.

The individual factor map (Figure 1b) shows that the first component separates raw from cooked vegetables. The cooked vegetables had higher IDF/SDF ratios. The second component separates cauliflower from Brussels sprouts and broccoli, indicating that cauliflower has less total DF than the other two vegetables tested. The lack of separation between vegetables subjected to two different thermal processes indicates that steam cooking and water cooking had a similar influence on changes in DF content.

3. Materials and Methods

3.1. Vegetable Material and Sample Preparation

The research material consisted of white cauliflower (*Brassica oleracea* L. var. *botrytis*), broccoli (*B. oleracea* L. var. *italica*), and Brussels sprouts (*B. oleracea* L. var. *gemmifera*). The vegetables were sourced from a local farmer with a regular harvest in early autumn. To achieve greater homogeneity and ensure consistency in the experiments, the vegetables were inspected to match specific criteria: uniformity in size, color (consistent maturity), and freshness (harvested within 48 h of analysis). Prior to the analysis, the quality was visually inspected to exclude any specimens with visible defects or signs of spoilage. These materials were chosen because they are widely consumed cruciferous vegetables known for their high nutritional value. Furthermore, their varying textures and compositions make them suitable for assessing the effects of different cooking methods on their quality and dietary fiber content.

The sample material was subjected to two methods of heat treatment. One was direct cooking in water, as traditionally carried out very often worldwide. The second procedure is also quite common: steam cooking, with contact with water vapor but a reduced possibility of compounds being leached out. The thermal treatment of vegetables was preceded by the removal of inedible parts and prior washing. In the case of cauliflower and broccoli, the vegetables were additionally divided into florets with a diameter of 7 cm.

The water cooking process was conducted with the use of an induction cooker (Hendi, Hamburg, Germany) and cookware made of stainless steel. Cooking in water was carried out at 100 °C for a time of 12–15 min, depending on the vegetable, until the samples were fully soft. Steam cooking was carried out in an Orange Vision 6× convection steam oven (Retigo, Rožnov pod Radhoštěm, Czech Republic) using full steam. The steaming process lasted 10–12 min, varying by vegetable type, and was terminated when the samples reached full softness. After cooking, the vegetables were cooled to room temperature, frozen at a temperature of -20 ± 2 °C in a shock cooling chamber (RedFox SHS-511, RM Gastro, Veselínad Lužnicí, Czech Republic), freeze-dried using a Christ Alpha 1–4 system (Martin Christ Gefriertrocknungsanlagen GmbH, Osterode am Harz, Germany), and ground in a Tecator Knifetec 1095 laboratory mill (Foss Tecator, Uppsala, Sweden) to obtain a homogeneous material (particle size $\leq$ 0.5 mm) for further analysis.

3.2. Analysis of Total Dietary Fiber, Soluble Dietary Fiber, and Insoluble Dietary Fiber

The dietary fiber content and the content of its fractions were determined using the enzymatic method according to the AOAC 991.43 Standard [41], employing a Total Dietary Fiber Assay Kit (Megazyme, Wicklow, Ireland). While no additional validation experiments were performed for this study, the accuracy of the results was ensured by adhering to the kit's validated protocols and incorporating reagent blanks to minimize analytical artifacts.

For the purpose of the analysis, 1 g of lyophilized samples were placed in incubation flasks, where the following enzymatic digestion steps were carried out sequentially in a shaking water bath (Memmert WNB14, Buchenbach, Germany):

1. α-Amylase treatment: The sample was suspended in 40 mL of MES-TRIS buffer (pH 8.2) and treated with 50 μL of α-amylase (thermostable). The mixture was incubated at 98–100 °C for 30 min with continuous shaking to solubilize and hydrolyze starch.
2. Protease treatment: After cooling to 60 °C, 100 μL of protease was added to digest proteins. The sample was incubated for 30 min at 60 °C in a shaking water bath.
3. Amyloglucosidase treatment: First, 5 mL of 0.561 M HCl was added, and the pH was adjusted to 4.0–4.6 using 1 M NaOH or 1 M HCl at 60 °C. Subsequently, 300 μL of amyloglucosidase was added while continuously mixing. The flasks were covered

with aluminum foil and incubated for 30 min at 60 °C in a shaking water bath to hydrolyze residual starch into glucose.

For the determination of DF, IDF, and SDF, the enzymatic digestate was filtered under vacuum using the Fibertec™ E filtration system (FOSS, Hillerød, Denmark). For IDF, the residue was first rinsed with warm water (2 × 10 mL, 70 °C) to remove soluble components and then sequentially washed with ethanol (78%, 2 × 15 mL; 95%, 2 × 15 mL) and acetone (2 × 15 mL). The filtrates were discarded, and the residues were dried overnight at 105 °C in a Venticell 55 Plus oven dryer (BMT, Brno, Czech Republic). For SDF, the combined filtrate and water washings from the IDF procedure were treated with 230 mL of preheated ethanol (95%, 60 °C) to precipitate soluble fiber. The precipitate was then filtered and subjected to the same rinsing (ethanol and acetone) and drying steps as described for IDF.

Subsequently, the protein content of the residue was determined by the Dumas combustion method [42] using a TruSpec N analyzer (LECO, St. Joseph, MI, USA). A nitrogen-to-protein conversion factor of 5.9 was applied. Ash content was determined by combusting the residue in a muffle furnace (Nabertherm, Lilienthal, Germany) at 525 °C for 5 h [43].

The dietary fiber content (X) in g/100 g of the analyzed food product was calculated using the formula:

$$X = \frac{R - A - P - B}{m} \cdot 100,$$

where:

- R—mass of the residue after filtration (mg);
- P—mass of ash in the sample (mg);
- A—mass of protein in the sample (mg);
- B—mass of the blank sample residue (mg);
- m—mass of the sample (mg).

The results were corrected for moisture content, determined according to ISO 712:2010 [44] using a Venticell 55 Plus oven dryer (BMT, Czech Republic) and expressed as g/100 g on a dry matter basis.

The method's reliability was verified using the TDF Controls KIT (Megazyme, Wicklow, Ireland). All analyses were performed in triplicate, and reagent blanks were included to account for potential analytical artifacts.

3.3. Statistical Analysis

Cooking was repeated four times. For each heat treatment and vegetable type, three replicate samples (1 g each) were analyzed, ensuring reliable measurements and repeatability. To account for variance due to the series of tests, differences between vegetables and types of processing were analyzed with linear mixed models with the series of tests as a random effect and vegetable types and cooking procedures as fixed effects. To compare the influence of thermal processes on selected cruciferous vegetables, a Principal Component Analysis (PCA) was performed. As a result, a two-dimensional sample map was prepared. All the statistical analyses were performed using statistical package R, version 4.4.1 [45]. A value of 0.05 was required for statistical significance.

4. Conclusions

The results of this study showed that the cooking process had a significant influence on the content of dietary fiber fractions in selected cruciferous vegetables. When considering the average impact of each process, both steam cooking and water cooking had a similar impact on changes in the concentrations of dietary fiber fractions. It can therefore be concluded that, when considering dietary fiber content, both processes can be equally well chosen as a thermal treatment for the cruciferous vegetables tested. With regard to nutritional–physiological aspects, we would need different tests to decide which processing condition might be preferable. However, to preserve the integrity of insoluble dietary fiber and support digestive health, consumers or the industry may consider raw or minimally cooked vegetables as a preferable option. On the other hand, moderate cooking may increase soluble dietary fiber content, which is beneficial for metabolic health. Tailoring cooking practices to specific health goals, such as maximizing insoluble dietary fiber for gut motility or enhancing soluble dietary fiber for improved metabolic function, could offer personalized dietary strategies.

It is often suggested that steam cooking is more preferential, particularly concerning the retention of water-soluble small molecules such as vitamin C or secondary metabolites like glucosinolates and polyphenols. Ideally, the cooking procedures preserve them as well and lead to a soft, easy-to-consume vegetable matrix while maintaining the quite complex structures of insoluble dietary fiber to the maximum extent. However, future studies should address the balance between preserving fiber content and minimizing nutrient losses in order to make more definitive recommendations.

Author Contributions: Conceptualization, M.H. and S.R.; methodology, K.N. and M.H.; formal analysis, M.H.; investigation, K.N.; resources, K.N.; writing—original draft preparation, K.N. and M.H.; writing—review and editing, S.R.; supervision, M.H. and S.R.; funding acquisition, M.H. All authors have read and agreed to the published version of the manuscript.

Funding: This research was subsidized by the Krakow University of Economics, project number: 50/ZJZ/2024/DOS.

Institutional Review Board Statement: Not applicable.

Informed Consent Statement: Not applicable.

Data Availability Statement: The data presented in this study are available on request from the corresponding author.

Conflicts of Interest: The authors declare no conflicts of interest.

References

1. Katagiri, R.; Goto, A.; Shimazu, T.; Yamaji, T.; Sawada, N.; Iwasaki, M.; Inoue, M.; Tsugane, S. Dietary fiber intake and risk of gastric cancer: The Japan Public Health Center based prospective study. *Int. J. Cancer* **2021**, *148*, 2664–2673. [CrossRef] [PubMed]
2. Ibrahim, O.; Menkovska, M. Dietary Fibers-Classification, Properties, Analysis and Function: A Review. *Adv. Biosci. Biotechnol.* **2022**, *13*, 527–544. [CrossRef]
3. Louis, P.; Flint, H.J. Formation of propionate and butyrate by the human colonic microbiota. *Environ. Microbiol.* **2017**, *19*, 29–41. [CrossRef]
4. O'Grady, J.; O'Connor, E.M.; Shanahan, F. Review article: Dietary fibre in the era of microbiome science. *Aliment. Pharm. Ther.* **2019**, *49*, 506–515. [CrossRef]
5. Raji, Z.; Karim, A.; Karam, A.; Khalloufi, S. A review on the heavy metal adsorption capacity of dietary fibers derived from agro-based wastes: Opportunities and challenges for practical applications in the food industry. *Trends Food Sci. Technol.* **2023**, *137*, 74–91. [CrossRef]
6. Alba, K.; MacNaughtan, W.; Laws, A.P.; Foster, T.J.; Campbell, G.M.; Kontogiorgos, V. Fractionation and characterisation of dietary fibre from blackcurrant pomace. *Food Hydrocolloid.* **2018**, *81*, 398–408. [CrossRef]
7. Zhong, L.; Fang, Z.; Wahlqvist, M.L.; Hodgson, J.M.; Johnson, S.K. Extrusion cooking increases soluble dietary fibre of lupin seed coat. *Food Sci. Technol.* **2018**, *99*, 547–554. [CrossRef]
8. Kalmpourtzidou, A.; Eilander, A.; Talsma, E.F. Global Vegetable Intake and Supply Compared to Recommendations: A Systematic Review. *Nutrients* **2020**, *12*, 1558. [CrossRef]
9. Favela-González, K.M.; Hernández-Almanza, A.Y.; De la Fuente-Salcido, N.M. The value of bioactive compounds of cruciferous vegetables (Brassica) as antimicrobials and antioxidants: A review. *J. Food Biochem.* **2020**, *44*, e13414. [CrossRef]
10. Morrison, I.M.; Burrows, S.E. The fibre yield, composition and cellulase degradability of brassica cultivars and chemically treated brassica cultivars. *Ind. Crops Prod.* **1994**, *2*, 171–177. [CrossRef]

11. Mandrich, L.; Caputo, E. Brassicaceae-Derived Anticancer Agents: Towards a Green Approach to Beat Cancer. *Nutrients* **2020**, *12*, 868. [CrossRef] [PubMed]
12. Rodríguez, R.; Jiménez, A.; Fernández-Bolaños, J.; Guillén, R.; Heredia, A. Dietary fibre from vegetable products as source of functional ingredients. *Trends Food Sci. Tech.* **2006**, *17*, 3–15. [CrossRef]
13. Ağagündüz, D.; Şahin, T.Ö.; Yılmaz, B.; Ekenci, K.D.; Duyar Özer, Ş.; Capasso, R. Cruciferous Vegetables and Their Bioactive Metabolites: From Prevention to Novel Therapies of Colorectal Cancer. *Evid. Based Complement. Alternat. Med.* **2022**, *11*, 1534083. [CrossRef] [PubMed]
14. Mehmood, A.; Zeb, A. Effects of different cooking techniques on bioactive contents of leafy vegetables. *Int. J. Gastron. Food Sci.* **2020**, *22*, 100246. [CrossRef]
15. Doniec, J.; Florkiewicz, A.; Duliński, R.; Filipiak-Florkiewicz, A. Impact of Hydrothermal Treatments on Nutritional Value and Mineral Bioaccessibility of Brussels Sprouts (*Brassica oleracea* var. *gemmifera*). *Molecules* **2022**, *27*, 1861. [CrossRef]
16. Kapusta-Duch, J.; Kusznierewicz, B.; Leszczyńska, T.; Borczak, B. Effect of cooking on the contents of glucosinolates and their degradation products in selected Brassica vegetables. *J. Funct. Food* **2016**, *23*, 412–422. [CrossRef]
17. Soares, A.; Carrascosa, C.; Raposo, A. Influence of different cooking methods on the concentration of glucosinolates and vitamin C in broccoli. *Food Bioprocess Technol.* **2017**, *10*, 1387–1411. [CrossRef]
18. Hanschen, F.S.; Lamy, E.; Schreiner, M.; Rohn, S. Reactivity and stability of glucosinolates and their breakdown products in foods. *Angew. Chem.* **2014**, *53*, 11430–11450. [CrossRef]
19. Wennberg, M.S.; Engqvist, G.M.; Nyman, E.M.G.-L. Effects of Boiling on Dietary Fiber Components in Fresh and Stored White Cabbage (Brassica oleracea var. *capitata*). *J. Food Sci.* **2003**, *68*, 1615–1621. [CrossRef]
20. Hedges, L.J.; Lister, C.E. *Nutritional Attributes of Brassica Vegetables*; Report No.: 1618; New Zealand Institute for Crop & Food Research Limited: Christchurch, New Zealand, 2002.
21. Kalala, G.; Kambashi, B.; Everaert, N.; Beckers, Y.; Richel, A.; Pachikian, B.; Neyrinck, A.M.; Delzenne, N.M.; Bindelle, J. Characterization of fructans and dietary fibre profiles in raw and steamed vegetables. *Int. J. Food Sci. Nutr.* **2018**, *69*, 682–689. [CrossRef]
22. Lafarga, T.; Bobo, G.; Viñas, I.; Collazo, C.; Aguiló-Aguayo, I. Effects of thermal and non-thermal processing of cruciferous vegetables on glucosinolates and its derived forms. *J. Food Sci. Techol.* **2018**, *55*, 1973–1981. [CrossRef] [PubMed]
23. Melim, C.; Lauro, M.R.; Pires, I.M.; Oliveira, P.J.; Cabral, C. The Role of Glucosinolates from Cruciferous Vegetables (Brassicaceae) in Gastrointestinal Cancers: From Prevention to Therapeutics. *Pharmaceutics* **2022**, *14*, 190. [CrossRef] [PubMed]
24. Kapusta-Duch, J.; Szeląg-Sikora, A.; Sikora, J.; Niemiec, M.; Gródek-Szostak, Z.; Kuboń, M.; Leszczyńska, T.; Borczak, B. Health-Promoting Properties of Fresh and Processed Purple Cauliflower. *Sustainability* **2019**, *11*, 4008. [CrossRef]
25. Khanum, F.; Swamy, M.S.; Sudarshana Krishna, K.R.; Santhanam, K.; Viswanathan, K.R. Dietary fiber content of commonly fresh and cooked vegetables consumed in India. *Plant Foods Hum. Nutr.* **2000**, *55*, 207–218. [CrossRef]
26. Núñez-Gómez, V.; González-Barrio, R.; Periago, M.J. Interaction between Dietary Fibre and Bioactive Compounds in Plant By-Products: Impact on Bioaccessibility and Bioavailability. *Antioxidants* **2023**, *12*, 976. [CrossRef]
27. Berndtsson, E. Content of Dietary Fibre and Phenolic Compounds in Broccoli Side Streams. Licentiate Thesis, Swedish University of Agricultural Sciences, Alnarp, Sweden, 2020. ISBN 978-91-576-9741-7.
28. Ferjančič, B.; Skrt, M.; Korošec, M.; Bertoncelj, J. Comparative analysis of dietary fibre determination by AOAC 991.43 and AOAC 2011.25 for frequently consumed foods in Slovenia. *Food Chem.* **2022**, *397*, 133753. [CrossRef]
29. Ozyurt, V.H.; Ötles, S. Effect of food processing on the physicochemical properties of dietary fibre. *Acta Sci. Pol. Technol. Aliment.* **2016**, *15*, 233–245. [CrossRef] [PubMed]
30. Nyman, M.; Pålsson, K.E.; Asp, N.G. Effects of Processing on Dietary Fibre in Vegetables. *Eur. J. Clin. Nutr.* **1995**, *49*, 29–36.
31. Rehman, Z.; Islam, M.; Shah, W. Effect of microwave and conventional cooking on insoluble dietary fibre components of vegetables. *Food Chem.* **2003**, *80*, 237–240. [CrossRef]
32. Mansour, A.; Shekib, L.; Elshimy, N.; Sharara, M. Biological Evaluation of Raw and Steamed Broccoli and Cauliflower as Sources of Dietary Fibers. *J. Food Dairy. Sci.* **2017**, *8*, 185–190. [CrossRef]
33. Puupponen-Pimiä, R.; Häkkinen, S.T.; Aarni, M.; Suortti, T.; Lampi, A.M.; Eurola, M.; Piironen, V.; Nuutila, A.M.; Oksman-Caldentey, K.M. Blanching and long-term freezing affect various bioactive compounds of vegetables in different ways. *J. Sci. Food Agr.* **2003**, *83*, 1389–1402. [CrossRef]
34. Yao, F.; Ma, J.; Cui, Y.; Huang, C.; Lu, R.; Hu, F.; Zhu, X.; Qin, P. Dietary intake of total vegetable, fruit, cereal, soluble and insoluble fiber and risk of all-cause, cardiovascular, and cancer mortality: Systematic review and dose–response meta-analysis of prospective cohort studies. *Front. Nutr.* **2023**, *10*, 1153165. [CrossRef] [PubMed]
35. Arayici, M.E.; Mert-Ozupek, N.; Yalcin, F.; Basbinar, Y.; Ellidokuz, H. Soluble and Insoluble Dietary Fiber Consumption and Colorectal Cancer Risk: A Systematic Review and Meta-Analysis. *Nutr. Cancer* **2021**, *74*, 2412–2425. [CrossRef] [PubMed]

36. McRorie, J.W., Jr.; McKeown, N.M. Understanding the Physics of Functional Fibers in the Gastrointestinal Tract: An Evidence -Based Approach to Resolving Enduring Misconceptions about Insoluble and Soluble Fiber. *J. Acad. Nutr. Diet.* **2017**, *117*, 251–264. [CrossRef] [PubMed]
37. El-Salhy, M.; Ystad, S.O.; Mazzawi, T.; Gundersen, D. Dietary fiber in irritable bowel syndrome (Review). *Int. J. Mol. Med.* **2017**, *40*, 607–613. [CrossRef] [PubMed] [PubMed Central]
38. Barber, T.M.; Kabisch, S.; Pfeiffer, A.F.H.; Weickert, M.O. The Health Benefits of Dietary Fibre. *Nutrients* **2020**, *12*, 3209. [CrossRef]
39. Thomson, C.; Garcia, A.L.; Edwards, C.A. Interactions between dietary fibre and the gut microbiota. *Proc. Nutr. Soc.* **2021**, *80*, 398–408. [CrossRef]
40. Mudgil, D. The Interaction Between Insoluble and Soluble Fiber. In *Dietary Fiber for the Prevention of Cardiovascular Disease*; Samaan, R.A., Ed.; Academic Press: Cambridge, MA, USA, 2017; pp. 35–59. [CrossRef]
41. *AOAC Official Method 991.43*; Total, Soluble, and Insoluble Dietary Fiber in Foods. Enzymatic-Gravimetric Method, MES-TRIS Buffer. AOAC International: Gaithersburg, MD, USA, 2000.
42. *ISO 16634-1:2008*; Food Products. Determination of the Total Nitrogen Content by Combustion According to the Dumas Principle and Calculation of the Crude Protein Content. International Organization for Standardization (ISO): Geneva, Switzerland, 2008.
43. *ISO 2171:2007*; Cereals, Pulses and by-Products. Determination of Ash Yield by Incineration. International Organization for Standardization (ISO): Geneva, Switzerland, 2007.
44. *ISO 712:2010*; Cereals and Cereal Products. Determination of the Moisture Content. Gravimetric Method. International Organization for Standardization (ISO): Geneva, Switzerland, 2010.
45. R Foundation for Statistical Computing. R Core Team: A language and Environment for Statistical Computing. Available online: https://www.R-project.org/ (accessed on 2 June 2024).

molecules

MDPI

Article

Influence of the Casein Genotype on Goat Milk Bioactivity: An In Silico Analysis of the Casein Peptidome

Aram Y. Rubio-Reyes [1], Iván Delgado-Enciso [2], Eduardo Casas [3], Estela Garza-Brenner [4] and Ana M. Sifuentes-Rincón [1,*]

[1] Laboratorio de Biotecnología Animal, Centro de Biotecnología Genómica, Instituto Politécnico Nacional, Reynosa 88710, Mexico; arubior2300@alumno.ipn.mx
[2] Facultad de Medicina, Universidad de Colima, Colima 28040, Mexico; ivan_delgado_enciso@ucol.mx
[3] National Animal Disease Center, USDA, ARS, Ames, IA 50010, USA; eduardo.casas@usda.gov
[4] Universidad Autónoma de Nuevo León, General Escobedo 66050, Mexico; egarzab@uanl.edu.mx
* Correspondence: asifuentes@ipn.mx; Tel.: + 8999243627 (ext. 87723)

Abstract: Goat caseins are highly polymorphic proteins that affect milk functional properties. In this study, an in silico approach was employed to analyze the influence of goat casein allelic variants on the quantity and bioactivity potential of peptides released after enzymatic hydrolysis. The reported protein sequences from the most frequent allelic variants in *Capra hircus* caseins (α-S1, β, α-S2, and κ-casein) were analyzed in the BIOPEP-UWM database to determine the frequency of occurrence of bioactive fragments from each casein. After specific hydrolysis with pepsin, trypsin, and chymotrypsin A, important differences in the peptide profile and bioactivity potential were observed within and between the casein allelic variants. The β-casein A and C alleles, α-S1-casein allele E, and α-S2-casein allele F presented the highest bioactivity potential, and some allele-specific peptides were also released, highlighting the impact of genotype on the predicted bioactivity. The inhibition of angiotensin-converting enzyme (ACE-I) and dipeptidyl peptidase IV (DPP-IV) activities was the most frequent bioactivity of the released peptides, suggesting possible antihypertensive and antidiabetic effects. Once confirmed by experimental studies, the use of goat casein genotyping could direct efforts to enhance the functional quality of goat milk.

Keywords: caseins; genotypes; bioactive peptides; polymorphism

1. Introduction

Milk proteins are considered reference macronutrients for determining the nutritional quality of dairy products [1]. Caseins have a significant economic impact because of their influence on the quality, quantity, coagulation capacity, and techno-functional properties of proteins, which are key aspects in the production of dairy byproducts [2].

In most mammals, four genes encoding caseins (*CSN1S1* (α-S1), *CSN2* (β), *CSN1S2* (α-S2), and *CSN3* (κ)) have been reported. These genes have highly polymorphic sequences, including single-nucleotide polymorphisms (SNPs), insertions, deletions, and even differences in splicing patterns [2,3]. Casein polymorphisms produce allelic variants that are related to the amount of casein produced; these variants also affect the fat content, micelle size, mineralization, and sensory characteristics of milk [2]. In some ruminants, such as cattle, casein polymorphisms are also related to bioactive peptide production, with the A1 allele of the β-casein gene exhibiting the strongest association. The A1 allele releases the β-casomorphin-7 bioactive peptide [4]. The molecular differentiation between the A1 and A2 alleles has been the basis for the development of new brands in the milk industry [5,6].

Studies of milk-derived bioactive peptides have been conducted via different approaches. Bioinformatic tools such as website-based databases have been widely used as efficient and cost-effective alternatives to search for bioactive peptides from a specific source [7].

In goats, the *CSN1S1* gene has at least twenty known alleles, the *CSN2* gene includes eight alleles, the *CSN1S2* gene consists of fourteen variants, and the *CSN3* gene has at least seventeen known polymorphisms, resulting in twenty-four DNA variants and fifteen protein variants [2,3]. The variability of goat casein genes has been studied worldwide for a variety of goat breeds and locations, and some alleles are usually reported as the most frequent. In the *CSN1S1* gene, the most frequent alleles are A, B, E, and F, with frequencies ranging from 0.5 to 0.70 [2,8,9]. In the *CSN2* gene, the A and C alleles are the most common, with frequencies greater than 0.70 [10]. Alleles A, B, C, and F are the most common (0.40–0.70) in the *CSN1S2* gene [2]. Finally, in the *CSN3* gene, the most frequent alleles are A, B, C, D, and E, with frequencies ranging from 0.20 to 0.70 [2].

Some studies have shown that the enzymatic hydrolysis of goat milk caseins releases bioactive peptides with opioid, immunomodulatory, antimicrobial, antithrombotic, growth-stimulating, and antihypertensive effects [11–13]; however, to our knowledge, no studies have associated the content and composition of bioactive peptides derived from the proteolysis of goat milk caseins with their specific allelic variants.

The aim of this study was to predict the genotype-specific bioactivity from goat caseins' allelic variants through an approach involving the casein allelic sequence data and in silico enzymatic digestion simulations using the BIOPEP-UWM database.

2. Results

2.1. Analysis of Caseins as a Source of Bioactive Peptides on the Basis of Specific Genotypes

Casein protein sequences were used to determine the parameter A values, and each allele was associated with potential bioactivities on the basis of its amino acid sequence. Differences between alleles of the same type of casein were identified, confirming the effect of allelic variants on the potential bioactivity of caprine casein.

As shown in Table 1, β-casein allele A presented the greatest total frequency of bioactive fragments (ΣA), whereas allele F of α-S1-casein presented the lowest value.

Table 1. Total frequency of the detected functional activities of bioactive fragments (∑A) in the most frequent allelic variants of goat caseins.

Casein Variant	ΣA *
α-S1-casein	
A	2.1447
B	2.1541
E	2.1216
F	1.6351
β-casein	
A	2.4500
C	2.4429
α-S2-casein	
A	1.9959
B	1.9735
C	1.9645
F	2.0094

Table 1. *Cont.*

Casein Variant	ΣA *
κ-casein	
A	2.1914
B	2.2038
C	2.2161
D	2.2286
E	2.2223

* A full description of each counted activity used to determine ΣA is presented in Appendix A.

2.2. *In Silico Proteolytic Release and Prediction of Bioactive Functions*

Figure 1 shows a comparison of the specific positions on each allelic protein variant that promotes in silico proteolysis and peptide release via pepsin (EC 3.4.23.1), trypsin (EC 3.4.21.4), and chymotrypsin A (EC 3.4.21.1). All the casein variants analyzed presented different peptide release profiles, with the release peptides varying in quantity, composition, and reported bioactivity. Briefly, α-S1-casein alleles A, B, and E released 48 peptides, whereas allele F released only 27 peptides. The alleles of β, α-S2, and κ-caseins released 53, 51, and 35 peptides, respectively, with variations in peptide composition identified within each allelic variant.

(A)

A M - K - L - L - IL - TCL - VAVAL - AR - PK - H - PIN - H - QGL - SPEVL - N - EN - L - L - R - F - [1 – 38]
B M - K - L - L - IL - TCL - VAVAL - AR - PK - H - PIN - H - QGL - SPEVL - N - EN - L - L - R - F - [1 – 38]
E M - K - L - L - IL - TCL - VAVAL - AR - PK - H - PIN - H - QGL - SPEVPN - EN - L - L - R - F - [1 – 38]
F M - K - L - L - IL - TCL - VAVAL - AR - PK - H - PIN - H - QGL - SPEVPN - EN - L - L - R - F - [1 – 38]

A VVAPF - PEVF - R - K - EN - IN - EL - SK - DIGSESTEDQAM - EDAK - QM - K - AGSSSSSEEIVPN [39 – 89]
B VVAPF - PEVF - R - K - EN - IN - EL - SK - DIGSESTEDQAM - EDAK - QM - K - AGSSSSSEEIVPN [39 – 89]
E VVAPF - PEVF - R - K - EN - IN - EL - SK - DIGSESTEDQAM - EDAK - QM - K - AGSSSSSEEIVPN [39 – 89]
F VVAPF - PEVF - R - K - EN - IN - EL - SK - DIGSESTEDQAM - EDAK - QM - K- AGSSCQVR - K [39 – 85]

A - SAQQK - Y - IQK - EDVPSER - Y - L - GY - L - EQL - L - R - L - K - K - Y - N - VPQL - EIVPK - [90 – 129]
B - SAEQK - Y - IQK - EDVPSER - Y - L - GY - L - EQL - L - R - L - K - K - Y - N - VPQL – EIVPK - [90 – 129]
E - SAEQK - Y - IQK - EDVPSER - Y - L - GY - L - EQL - L - K - L - K - K - Y - N - VPQL - EIVPK - [90 – 129]
F - L - F - PIVL - SR - STF - K - R - K - M - CPL - SVTW - VIW - N - SF - SD [86 – 115]

A QL - DAY - PSGAW - Y - Y - L - PL - GTQY - TDAPSF - SDIPN - PIGSEN - SGK - TTM - PL - W [170 – 214]
B QL - DAY - PSGAW - Y - Y - L - PL - GTQY - TDAPSF - SDIPN - PIGSEN - SGK - TTM - PL - W [170 – 214]
E QL - DAY - PSGAW - Y - Y - L - PL - GTQY - TDAPSF - SDIPN - PIGSEN - SGK - AAM - PL - W [170 – 214]
F

(B)

A - VL - PVPQK - AVPQR - DM - PIQAF - L - L - Y - QEPVL - GPVR - GPF - PIL - V [185 – 222]
C - VL - PVPQK - VVPQR - DM - PIQAF - L - L - Y - QEPVL - GPVR - GPF - PIL [185 – 221]

(C)

A M - K - F - F - IF - TCL - L - AVAL - AK - H - K - M - EH - VSSSEEPIN - IF - QEIY - K - QEK - N - [1 – 41]
B M - K - F - F - IF - TCL - L - AVAL - AK - H - K - M - EH - VSSSEEPIN - IF - QEIY - K - QEK - N - [1 – 41]
C M - K - F - F - IF - TCL - L - AVAL - AK - H - K - M - EH - VSSSEEPIN - IF - QEIY - K - QEK - N - [1 – 41]
F M - K - F - F - IF - TCL - L - AVAL - AK - H - K - M - EH - ISSSEEPIN - IF - QEIY - K - QEK - N - [1 – 41]

A M - AIH - PR - K - EK - L - CTTSCEEVVR - N - AN - EEEY - SIR - SSSEESAEVAPEEIK - ITVDDK [42 – 92]
B M - AIH - PR - K - EK - L - CTTSCEEVVR - N - AN - EEEY - SIR - SSSEESAKVAPEEIK - ITVDDK [42 – 92]
C M - AIH - PR - K - EK - L - CTTSCEEVVR - N - AN - EEEY - SIR - SSSEESAEVAPEEIK - ITVDDK [42 – 92]
F M - AIH - PR - K - EK - L - CTTSCEEVVR - N - AN - EEEY - SIR - SSSEESAEVAPEEIK - ITVDDK [42 – 92]

A N - AGAF - TPTVN - R - EQL - STSEEN - SK - K - TIDM - ESTEVF - TK - K - TK - L - TEEEK - N [131 – 175]
B N - AGAF - TPTVN - R - EQL - STSEEN - SK - K - TIDM - ESTEVF - TK - K - TK - L - TEEEK - N [131 – 175]
C N - AGAF - TPTVN - R - EQL - STSEEN - SK - K - TIDM - ESTEVF - TK - K - TK - L - TEEEK - N [131 – 175]
F N - AGPF - TPTVN - R - EQL - STSEEN - SK - K - TIDM - ESTEVF - TK - K - TK - L - TEEEK - N [131 – 175]

A - R - L - N - F - L - K - K - ISQY - Y - QK - F - AW - PQY - L - K - TVDQH - QK - AM - K - PW - [176 – 209]
B - R - L - N - F - L - K - K - ISQY - Y - QK - F - AW - PQY - L - K - TVDQH - QK - AM - K - PW - [176 – 209]
C - R - L - N - F - L - K - IISQY - Y - QK - F - AW - PQY - L - K - TVDQH - QK - AM - K - PW - [176 – 209]
F - R - L - N - F - L - K - K - ISQY - Y - QK - F - AW - PQY - L - K - TVDQH - QK - AM - K – PW - [176 – 209]

Figure 1. *Cont.*

(D)

A CCEK - DER - F - F - DDK - IAK - Y - IPIQY - VL - SR - Y - PSY - GL - N - Y - Y - QQR - PVAL - [1 − 41]
B CCEK - DER - F - F - DDK - IAK - Y - IPIQY - VL - SR - Y - PSY - GL - N - Y - Y - QQR - PVAL - [1 − 41]
C CCEK - DER - F - F - DDK - IAK - Y - IPIQY - VL - SR - Y - PSY - GL - N - Y - Y - QQR - PVAL - [1 − 41]
D CCEK - DER - F - F - DDK - IAK - Y - IPIQY - VL - SR - Y - PSY - GL - N - Y - Y - R - QR - PVAL - [1 − 41]
E CCEK - DER - F - F - DDK - IAK - Y - IPIQY - VL - SR - Y - PSY - GL - N - Y - Y - QQR - PVAL - [1 − 41]

A IN - N - QF - L - PY - PY - Y - AK - PVAVR - SPAQTL - QW - QVL - PN - TVPAK - SCQDQPTTL - [42 − 86]
B IN - N - QF - L - PY - PY - Y - AK - PVAVR - SPAQTL - QW - QVL - PN - TVPAK - SCQDQPTTL - [42 − 86]
C IN - N - QF - L - PY - PY - Y - AK - PIAVR - SPAQTL - QW - QVL - PN - TVPAK - SCQDQPTTL - [42 − 86]
D IN - N - QF - L - PY - PY - Y - AK - PIAVR - SPAQTL - QW - QVL - PN - TVPAK - SCQDQPTTL - [42 − 86]
E IN - N - QF - L - PY - PY - Y - AK - PVAVR - SPAQTL - QW - QVL - PN - TVPAK - SCQGQPTTL - [42 − 86]

A AR - H - PH - PH - L - SF - M - AIPPK - K - DQDK - TEVPAIN - TIASAEPTVH - STPTTEAIVN - [87 − 134]
B AR - H - PH - PH - L - SF - M - AIPPK - K - DQDK - TEIPAIN - TIASAEPTVH - STPTTEAIVN - [87 − 134]
C AR - H - PH - PH - L - SF - M - AIPPK - K - DQDK - TEIPAIN - TIASAEPTVH - STPTTEAIVN - [87 − 134]
D AR - H - PH - PH - L - SF - M - AIPPK - K - DQDK - TEIPAIN - TIASAEPTVH - STPTTEAIVN - [87 − 134]
E AR - H - PH - PH - L - SF - M - AIPPK - K - DQDK - TEIPAIN - TIASAEPTVH - STPTTEAIVN - [87 − 134]

A TVDN - PEASSESIASASETN - TAQVTSTEV [135 − 162]
B TVDN - PEASSESIASASETN - TAQVTSTEV [135 − 162]
C TVDN - PEASSESIVSAPETN - TAQVTSTEV [135 − 162]
D TVDN - PEASSESIASAPETN - TAQVTSTEV [135 − 162]
E TVDN - PEASSESIASASETN - TAQVTSTEV [135 − 162]

Figure 1. Comparison of in silico proteolysis results using pepsin, trypsin, and chymotrypsin in goat casein alleles. Only the positions where there were differences in the quantity and type of released peptides occur are shown: (**A**) α-S1-casein alleles, (**B**) β-casein alleles, (**C**) α-S2-casein alleles, and (**D**) κ-casein alleles. Allele-specific peptides are highlighted in yellow. A comparison of the complete proteolysis profile for each casein is presented in Appendix B.

Once the peptides were released, the potential bioactivity index was predicted, and considering a 0.5 threshold value and peptide length of 2–6 amino acids, 35 potential bioactive peptides were found, 32 of which were registered in the BIOPEP-UWM database (Table 2). Regarding their distribution, 14 bioactive peptides were identified in the alleles of α-S1-casein, with distributions of 9, 9, 10, and 6 peptides in alleles A, B, E, and F, respectively. For α-S2-casein, 10 bioactive peptides were found, with 9 present in alleles A, B, and C and 9 present in allele F, differing only by the AGAF peptide in alleles A, B, and C and AGPF in allele F. Finally, in the alleles of β-casein and κ-casein, 9 and 7 bioactive peptides were identified, respectively.

Twenty-eight peptides exhibited two or more bioactive functions. Those released due to amino acid changes resulting from the allelic variant were particularly relevant, as they highlighted the impact of the genotype on the predicted bioactivity of the identified peptides. In the specific case of α-S1-casein, the STF peptide was identified in the F allele and is associated with pancreatic lipase inhibitory activity, a function exclusive to this allele among all analyzed caseins. In the E allele, the amino acid substitution of T to A at positions 209 and 210 in the amino acid sequence releases the AAM peptide, which is considered potentially bioactive (compared with the alleles A and B peptide, TTM). This peptide stands out for its potential multifunctionality, with unique bioactivities such as antibacterial effects, inhibition of D-Ala-D-Ala dipeptidase activity, hypotensive effects, and inhibition of cytosolic alanyl aminopeptidase activity.

In α-S2-casein, an amino acid substitution of A to P at position 134 in allele F (as shown in the sequence alignment) resulted in the AGPF peptide, which exhibited greater bioactivity potential than the AGAF peptide released by alleles A, B, and C. This amino acid change altered the bioactivity profile of the peptides: the AGAF peptide may present effects such as inhibition of alanine carboxypeptidase activity, inhibition of tripeptidyl peptidase II activity, and CaMPDE inhibition, the last of which is exclusive to this allele. On the other hand, the AGPF peptide has a distinct bioactivity profile, including antiamnestic activity, ACE2 and neprilysin inhibition, antithrombotic activity, and regulatory functions.

Table 2. Bioactive fragments released through in silico proteolysis of goat casein alleles using pepsin, trypsin, and chymotrypsin.

Peptide	Peptide Ranker *	Bioactive Activity	α-S1-Casein				β-Casein		α-S2-Casein				κ-Casein				
			A	B	E	F	A	C	A	B	C	F	A	B	C	D	E
QGL	0.533495	ACE-I; DPP-IV-I	✓	✓	✓	✓											
QM	0.607122	-	✓	✓	✓	✓											
STF	0.58977	ACE-I; H; DPP-IV-I; DPP-III-I; R-I; P-L-I				+											
CPL	0.916551	ACE-I; DPP-IV-I; X-P-I; L-I				+											
VIW	0.610494	ACE-I; DPP-IV-I				+											
SF	0.948796	ACE-I; DPP-IV-I; R-I				✓							✓	✓	✓	✓	✓
GY	0.741592	ACE-I; DPP-IV-I; DPP-III-I	✓	✓	✓												
SM	0.628268	DPP-III-I	✓	✓	✓												
QPM	0.810167	ACE-I; DPP-IV-I	✓	✓	✓												
PQL	0.527882	ACE-I; DPP-IV-I	✓	✓	✓												
QF	0.946135	DPP-IV-I; R-I	✓	✓	✓				✓	✓	✓	✓	✓	✓	✓	✓	✓
PSGAW	0.870583	ACE-I; AO; I; DPP-IV-I; A-C-I	✓	✓	✓												
PL	0.811148	ACE-I; DPP-IV-I; X-P-I; L-I	✓	✓	✓		✓	✓									
AAM	0.55858	ACE-I; A-B; H; DPP-IV-I; I-TPP-II; I-C-A-AP; D-A-D-DP-I			+												
ACL	0.746733	-					✓	✓									
PF	0.99343	DPP-IV-I; DPP-III-I; ACE2-I					✓	✓									
PVEPF	0.604782	ACE-I; AO; DPP-IV-I; A-G-I; DPP-III-I; ACE2-I; N-I					✓	✓									
QPPQPL	0.823819	ACE-I; DPP-IV-I; A-G-I; X-P-I; L-I					✓	✓									
DM	0.607466	ACE-I					✓	✓									
PIQAF	0.749093	ACE-I; DPP-IV-I; I-TPP-II					✓	✓									
GPF	0.989324	AAM; ACE-I; AT; RL; AO; H; DPP-IV-I; DPP-III-I; ACE2-I; N-I					✓	✓									
PIL	0.641797	ACE-I; S; NP; DPP-IV-I					✓	✓									
IF	0.949173	ACE-I							✓	✓	✓	✓					
PR	0.787626	ACE-I; DPP-III-I							✓	✓	✓	✓					
PY	0.736696	NP; A-I; DPP-IV-I; PL-A2-I							✓	✓	✓	✓	✓	✓	✓	✓	✓
PW	0.992911	AO; DPP-IV-I							✓	✓	✓	✓					
AGAF	0.873661	ACE-I; AO; DPP-IV-I; CaMPDE-I; I-TPP-II; A-C-I							✓	✓	✓						
AGPF	0.969222	AAM; ACE-I; AT; RL; AO; DPP-IV-I; DPP-III-I; ACE2-I; N-I										+					
AW	0.9669	ACE-I; AO; DPP-IV-I							✓	✓	✓	✓					
AM	0.74549	-							✓	✓	✓	✓					
AIPY	0.613395	ACE-I; NP; A-I; DPP-IV-I; PL-A2-I							✓	✓	✓	✓					
GL	0.808777	ACE-I; DPP-IV-I											✓	✓	✓	✓	✓
QW	0.928524	DPP-IV-I											✓	✓	✓	✓	✓
PH	0.541688	ACE-I; DPP-IV-I; AO											✓	✓	✓	✓	✓
AIPPK	0.575607	A-A-I; ACE-I; AT; AO; A-I; DPP-IV-I; A-G-I; ACE2-I											✓	✓	✓	✓	✓

* Full list of the bioactive potential index is presented in Appendix C. ✓: Peptide released. +: Potentially bioactive peptide released on a single allele. ACE inhibitor: ACE-I. ACE2 inhibitor: ACE2-I. Alanine carboxypeptidase inhibitor: A-C-I. Alpha-amylase inhibitor: A-A-I. Alpha-glucosidase inhibitor: A-G-I. Anti inflammatory: A-I. Antiamnestic: AAM. Antibacterial: A-B. Antioxidative: AO. Antithrombotic: AT. CaMPDE inhibitor: CaMPDE-I. D-Ala-D-Ala dipeptidase inhibitor: D-A-D-DP-I. Dipeptidyl peptidase III inhibitor: DPP-III-I. Dipeptidyl peptidase IV inhibitor: DPP-IV-I. Hypotensive: H. Inhibitor: I. Inhibitor of cytosol alanyl aminopeptidase: I-C-A-AP. Inhibitor of tripeptidyl peptidase II: I-TPP-II. Lactocepin inhibitor: L-I. Neuropeptide: NP. Neprilysin inhibitor: N-I. Pancreatic lipase inhibitor: P-L-I. Phospholipase A2 inhibitor: PL-A2-I. Regulating: RL. Renin inhibitor: R-I. Stimulating: S. Xaa-pro inhibitor: X-P-I.

Finally, Figure 2 illustrates the expected bioactivity potential of all the goat casein alleles on the basis of peptides released through in silico hydrolysis with pepsin, trypsin, and chymotrypsin. The color variations in the heatmap clearly show that the predominant effects of all the caseins include the inhibition of angiotensin-converting enzyme (ACE-I) and dipeptidyl peptidase IV (DPP-IV-I) activities. Differences in the bioactivity of each allele within a specific casein were also observed, and the alleles with lower expected bioactivity potential are represented by lighter tones. For example, in α-S1-casein, a reduction in ACE, DPP-IV, dipeptidyl peptidase III, and renin inhibition was observed in some alleles. Similarly, in α-S2-casein, lower antioxidant activity and reduced dipeptidyl peptidase III inhibition were identified. In contrast, in β-casein and κ-casein, no significant variations in bioactivities were found among the alleles.

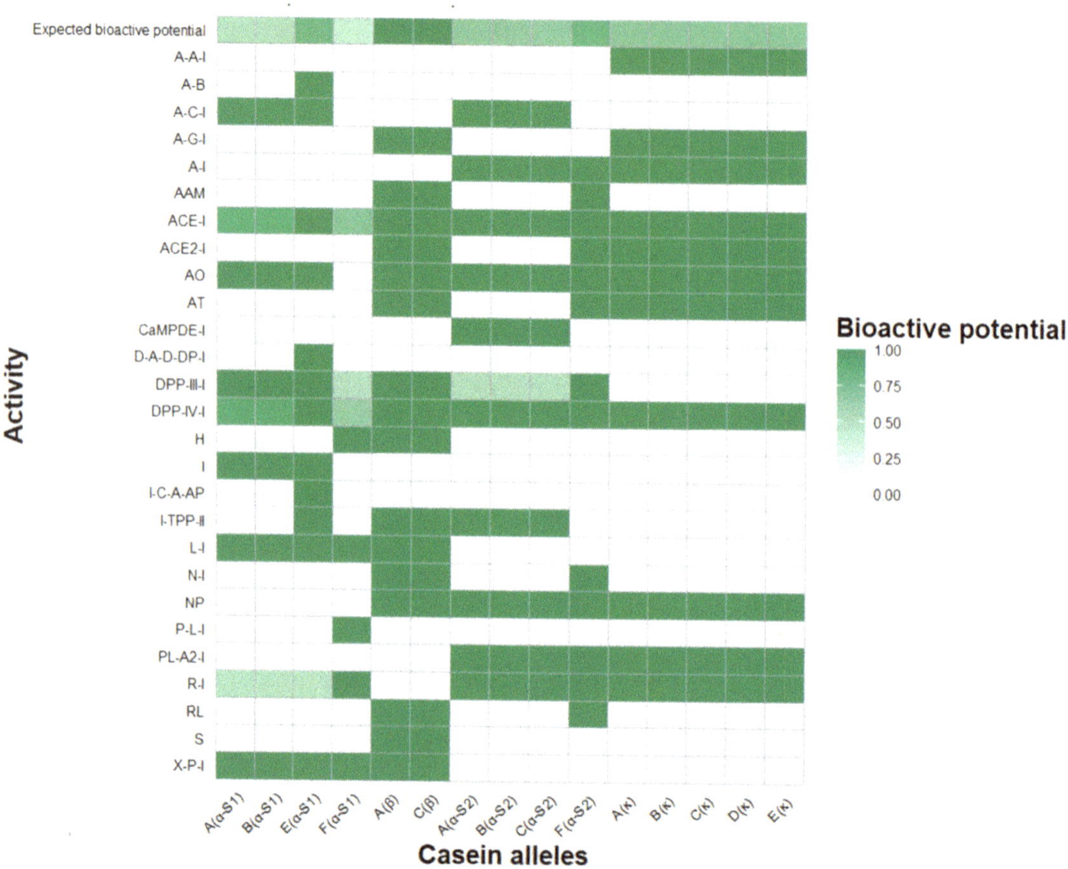

Figure 2. Expected bioactive potential of goat casein alleles, where white indicates the absence of activity, while colored shades represent different levels of bioactive activity. A(α-S1): α-S1-casein allele A. B(α-S1): α-S1-casein allele B. E(α-S1): α-S1-casein allele E. F(α-S1): α-S1-casein allele F. A(β): β-casein allele A. C(β): β-casein allele C. A(α-S2): α-S2-casein allele A. B(α-S2): α-S2-casein allele B. C(α-S2): α-S2-casein allele C. F(α-S2): α-S2-casein allele F. A(κ): κ-casein allele A. B(κ): κ-casein allele B. C(κ): κ-casein allele C. D(κ): κ-casein allele D. E(κ): κ-casein allele E. ACE inhibitor: ACE-I. ACE2 inhibitor: ACE2-I. Alanine carboxypeptidase inhibitor: A-C-I. Alpha-amylase inhibitor: A-A-I. Alpha-glucosidase inhibitor: A-G-I. Anti inflammatory: A-I. Antiamnestic: AAM. Antibacterial: A-B. Antioxidative: AO. Antithrombotic: AT. CaMPDE inhibitor: CaMPDE-I. D-Ala-D-Ala dipeptidase inhibitor: D-A-D-DP-I. Dipeptidyl peptidase III inhibitor: DPP-III-I. Dipeptidyl peptidase IV inhibitor: DPP-IV-I. Hypotensive: H. Inhibitor: I. Inhibitor of cytosol alanyl aminopeptidase: I-C-A-AP. Inhibitor of tripeptidyl peptidase II: I-TPP-II. Lactocepin inhibitor: L-I. Neuropeptide: NP. Neprilysin inhibitor: N-I. Pancreatic lipase inhibitor: P-L-I. Phospholipase A2 inhibitor: PL-A2-I. Regulating: RL. Renin inhibitor: R-I. Stimulating: S. Xaa-pro inhibitor: X-P-I.

After evaluating the bioactivity potential of each casein allele, it could be inferred that β-casein alleles A and C have the potential to exhibit the highest bioactivity, with a greater probability of displaying a more comprehensive bioactive profile. The α-S1-casein allele E has the potential to exhibit greater bioactivity than alleles A, B, and F do, with the latter being the least functional of all caseins. In α-S2-casein, allele F stands out as the most functional allele compared with alleles A, B, and C. For κ-casein, all the alleles share the same theoretical bioactivity profile.

3. Discussion

The results obtained in this study allowed the identification of changes in bioactive peptide release due to variations in the protein sequences of allelic variants of caseins. In recent decades, several studies have reported the release of bioactive peptides from goat milk and goat dairy products [13,14]. However, the effects of allelic variants on the release of these peptides in goat caseins have not been evaluated in vivo or in silico. Here, after the total frequency of bioactive fragment occurrence (ΣA) was calculated, differences were identified among the four types of caseins, as well as among alleles of the same casein type, indicating a high probability that genotype significantly influences the release of bioactive peptides.

Different studies in cattle and other species have shown that a higher ΣA value indicates a greater probability of bioactive peptides being released from the analyzed sequence [15]. Lin et al. [16] and Gu et al. [17] evaluated the potential for bioactive peptide release in yak and buffalo milk, respectively, via the A parameter. In both cases, β-casein presented higher ΣA values than did α-S1, α-S2, and κ-casein, similar to the results obtained in this study. However, the ΣA value in the goat caseins analyzed in this study was even greater than that reported for yak and buffalo milk caseins, suggesting that goat caseins have greater potential for releasing bioactive peptides.

The release of bioactive peptides from proteins through enzymatic hydrolysis depends on the specificity of proteases in recognizing and cleaving peptide bonds within the protein. The type of enzymes used and the hydrolysis conditions vary depending on the nature of the precursor protein, thereby influencing the release and activity of bioactive peptides [18–20]. In this context, the enzymatic hydrolysis of dairy proteins has been widely applied to improve their solubility in water and release peptides with potential biological effects [21]. Different studies in goats and other species have proposed the use of pepsin, trypsin, and chymotrypsin as hydrolytic proteases because of their specificity for cleaving peptide bonds. Trypsin is specific for lysine and arginine residues, whereas chymotrypsin is specific for aromatic amino acid chains such as tryptophan, phenylalanine, and tyrosine [7,22]. Pepsin is the principal enzyme involved in protein digestion in the gastric phase and is a widely used digestive protease for milk and other food proteins [23].

The in silico analysis of pepsin, trypsin, and chymotrypsin confirmed that goat milk caseins, depending on their genotype, are suitable precursors for the release of bioactive peptides. The predictive tool allowed the identification of differences in the quantity and composition of the peptides released, highlighting the impact of genetic variations on the peptide profile.

A clear example of this variability was observed in α-S1-casein hydrolysis. In this study, the E allele presented the most extensive peptide profile, whereas the F allele presented a reduced profile because of the lack of recognition sites. This could be explained by the loss and modification of amino acids reported for this allele due to a cytosine deletion in exon 9, along with 11- and 3-base pair insertions in intron 9, of the *CSN1S1* gene. These alterations cause frameshifts that eliminate exons 9, 10, and 11 [2,24,25]. Consequently, this allele releases the peptide STF, which exhibits pancreatic lipase inhibitory activity, suggesting a possible antiobesity effect [26].

Moreover, single or double amino acid substitutions in casein genes modified the bioactivity of the released peptides. In α-S2-casein, the substitution of A for P at position 134 of the F allele resulted in the peptide AGPF, whereas in the A, B, and C alleles, the peptide AGAF was released. This amino acid change produced different functional profiles;

the AGAF peptide has unique CaMPDE inhibitory activity, which could be useful in the treatment of atherosclerosis and cancer [27], whereas in α-S1-casein, the replacement of the amino acid sequence TTM (A allele) with AAM at positions 209 and 210 in the E allele converted a previously nonbioactive fragment into a peptide with a high probability of bioactivity. This peptide exhibited unique bioactivities among the four types of casein, such as antibacterial activity, hypotensive effects, and inhibition of cytosolic alanyl aminopeptidase and D-Ala-D-Ala dipeptidase activities, the last of which potentially contribute to antimicrobial effects [28].

The high probability of the peptides inhibiting angiotensin-converting enzyme (ACE-I) and dipeptidyl peptidase IV (DPP-IV-I) activities could provide opportunities for the development of functional foods with antihypertensive and antidiabetic effects, respectively [29–31].

According to the BIOPEP-UWM database, the enzymes used in this study have a preferential cleavage site within the casein sequences. Pepsin cleaves at the C-terminal end after residues such as phenylalanine (Phe) and leucine (Leu), trypsin cleaves at the C-terminal end after residues such as lysine (Lys) and arginine (Arg), while chymotrypsin cleaves at the C-terminal end after residues such as tyrosine (Tyr), tryptophan (Trp), phenylalanine (Phe), leucine (Leu), asparagine (Asn), histidine (His), and methionine (Met); at the N-terminal end, the enzyme preferentially cleaves isoleucine (Ile).

Other in silico studies have evaluated combinations of different enzymes to release bioactive peptides from goat caseins. Wu et al. [32] used the BIOPEP-UWM database to simulate the hydrolysis of goat milk β-casein with pepsin (EC: 3.4.23.1), chymotrypsin A (EC: 3.4.21.1), and trypsin (EC: 3.4.21.4), identifying 51 peptides. In our study of β-casein, we identified 53 peptides, confirming that the high polymorphism of caseins may modify enzyme recognition sites.

In this study, we identified a greater number of bioactivities for the allelic variants of β-casein than for those of α-S1-casein, α-S2-casein, and κ-casein. According to reported studies, most of the biofunctionalities identified in milk from different species have been associated primarily with peptides derived from β-casein, followed by these three caseins, which is consistent with the results obtained in this in silico study [13]. This could be related to the structure of β-casein and its susceptibility to enzymatic hydrolysis, facilitating the release of peptides with well-documented biological effects. Our results suggest that while β-casein, α-S1, and α-S2 may represent promising sources of bioactive peptides, experimental studies are needed to confirm their functionality and compare their impact with peptides derived from β-casein.

Integrating genomic and bioinformatic tools represents a promising strategy for the development of dairy products with health benefits. However, this type of analysis has limitations. In silico proteolysis does not guarantee that the predicted peptides can be experimentally reproduced, as proteins may not undergo complete hydrolysis [33], and also, the predictive power of the method depends on the cleavage sites reported for proteases, which may not accurately reflect their actual behavior, as the bioactivities of peptides are predicted based on sequence similarity to previously characterized fragments [16]. Despite these considerations, the obtained results have important practical applications in the discovery of bioactive peptides, such as directing more cost-effective experimental designs to test and validate the in silico results.

Future work could include the in vitro hydrolysis of genotype-specific precursor proteins or even the direct synthesis of the most promising bioactive peptides, followed by experimental evaluation of their biological effects [34].

Finally, considering that casein allelic variant genotyping is a practical tool available for most producers, once the bioactive potential of the casein allelic variants is confirmed, genotyping goat populations could guide breeding strategies aimed at enhancing the functional properties of dairy products by selecting those carriers of the casein haplotypes that have higher bioactive potential.

4. Materials and Methods

4.1. Analysis of Capra Hircus Caseins as a Source of Bioactive Peptides

The protein sequences of *Capra hircus* caseins were selected from the NCBI database (https://www.ncbi.nlm.nih.gov/ accessed on 7 April 2025). Because some protein sequences from allelic variants reported as high-frequency alleles in goats are not available in the NCBI database, hypothetical sequences were generated on the basis of the reference alleles of each casein and by substituting the amino acid composition at the positions described in the literature [2]. The studied allelic variants were as follows: for α-S1 casein, alleles A (NP_001424592.1, reference allele), B (hypothetical sequence), E (X72221.1), and F (AJ504711.2); for β-casein, alleles A (AJ011018.3) and C (AY563136.1, reference allele); for α-S2 casein, alleles A (XP_013820127.2, reference allele), B (hypothetical sequence), and C (hypothetical sequence) and F (AJ289716.1); and for κ-casein, alleles A (AF485339.1), B (AF485340.1, reference allele), C (AF485341.1), D (AY090465.1), and E (AF486523.1). Alignment, comparison, and analysis of casein protein sequences were performed via MEGA XI software v 11.0.13 [35]. Once aligned, positions with amino acid changes due to allelic variations in each type of casein were identified. The workflow of the analysis is shown in Figure 3.

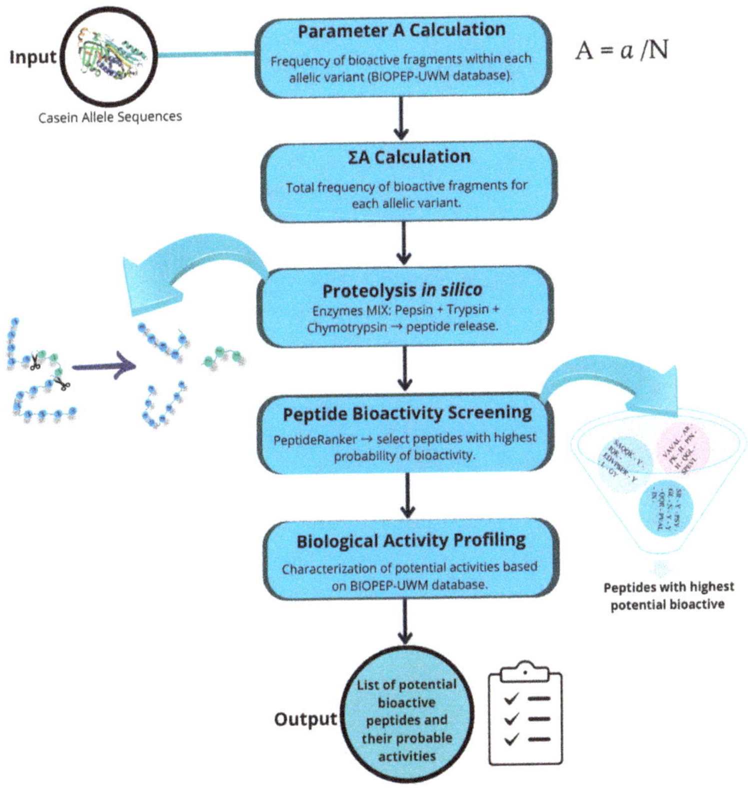

Figure 3. Workflow of the in silico analysis of bioactive peptide release from casein allelic variants.

The potential of the selected casein allele sequences to release bioactive peptides was determined via the BIOPEP-UWM database (https://biochemia.uwm.edu.pl/biopep-uwm/ accessed on 22 April 2025), which contains 5213 known bioactive peptides and 93 biological activities. The BIOPEP-UWM not only simulates proteolytic digestion but also provides curated information from the scientific literature about peptide sequences, protein sources, extraction methods, and evidence of bioactivity. It also integrates data from other specialized databases [36,37].

Using the "calculations" tool available in this database, the A parameter was determined (a quantitative value that characterizes proteins as potential precursors of bioactive peptides). This parameter represents the frequency of the occurrence of bioactive fragments within a protein sequence, considering all bioactive peptides present and their possible bioactivity. This parameter was calculated via the following equation:

$$A = a/N$$

where

a = Number of fragments with a specific activity in a protein sequence;
N = Total number of amino acid residues in the protein.

The total frequency of bioactive fragments in the sequences of each casein allele (α-S1, β-casein, α-S2, and κ-casein) ($\sum A$) was subsequently determined. This is an unweighted summed value that indicates the number of bioactive fragments (with any biological activity reported in the BIOPEP-UWM database) identified in the analyzed sequence [16,36].

4.2. *In Silico Proteolytic Release and Prediction of Bioactive Functions*

For proteolytic release, in silico hydrolysis of each casein/allelic sequence was executed via the BIOPEP-UWM database with the "ENZYME(S) ACTION" tool. The release of bioactive peptides was simulated via the simultaneous action of pepsin (EC 3.4.23.1), trypsin (EC 3.4.21.4) and chymotrypsin A (EC 3.4.21.1) [36,37]. Cleavage sites were assigned based on the default specificity parameters provided by the BIOPEP-UWM platform for each enzyme. These rules define the expected hydrolysis patterns according to enzymatic cleavage preferences previously determined. The simulation considered overlapping peptides resulting from successive cleavage events, which were included in the output.

The potential bioactivity index of the fragments released by proteolysis was evaluated via PeptideRanker software http://distilldeep.ucd.ie/PeptideRanker/ (accessed on 24 April 2025), which predicts how likely the peptide is to be bioactive, on the basis of a novel N-to-1 type neural network. PeptideRanker assigns score values ranging from 0 to 1, where a value greater than 0.5 indicates a high probability of bioactivity; only peptides that exceeded this threshold were considered for evaluating their potential biological activity profile via the "profiles of potential biological activity" tool available in the BIOPEP-UWM bioactive peptide database. The profile of potential biological activity refers to the nature and location of bioactive fragments within a protein or peptide sequence. This concept is based on the premise that the same bioactive fragment, particularly if it is short (2–3 amino acid residues), is not unique to a single protein but can be found in multiple sequences, forming what are known as conserved or common subsequences [36,38,39].

A heatmap was generated in RStudio V.2024.9.1.394 [40] to visualize the assigned bioactivities from each casein allele on the basis of the number of identified bioactive peptides. As different peptides were found to have the same bioactivity, for each gene and allelic variant, a matrix containing the sum values of each bioactivity was then created, and the color gradient in the heatmap was proportional to the intensity of the activity, where white indicates the absence of activity, whereas colored shading represents different levels of bioactive activity.

5. Conclusions

In silico analysis revealed that the most frequent allelic variants of the four casein genes impact the bioactive properties of goat milk, altering the number and composition of peptides released after hydrolysis with different digestive enzymes.

Specific and unique bioactive peptides were found to be α-S2-casein F allelic variants and between α-S1-casein E and F allelic variants. Compared with the other analyzed alleles of the casein genes, the β-casein A and C alleles, α-S1-casein E allele, and α-S2-casein F allele presented greater bioactivity potential.

Additional experimental studies are needed to validate the in silico results and, thus, use casein genotyping to select carriers with allelic variants of goat milk caseins with favorable bioactivities.

Author Contributions: Conceptualization, A.M.S.-R. and A.Y.R.-R.; methodology and formal analysis, A.Y.R.-R.; investigation, A.Y.R.-R. and A.M.S.-R.; writing—original draft preparation, A.Y.R.-R. and A.M.S.-R.; writing—review and editing, A.Y.R.-R., A.M.S.-R., E.C., E.G.-B. and I.D.-E.; supervision, project administration and funding acquisition, A.M.S.-R. All authors have read and agreed to the published version of the manuscript.

Funding: The authors want to thank the Instituto Politécnico Nacional via project SIP 20241271.

Institutional Review Board Statement: Not applicable.

Informed Consent Statement: Not applicable.

Data Availability Statement: Data available on request from the authors.

Acknowledgments: The authors want to thank SECIHTI for support through the master's degree program scholarship (A.Y.R.-R.) and the Instituto Politécnico Nacional via SIP project 20241271 (A.M.S.-R.). The authors also acknowledge Ing. Wilfrido Du Solier Espinosa for the collaboration in the agreement IPN-RANCHO CABRIO, S.P.R. DE R.L.

Conflicts of Interest: The authors declare no conflicts of interest.

Appendix A

Table A1. Frequency of bioactive peptide occurrence (parameter A) in the different variants of α-S1, β, α-S2 and κ-Casein.

∑ Functional Detected Activities	α-S1-Casein				B-Casein		α-S2-Casein				κ-Casein				
	Allele A	**Allele B**	**Allele E**	**Allele F**	**Allele A**	**Allele C**	**Allele A**	**Allele B**	**Allele C**	**Allele F**	**Allele A**	**Allele B**	**Allele C**	**Allele D**	**Allele E**
Alpha-amylase inhibitor	0.0093	0.0093	0.0093	0	0	0	0.0045	0.0045	0.0045	0.0045	0.0062	0.0062	0.0062	0.0062	0.0062
ACE 2 activator	0	0	0	0	0	0	0	0	0	0	0.0062	0.0062	0.0062	0.0062	0.0062
ACE inhibitor	0.5794	0.5794	0.5841	0.4609	0.6441	0.638	0.4888	0.4843	0.4798	0.4888	0.5802	0.5864	0.5864	0.5926	0.6049
ACE2 inhibitor	0.0047	0.0047	0.0047	0.0087	0.0315	0.0317	0	0	0	0.0045	0.0062	0.0062	0.0062	0.0062	0.0062
Activating ubiquitin-mediated proteolysis	0.0093	0.0093	0.0093	0.0087	0.0135	0.0136	0.009	0.009	0.009	0.009	0.0062	0.0062	0.0062	0.0062	0.0062
Alanine carboxypeptidase inhibitor	0.0047	0.0047	0.0047	0	0.0045	0.0045	0.009	0.009	0.009	0.0045	0.0062	0.0062	0.0062	0.0062	0.0062
Alpha-glucosidase inhibitor	0.0374	0.0374	0.0327	0.0261	0.0405	0.0407	0.0179	0.0179	0.0179	0.0179	0.0494	0.0494	0.0556	0.0556	0.0494
Anti inflammatory	0	0	0	0	0.0045	0.0045	0.0135	0.0135	0.0135	0.0135	0.0185	0.0185	0.0185	0.0185	0.0185
Anti-apoptotic	0	0	0	0	0.0045	0.0045	0	0	0	0	0	0	0	0	0
Antiamnestic	0.0047	0.0047	0.0047	0	0.018	0.0181	0.0045	0.0045	0.0045	0.009	0.0123	0.0123	0.0123	0.0123	0.0123
Antibacterial	0.0093	0.0093	0.0047	0	0.009	0.009	0.0179	0.0179	0.009	0.0179	0.0185	0.0185	0.0185	0.0185	0.0185
Anticancer	0.0187	0.0187	0.0187	0.0087	0.009	0.009	0.009	0.009	0.0045	0.009	0	0	0	0	0
Antidiabetic	0.0047	0.0047	0.0047	0	0.009	0.009	0.0045	0.0045	0.0045	0.0045	0	0	0	0	0
Antifungal	0.0047	0.0047	0	0	0	0	0	0	0	0	0	0	0	0	0
Antioxidative	0.243	0.243	0.2336	0.0783	0.1622	0.1629	0.139	0.139	0.139	0.139	0.1914	0.1914	0.1914	0.1914	0.1914
Antithrombotic	0	0	0	0	0.0135	0.0136	0.009	0.009	0.009	0.0135	0.037	0.037	0.037	0.037	0.037
Antiviral	0	0	0	0	0	0	0	0	0	0	0.0062	0.0062	0.0062	0.0062	0.0062
Bacterial permease ligand	0.0047	0.0047	0.0047	0	0.0045	0.0045	0.0135	0.0135	0.009	0.0135	0.0062	0.0062	0.0062	0.0062	0.0062
Binding	0.0047	0.0047	0.0047	0	0.0045	0.0045	0	0	0	0	0	0	0	0	0
Calpain 1 inhibitor	0.0047	0.0047	0.0047	0.0087	0	0	0.0045	0.0045	0.0045	0.0045	0	0	0	0	0
CaMPDE inhibitor	0	0	0	0	0.0045	0.0045	0.0224	0.0224	0.0224	0.0179	0	0	0	0	0
Cathepsin B inhibitor	0	0	0	0	0.0045	0.0045	0	0	0	0	0	0	0	0	0
Citrate lyase deacetylase inhibitor	0.0093	0.0093	0.0093	0	0.0135	0.0136	0.0404	0.0404	0.0404	0.0404	0	0	0	0	0
Contracting	0	0	0	0	0	0	0	0	0	0	0.0247	0.0247	0.0247	0.0247	0.0247
D-Ala-D-Ala dipeptidase inhibitor	0	0	0.0047	0	0	0	0	0	0	0	0	0	0	0	0
Dipeptidyl peptidase III inhibitor	0.1075	0.1075	0.1075	0.0957	0.0946	0.0905	0.0717	0.0717	0.0717	0.0762	0.0741	0.0741	0.0802	0.0864	0.0741
Dipeptidyl peptidase IV inhibitor	0.6168	0.6168	0.6075	0.5826	0.8514	0.8462	0.6771	0.6682	0.6771	0.6771	0.7778	0.784	0.7778	0.7778	0.7778
Glutamate carboxypeptidase II inhibitor	0.028	0.0327	0.0327	0.0087	0.0225	0.0226	0.0583	0.0538	0.0583	0.0583	0.0185	0.0185	0.0185	0.0185	0.0185
Glutamate carboxypeptidase inhibitor	0.0093	0.0093	0.0093	0	0.0225	0.0226	0.0404	0.0404	0.0404	0.0404	0	0	0	0	0
HMG-CoA reductase inhibitor	0	0	0	0	0	0	0	0	0	0	0.0062	0.0062	0.0062	0.0062	0.0062
Hypotensive	0.0187	0.0187	0.0234	0.0087	0.0225	0.0226	0.009	0.009	0.009	0.0135	0.0185	0.0185	0.0185	0.0185	0.0185
Hypouricemic	0.0327	0.0327	0.0234	0.0348	0.036	0.0362	0.0179	0.0179	0.0179	0.0179	0.0494	0.0494	0.0494	0.0494	0.0494
Immunomodulating	0.0047	0.0047	0	0	0	0	0	0	0	0	0	0	0	0	0
Immunostimulating	0.0047	0.0047	0.0047	0	0.009	0.009	0	0	0	0	0.0062	0.0062	0.0062	0.0062	0.0062
Inhibitor	0.0047	0.0047	0.0047	0	0	0	0	0	0	0	0.0062	0.0062	0.0062	0.0062	0.0062
Inhibitor of cytosol alanyl aminopeptidase	0.014	0.014	0.0187	0.0174	0.0045	0.0045	0.0045	0.0045	0.0045	0.0045	0	0	0	0	0
Inhibitor of tripeptidyl peptidase II	0.0374	0.0374	0.0421	0.0522	0.0315	0.0362	0.0269	0.0269	0.0269	0.0224	0.0185	0.0185	0.0185	0.0185	0.0185
Lactocepin inhibitor	0.028	0.028	0.028	0.0261	0.045	0.0452	0.0045	0.0045	0.0045	0.0045	0.0123	0.0123	0.0123	0.0123	0.0123
Leucyltransferase inhibitor	0.0047	0.0047	0.0047	0.0087	0.0045	0.0045	0	0	0	0	0.0062	0.0062	0.0062	0.0062	0.0062
Lipoxygenase inhibitor	0	0	0	0	0.009	0.009	0	0	0	0	0	0	0	0	0
Neprilysin 2 inhibitor	0.0047	0.0047	0.0047	0.0087	0	0	0.0045	0.0045	0.0045	0.0045	0	0	0	0	0
Neprilysin inhibitor	0.0327	0.0374	0.0374	0.0348	0.0586	0.0633	0.0314	0.0269	0.0269	0.0359	0.0617	0.0617	0.0617	0.0617	0.0617
Neurolysin inhibitor	0.0047	0.0047	0.0047	0.0087	0	0	0	0	0	0	0.0062	0.0062	0.0062	0.0062	0.0062
Neuropeptide	0.0374	0.0374	0.0374	0.0174	0.018	0.0181	0.0224	0.0224	0.0224	0.0224	0.0185	0.0185	0.0185	0.0247	0.0247
Opioid	0.014	0.014	0.014	0	0.0135	0.0136	0.0045	0.0045	0.0045	0	0	0	0	0	0

Table A1. *Cont.*

∑ Functional Detected Activities	α-S1-Casein				B-Casein		α-S2-Casein				κ-Casein				
	Allele A	Allele B	Allele E	Allele F	Allele A	Allele C	Allele A	Allele B	Allele C	Allele F	Allele A	Allele B	Allele C	Allele D	Allele E
Opioid agonist	0.0047	0.0047	0.0047	0	0	0	0	0	0	0	0	0	0	0	0
Opioid antagonist	0	0	0	0	0	0	0	0	0	0	0.0247	0.0247	0.0247	0.0247	0.0247
Osteoanabolic	0.0093	0.0093	0.0093	0	0.0045	0.0045	0	0	0	0	0.0123	0.0123	0.0123	0.0123	0.0123
Pancreatic lipase inhibitor	0	0	0	0.0087	0.0045	0.0045	0.0045	0.0045	0.0045	0.0045	0	0	0	0	0
Peptidylprolyl isomerase inhibitor	0.0093	0.0093	0.0093	0.0087	0	0	0.0045	0.0045	0.0045	0.0045	0	0	0.0062	0.0062	0
Phospholipase A2 inhibitor	0	0	0	0	0	0	0.009	0.009	0.009	0.009	0.0123	0.0123	0.0123	0.0123	0.0123
Pseudolysin inhibitor	0	0	0	0	0	0	0.0045	0.0045	0.0045	0.0045	0.0062	0.0062	0.0062	0.0062	0.0062
Regulating	0.0047	0.0047	0.0047	0	0.036	0.0362	0.0045	0.0045	0.0045	0.009	0	0	0	0	0
Renin inhibitor	0.028	0.028	0.0234	0.0261	0.0315	0.0317	0.0448	0.0448	0.0448	0.0448	0.0185	0.0185	0.0185	0.0185	0.0185
Stimulating	0.0888	0.0888	0.0841	0.0696	0.1036	0.0995	0.0852	0.0852	0.0897	0.0852	0.037	0.037	0.037	0.0309	0.037
Thymidylate synthase inhibitor	0.0093	0.0093	0.0093	0	0.0135	0.0136	0.0404	0.0404	0.0404	0.0404	0	0	0	0	0
Toxic	0.0093	0.0093	0.0093	0.0087	0	0	0.009	0.009	0.0045	0.009	0	0	0	0	0
Tubulin-tyrosine ligase inhibitor	0.014	0.014	0.014	0	0	0	0.009	0.009	0.009	0.009	0.0247	0.0247	0.0247	0.0247	0.0247
Xaa-pro inhibitor	0.0093	0.0093	0.0093	0.0087	0.018	0.0181	0	0	0	0	0	0	0	0	0
∑A	2.1447	2.1541	2.1216	1.6351	2.4500	2.4429	1.9959	1.9735	1.9645	2.0094	2.1914	2.2038	2.2161	2.2286	2.2223

Appendix B

(A)

A M - K - L - L - IL - TCL - VAVAL - AR - PK - H - PIN - H - QGL - SPEVL - N - EN - L - L - R - F -
B M - K - L - L - IL - TCL - VAVAL - AR - PK - H - PIN - H - QGL - SPEVL - N - EN - L - L - R - F -
E M - K - L - L - IL - TCL - VAVAL - AR - PK - H - PIN - H - QGL - SPEVPN - EN - L - L - R - F -
F M - K - L - L - IL - TCL - VAVAL - AR - PK - H - PIN - H - QGL - SPEVPN - EN - L - L - R - F -

A VVAPF - PEVF - R - K - EN - IN - EL - SK - DIGSESTEDQAM - EDAK - QM - K - AGSSSSSEEIVPN
B VVAPF - PEVF - R - K - EN - IN - EL - SK - DIGSESTEDQAM - EDAK - QM - K - AGSSSSSEEIVPN
E VVAPF - PEVF - R - K - EN - IN - EL - SK - DIGSESTEDQAM - EDAK - QM - K - AGSSSSSEEIVPN
F VVAPF - PEVF - R - K - EN - IN - EL - SK - DIGSESTEDQAM - EDAK - QM - K- AGSSCQVR - K

A - SAQQK - Y - IQK - EDVPSER - Y - L - GY - L - EQL - L - R - L - K - K - Y - N - VPQL - EIVPK -
B - SAEQK - Y - IQK - EDVPSER - Y - L - GY - L - EQL - L - R - L - K - K - Y - N - VPQL – EIVPK -
E - SAEQK - Y - IQK - EDVPSER - Y - L - GY - L - EQL - L - K - L - K - K - Y - N - VPQL - EIVPK -
F - L - F - PIVL - SR - STF - K - R - K - M - CPL - SVTW - VTW - N - SF - SD

A SAEEQL - H - SM - K - EGN - PAH - QK - QPM - IAVN - QEL - AY - F - Y - PQL - F - R - QF - Y -
B SAEEQL - H - SM - K - EGN - PAH - QK - QPM - IAVN - QEL - AY - F - Y - PQL - F - R - QF - Y -
E SAEEQL - H - SM - K - EGN - PAH - QK - QPM - IAVN - QEL - AY - F - Y - PQL - F - R - QF - Y -
F

A QL - DAY - PSGAW - Y - Y - L - PL - GTQY - TDAPSF - SDIPN - PIGSEN - SGK - TTM - PL - W
B QL - DAY - PSGAW - Y - Y - L - PL - GTQY - TDAPSF - SDIPN - PIGSEN - SGK - TTM - PL - W
E QL - DAY - PSGAW - Y - Y - L - PL - GTQY - TDAPSF - SDIPN - PIGSEN - SGK - AAM - PL - W
F

(B)

A M - K - VL - IL - ACL - VAL - AL - AR - EQEEL - N - VVGETVESL - SSSEESITH - IN - K - K - IEK
C M - K - VL - IL - ACL - VAL - AL - AR - EQEEL - N - VVGETVESL - SSSEESITH - IN - K - K - IEK

A - F - QSEEQQQTEDEL - QDK - IH - PF - AQAQSL - VY - PF - TGPIPN - SL - PQN - IL - PL -
C - F - QSEEQQQTEDEL - QDK - IH - PF - AQAQSL - VY - PF - TGPIPN - SL - PQN - IL - PL -

A TQTPVVVPPF - L - QPEIM - GVPK - VK - ETM - VPK - H - K - EM - PF - PK - Y - PVEPF - TESQSL
C TQTPVVVPPF - L - QPEIM - GVPK - VK - ETM - VPK - H - K - EM - PF - PK - Y - PVEPF - TESQSL

A - TL - TDVEK - L - H - L - PL - PL - VQSW - M - H - QPPQPL - SPTVM - F - PPQSVL - SL - SQPK
C - TL - TDVEK - L - H - L - PL - PL - VQSW - M - H - QPPQPL - SPTVM - F - PPQSVL - SL - SQPK

A - VL - PVPQK - AVPQR - DM - PIQAF - L - L - Y - QEPVL - GPVR - GPF - PIL - V
C - VL - PVPQK - VVPQR - DM - PIQAF - L - L - Y - QEPVL - GPVR - GPF - PIL

(C)

A M - K - F - F - IF - TCL - L - AVAL - AK - H - K - M - EH - VSSSEEPIN - IF - QEIY - K - QEK - N -
B M - K - F - F - IF - TCL - L - AVAL - AK - H - K - M - EH - VSSSEEPIN - IF - QEIY - K - QEK - N -
C M - K - F - F - IF - TCL - L - AVAL - AK - H - K - M - EH - VSSSEEPIN - IF - QEIY - K - QEK - N -
F M - K - F - F - IF - TCL - L - AVAL - AK - H - K - M - EH - ISSSEEPIN - IF - QEIY - K - QEK - N -

A M - AIH - PR - K - EK - L - CTTSCEEVVR - N - AN - EEEY - SIR - SSSEESAEVAPEEIK - ITVDDK
B M - AIH - PR - K - EK - L - CTTSCEEVVR - N - AN - EEEY - SIR - SSSEESAKVAPEEIK - ITVDDK
C M - AIH - PR - K - EK - L - CTTSCEEVVR - N - AN - EEEY - SIR - SSSEESAEVAPEEIK - ITVDDK
F M - AIH - PR - K - EK - L - CTTSCEEVVR - N - AN - EEEY - SIR - SSSEESAEVAPEEIK - ITVDDK

A - H - Y - QK - AL - N - EIN - QF - Y - QK - F - PQY - L - QY - PY - QGPIVL - N - PW - DQVK - R -
B - H - Y - QK - AL - N - EIN - QF - Y - QK - F - PQY - L - QY - PY - QGPIVL - N - PW - DQVK - R -
C - H - Y - QK - AL - N - EIN - QF - Y - QK - F - PQY - L - QY - PY - QGPIVL - N - PW - DQVK - R -
F - H - Y - QK - AL - N - EIN - QF - Y - QK - F - PQY - L - QY - PY - QGPIVL - N - PW - DQVK - R -

A N - AGAF - TPTVN - R - EQL - STSEEN - SK - K - TIDM - ESTEVF - TK - K - TK - L - TEEEK - N
B N - AGAF - TPTVN - R - EQL - STSEEN - SK - K - TIDM - ESTEVF - TK - K - TK - L - TEEEK - N
C N - AGAF - TPTVN - R - EQL - STSEEN - SK - K - TIDM - ESTEVF - TK - K - TK - L - TEEEK - N
F N - AGPF - TPTVN - R - EQL - STSEEN - SK - K - TIDM - ESTEVF - TK - K - TK - L - TEEEK - N

A - R - L - N - F - L - K - K - ISQY - Y - QK - F - AW - PQY - L - K - TVDQH - QK - AM - K - PW -
B - R - L - N - F - L - K - K - ISQY - Y - QK - F - AW - PQY - L - K - TVDQH - QK - AM - K - PW -
C - R - L - N - F - L - K - IISQY - Y - QK - F - AW - PQY - L - K - TVDQH - QK - AM - K - PW -
F - R - L - N - F - L - K - K - ISQY - Y - QK - F - AW - PQY - L - K - TVDQH - QK - AM - K – PW -

A TQPK - TN - AIPY - VR - Y - L
B TQPK - TN - AIPY - VR - Y - L
C TQPK - TN - AIPY - VR - Y - L
F TQPK - TN - AIPY - VR - Y - L

(D)

A CCEK - DER - F - F - DDK - IAK - Y - IPIQY - VL - SR - Y - PSY - GL - N - Y - Y - QQR - PVAL -
B CCEK - DER - F - F - DDK - IAK - Y - IPIQY - VL - SR - Y - PSY - GL - N - Y - Y - QQR - PVAL -
C CCEK - DER - F - F - DDK - IAK - Y - IPIQY - VL - SR - Y - PSY - GL - N - Y - Y - QQR - PVAL -
D CCEK - DER - F - F - DDK - IAK - Y - IPIQY - VL - SR - Y - PSY - GL - N - Y - Y - R - QR - PVAL -
E CCEK - DER - F - F - DDK - IAK - Y - IPIQY - VL - SR - Y - PSY - GL - N - Y - Y - QQR - PVAL -

A IN - N - QF - L - PY - PY - Y - AK - PVAVR - SPAQTL - QW - QVL - PN - TVPAK - SCQDQPTTL -
B IN - N - QF - L - PY - PY - Y - AK - PVAVR - SPAQTL - QW - QVL - PN - TVPAK - SCQDQPTTL -
C IN - N - QF - L - PY - PY - Y - AK - PIAVR - SPAQTL - QW - QVL - PN - TVPAK - SCQDQPTTL -
D IN - N - QF - L - PY - PY - Y - AK - PIAVR - SPAQTL - QW - QVL - PN - TVPAK - SCQDQPTTL -
E IN - N - QF - L - PY - PY - Y - AK - PVAVR - SPAQTL - QW - QVL - PN - TVPAK - SCQGQPTTL -

A AR - H - PH - PH - L - SF - M - AIPPK - K - DQDK - TEVPAIN - TIASAEPTVH - STPTTEAIVN -
B AR - H - PH - PH - L - SF - M - AIPPK - K - DQDK - TEIPAIN - TIASAEPTVH - STPTTEAIVN -
C AR - H - PH - PH - L - SF - M - AIPPK - K - DQDK - TEIPAIN - TIASAEPTVH - STPTTEAIVN -
D AR - H - PH - PH - L - SF - M - AIPPK - K - DQDK - TEIPAIN - TIASAEPTVH - STPTTEAIVN -
E AR - H - PH - PH - L - SF - M - AIPPK - K - DQDK - TEIPAIN - TIASAEPTVH - STPTTEAIVN -

A TVDN - PEASSESIASASETN - TAQVTSTEV
B TVDN - PEASSESIASASETN - TAQVTSTEV
C TVDN - PEASSESIVSAPETN - TAQVTSTEV
D TVDN - PEASSESIASAPETN - TAQVTSTEV
E TVDN - PEASSESIASASETN - TAQVTSTEV

Figure A1. Comparison of in silico proteolysis results using pepsin, trypsin, and chymotrypsin in goat casein alleles: (**A**) α-S1-casein alleles, (**B**) β-casein alleles, (**C**) α-S2-casein alleles, and (**D**) κ-casein alleles. Peptides unique to each allele are highlighted in yellow.

Appendix C

Table A2. Results of the bioactivity index of peptides released by in silico enzymatic hydrolysis using Peptide Ranker software.

No	Peptide	Activity Prediction	No	Peptide	Activity Prediction	No	Peptide	Activity Prediction
1	IL	0.392515	59	TTM	0.137765	117	AN	0.156915
2	TCL	0.47708	60	AAM	0.55858	118	EEEY	0.0347581
3	VAVAL	0.114473	61	VL	0.126025	119	SIR	0.292181
4	AR	0.394584	62	ACL	0.746733	120	SSSEESAEVAPEEIK	0.128476
5	PK	0.325772	63	VAL	0.127235	121	ITVDDK	0.0507604
6	PIN	0.392694	64	AL	0.43789	122	EIN	0.0574424
7	QGL	0.533495	65	EQEEL	0.0476195	123	PQY	0.465473
8	SPEVL	0.240941	66	VVGETVESL	0.044042	124	QY	0.233017
9	SPEVPN	0.288857	67	SSSEESITH	0.123839	125	PY	0.736696
10	EN	0.0363788	68	IEK	0.0431926	126	QGPIVL	0.474397
11	VVAPF	0.482403	69	QSEEQQQTEDEL	0.0562204	127	PW	0.992911
12	PEVF	0.416246	70	QDK	0.0742183	128	DQVK	0.0569847
13	IN	0.152106	71	IH	0.213873	129	AGAF	0.873661
14	EL	0.0728272	72	PF	0.99343	130	AGPF	0.969222
15	SK	0.0732708	73	AQAQSL	0.187449	131	TPTVN	0.0691266
16	DIGSESTEDQAM	0.118262	74	VY	0.0989681	132	STSEEN	0.0452869
17	EDAK	0.0508357	75	TGPIPN	0.416883	133	TIDM	0.226127
18	QM	0.607122	76	SL	0.330018	134	ESTEVF	0.118496
19	AGSSSSSEEIVPN	0.150856	77	PQN	0.285353	135	TEEEK	0.0196166
20	AGSSCQVR	0.361516	78	TQTPVVVPPF	0.213655	136	ISQY	0.183534
21	PIVL	0.3331	79	QPEIM	0.368217	137	AW	0.9669
22	SR	0.308189	80	GVPK	0.24186	138	TVDQH	0.048737
23	STF	0.58977	81	VK	0.03329	139	AM	0.74549
24	CPL	0.916551	82	ETM	0.0952962	140	TQPK	0.117696
25	SVTW	0.38436	83	VPK	0.135867	141	TN	0.0512668
26	VIW	0.610494	84	EM	0.194256	142	AIPY	0.613395
27	SF	0.948796	85	PVEPF	0.604782	143	VR	0.114691
28	SD	0.102577	86	TESQSL	0.0615565	144	CCEK	0.328494
29	SAQQK	0.115388	87	TL	0.144542	145	DER	0.0799595
30	SAEQK	0.0721709	88	TDVEK	0.0283043	146	DDK	0.0807603
31	IQK	0.0864674	89	VQSW	0.328419	147	IAK	0.112126
32	EDVPSER	0.0960623	90	QPPQPL	0.823819	148	IPIQY	0.360781
33	GY	0.741592	91	SPTVM	0.441571	149	PSY	0.46941
34	EQL	0.0721403	92	PPQSVL	0.447296	150	GL	0.808777
35	VPQL	0.306426	93	SQPK	0.227354	151	QQR	0.201093
36	EIVPK	0.0893465	94	PVPQK	0.223551	152	PVAL	0.277634
37	SAEEQL	0.104281	95	AVPQR	0.253856	153	PVAVR	0.134071
38	SM	0.628268	96	VVPQR	0.140161	154	PIAVR	0.239292
39	EGN	0.094901	97	DM	0.607466	155	SPAQTL	0.459196
40	PAH	0.432769	98	PIQAF	0.749093	156	QW	0.928524
41	QK	0.0619833	99	QEPVL	0.19215	157	QVL	0.120783
42	QPM	0.810167	100	GPVR	0.488393	158	PN	0.480465
43	IAVN	0.0822104	101	GPF	0.989324	159	TVPAK	0.0926354
44	QEL	0.0839476	102	PIL	0.641797	160	SCQDQPTTL	0.428259
45	AY	0.346246	103	IF	0.949173	161	PH	0.541688
46	PQL	0.527882	104	AVAL	0.158386	162	AIPPK	0.575607
47	QF	0.946135	105	AK	0.0979062	163	DQDK	0.0824949
48	QL	0.2924	106	EH	0.0533694	164	TEVPAIN	0.0754348
49	DAY	0.234477	107	VSSSEEPIN	0.148998	165	TEIPAIN	0.108978
50	PSGAW	0.870583	108	ISSSEEPIN	0.19248	166	TIASAEPTVH	0.0919084
51	PL	0.811148	109	QEIY	0.12052	167	STPTTEAIVN	0.0575411
52	GTQY	0.184477	110	QEK	0.0353735	168	TVDN	0.0382016
53	TDAPSF	0.417727	111	AIH	0.212314	169	PEASSESIASASETN	0.131678
54	SDIPN	0.394725	112	PR	0.787626	170	PEASSESIVSAPETN	0.126334
55	PIGSEN	0.146949	113	EK	0.0247356	171	TAQVTSTEV	0.0300416
56	SGK	0.220066	114	CTTSCEEVVR	0.0950641	172	SCQGQPTTL	0.424559
57	SSSEESAKVAPEEIK	0.167177	115	IISQY	0.162259			
58	TK	0.0329947	116	QR	0.274416			

References

1. Nayik, G.A.; Jagdale, Y.D.; Gaikwad, S.A.; Devkatte, A.N.; Dar, A.H.; Ansari, M.J. Nutritional profile, processing and potential products: A comparative review of goat milk. *Dairy* **2022**, *3*, 622–647. [CrossRef]

2. Rahmatalla, S.A.; Arends, D.; Brockmann, G.A. Genetic and protein variants of milk caseins in goats. *Front. Genet.* **2022**, *13*, 995349. [CrossRef] [PubMed]
3. Marletta, D.; Criscione, A.; Bordonaro, S.; Guastella, A.M.; d'Urso, G. Casein polymorphism in goat's milk. *Dairy Sci. Technol.* **2007**, *87*, 491–504. [CrossRef]
4. Pal, S.; Woodford, K.; Kukuljan, S.; Ho, S. Milk intolerance, beta-casein and lactose. *Nutrients* **2015**, *7*, 7285–7297. [CrossRef]
5. Dantas, A.; Kumar, H.; Prudencio, E.S.; de Avila Junior, L.B.; Orellana-Palma, P.; Dosoky, N.S.; Kumar, D. An approach on detection, quantification, technological properties, and trends market of A2 cow milk. *Food Res. Int.* **2023**, *167*, 112690. [CrossRef]
6. Giribaldi, M.; Lamberti, C.; Cirrincione, S.; Giuffrida, M.G.; Cavallarin, L. A2 milk and BCM-7 peptide as emerging parameters of milk quality. *Front. Nutr.* **2022**, *9*, 842375. [CrossRef]
7. Kashung, P.; Karuthapandian, D. Milk-derived bioactive peptides. *Food Prod. Process Nutr.* **2025**, *7*, 6. [CrossRef]
8. Ouafi, A.T.; Babilliot, J.M.; Leroux, C.; Martin, P. Genetic diversity of the two main Moroccan goat breeds: Phylogenetic relationships with four breeds reared in France. *Small Rumin. Res.* **2002**, *45*, 225–233. [CrossRef]
9. Maga, E.A.; Daftari, P.; Kültz, D.; Penedo, M.C.T. Prevalence of αs1-casein genotypes in American dairy goats. *J. Anim. Sci.* **2009**, *87*, 3464–3469. [CrossRef]
10. Chessa, S.; Budelli, E.; Chiatti, F.; Cito, A.M.; Bolla, P.; Caroli, A. Predominance of β-casein (CSN2) C allele in goat breeds reared in Italy. Journal of dairy science. *J. Dairy Sci.* **2005**, *88*, 1878–1881. [CrossRef]
11. Ibrahim, H.R.; Ahmed, A.S.; Miyata, T. Novel angiotensin-converting enzyme inhibitory peptides from caseins and whey proteins of goat milk. *J. Adv. Res.* **2017**, *8*, 63–71. [CrossRef] [PubMed]
12. Sharma, G.; Rout, P.K.; Kaushik, R.; Singh, G. Identification of bioactive peptides in goat milk and their health application. *J. Adv. Dairy Res.* **2017**, *5*, 1000191. [CrossRef]
13. Guha, S.; Sharma, H.; Deshwal, G.K.; Rao, P.S. A comprehensive review on bioactive peptides derived from milk and milk products of minor dairy species. *Food Prod. Process. Nutr.* **2021**, *3*, 2. [CrossRef]
14. Dos Santos, W.M.; Gomes, A.C.G.; de Caldas Nobre, M.S.; de Souza Pereira, Á.M.; dos Santos Pereira, E.V.; dos Santos, K.M.O.; Buriti, F.C.A. Goat milk as a natural source of bioactive compounds and strategies to enhance the amount of these beneficial components. *Int. Dairy J.* **2023**, *137*, 105515. [CrossRef]
15. Dave, L.A.; Montoya, C.A.; Rutherfurd, S.M.; Moughan, P.J. Gastrointestinal endogenous proteins as a source of bioactive peptides-an in silico study. *PLoS ONE* **2014**, *9*, e98922. [CrossRef]
16. Lin, K.; Zhang, L.W.; Han, X.; Xin, L.; Meng, Z.X.; Gong, P.M.; Cheng, D.Y. Yak milk casein as potential precursor of angiotensin I-converting enzyme inhibitory peptides based on in silico proteolysis. *Food Chem.* **2018**, *254*, 340–347. [CrossRef] [PubMed]
17. Gu, Y.; Li, X.; Qi, X.; Ma, Y.; Chan, E.C.Y. In silico identification of novel ACE and DPP-IV inhibitory peptides derived from buffalo milk proteins and evaluation of their inhibitory mechanisms. *Amino Acids* **2023**, *55*, 161–171. [CrossRef]
18. Sundarraj, A.A.; Rajathi, A.A.; Vishaal, S.C.; Rohit, D.; Prakash, M.S.; Sam, A.A.; Seihenbalg, S.S. Food biotechnology applications in dairy and dairy products. *J. Pharm. Res.* **2018**, *12*, 520–525.
19. Balthazar, C.F.; Pimentel, T.C.; Ferrão, L.L.; Almada, C.N.; Santillo, A.; Albenzio, M.; Cruz, A.G. Sheep milk: Physicochemical characteristics and relevance for functional food development. *Compr. Rev. Food Sci. Food Saf.* **2017**, *16*, 247–262. [CrossRef]
20. Nongonierma, A.B.; FitzGerald, R.J. Strategies for the discovery and identification of food protein-derived biologically active peptides. *Trends Food Sci. Technol.* **2017**, *69*, 289–305. [CrossRef]
21. Cui, Q.; Duan, Y.; Zhang, M.; Liang, S.; Sun, Y.; Cheng, J.; Guo, M. Peptide profiles and antioxidant capacity of extensive hydrolysates of milk protein concentrate. *J. Dairy Sci.* **2022**, *105*, 7972–7985. [CrossRef] [PubMed]
22. Giacometti, J.; Buretić-Tomljanović, A. Peptidomics as a tool for characterizing bioactive milk peptides. *Food Chem.* **2017**, *230*, 91–98. [CrossRef]
23. Yang, M.; Yang, Z.; Everett, D.W.; Gilbert, E.P.; Singh, H.; Ye, A. Digestion of food proteins: The role of pepsin. *Crit. Rev. Food Sci. Nutr.* **2025**, 1–22. [CrossRef]
24. Martin, P.; Ollivier-Bousquet, M.; Grosclaude, F. Genetic polymorphism of caseins: A tool to investigate casein micelle organization. *Int. Dairy J.* **1999**, *9*, 163–171. [CrossRef]
25. Ramunno, L.; Cosenza, G.; Rando, A.; Pauciullo, A.; Illario, R.; Gallo, D.; Masina, P. Comparative analysis of gene sequence of goat CSN1S1 F and N alleles and characterization of CSN1S1 transcript variants in mammary gland. *Gene* **2005**, *345*, 289–299. [CrossRef]
26. Lunagariya, N.A.; Patel, N.K.; Jagtap, S.C.; Bhutani, K.K. Inhibitors of pancreatic lipase: State of the art and clinical perspectives. *EXCLI J.* **2014**, *13*, 897–921. [PubMed]
27. Udenigwe, C.C.; Aluko, R.E. Multifunctional cationic peptide fractions from flaxseed protein hydrolysates. *Plant Foods Hum. Nutr.* **2012**, *67*, 1–9. [CrossRef] [PubMed]
28. Lv, M.; Zhang, Y.J.; Zhou, F.; Ge, Y.; Zhao, M.H.; Liu, Y.; Yang, K.W. Real-time monitoring of D-Ala-D-Ala dipeptidase activity of VanX in living bacteria by isothermal titration calorimetry. *Anal. Biochem.* **2019**, *578*, 29–35. [CrossRef]

29. Nongonierma, A.B.; Cadamuro, C.; Le Gouic, A.; Mudgil, P.; Maqsood, S.; FitzGerald, R.J. Dipeptidyl peptidase IV (DPP-IV) inhibitory properties of a camel whey protein enriched hydrolysate preparation. *Food Chem.* **2019**, *279*, 70–79. [CrossRef]
30. Daliri, E.B.M.; Lee, B.H.; Oh, D.H. Current trends and perspectives of bioactive peptides. *Crit. Rev. Food Sci. Nutr.* **2018**, *5813*, 2273–2284. [CrossRef]
31. Singh, B.P.; Aluko, R.E.; Hati, S.; Solanki, D. Bioactive peptides in the management of lifestyle-related diseases: Current trends and future perspectives. *Crit. Rev. Food Sci. Nutr.* **2022**, *62*, 4593–4606. [CrossRef]
32. Wu, Y.; Zhang, J.; Mu, T.; Zhang, H.; Cao, J.; Li, H.; Zhao, K. Selection of goat β-casein derived ACE-inhibitory peptide SQPK and insights into its effect and regulatory mechanism on the function of endothelial cells. *Int. J. Biol. Macromol.* **2023**, *253*, 127312. [CrossRef] [PubMed]
33. Udenigwe, C.C. Bioinformatics approaches, prospects and challenges of food bioactive peptide research. *Trends Food Sci Technol.* **2014**, *36*, 137–143. [CrossRef]
34. Srinivas, S.; Prakash, V. Bioactive peptides from bovine milk α-casein: Isolation, characterization and multifunctional properties. *Int. J. Pept. Res. Ther.* **2010**, *16*, 7–15. [CrossRef]
35. Tamura, K.; Stecher, G.; Kumar, S. MEGA11: Molecular evolutionary genetics analysis version 11. *Mol. Biol. Evol.* **2021**, *38*, 3022–3027. [CrossRef]
36. Minkiewicz, P.; Iwaniak, A.; Darewicz, M. BIOPEP-UWM database of bioactive peptides: Current opportunities. *Int. J. Mol. Sci.* **2019**, *20*, 5978. [CrossRef] [PubMed]
37. Minkiewicz, P.; Dziuba, J.; Iwaniak, A.; Dziuba, M.; Darewicz, M. BIOPEP database and other programs for processing bioactive peptide sequences. *J. AOAC Int.* **2008**, *91*, 965–980. [CrossRef]
38. Minkiewicz, P.; Darewicz, M.; Iwaniak, A.; Sokołowska, J.; Starowicz, P.; Bucholska, J.; Hrynkiewicz, M. Common amino acid subsequences in a universal proteome—Relevance for food science. *Int. J. Mol. Sci.* **2015**, *16*, 20748–20773. [CrossRef]
39. Dziuba, J.; Minkiewicz, P.; Nałecz, D.; Iwaniak, A. Database of biologically active peptide sequences. *Food/Nahrung* **1999**, *43*, 190–195. [CrossRef]
40. Posit team. *RStudio: Integrated Development Environment for R*; Posit Software, PBC: Boston, MA, USA, 2024. Available online: http://www.posit.co/ (accessed on 25 April 2025).

molecules

MDPI

Review

The Role of *Wolfiporia cocos* (F. A. *Wolf*) Ryvarden and Gilb. Polysaccharides in Regulating the Gut Microbiota and Its Health Benefits

Yong Lai [1,†], Xin Lan [2,†], Zhicheng Chen [3], Guanhua Lou [1], Ying Li [1], Chang Liu [1], Jianan Feng [1], Xi Li [1,*] and Yu Wang [1,*]

1 Institute of Traditional Chinese Medicine of Sichuan Academy of Chinese Medicine Sciences, Chengdu 610031, China; yonglai3210@163.com (Y.L.); louguanhua@sc2zzy.com (G.L.); liying@sc2zzy.com (Y.L.); liuchang@sc2zzy.com (C.L.); fengjianan@sc2zzy.com (J.F.)

2 School of Basic Medical Sciences, Southwest Medical University, Luzhou 646000, China; lanxin202202@163.com

3 School of Clinic Medical Sciences, Southwest Medical University, Luzhou 646000, China; 15281207768@163.com

* Correspondence: lixi@sc2zzy.com (X.L.); wyontheway01@163.com (Y.W.)

† These authors contributed equally to this work.

Abstract: *Wolfiporia cocos* (F. A. *Wolf*) Ryvarden and Gilb. is a widely used herb in China, belonging to the large fungi of the family Polyporaceae. *P. cocos*; it consists of a variety of biologically active ingredients such as polysaccharides, triterpenes, and sterols, and is considered a treasure in traditional Chinese medicine (TCM). Notably, *P. cocos* polysaccharides, as the most prominent constituent, are of interest for their superior anti-obesity, anti-tumor, anti-inflammatory, antioxidant, and immunomodulatory activities. *P. cocos* polysaccharides can be divided into water-soluble polysaccharides and water-insoluble polysaccharides, which may contribute to their diverse biological functions. Numerous scholars have focused on the extraction process, structural identification, and classical pharmacological pathways of *P. cocos* polysaccharides, but there are few systematic reviews on *P. cocos* polysaccharides regulating the gut microbiota. Natural products and their active ingredients are closely related to intestinal health, and further exploration of these mechanisms is warranted. This review summarizes the recent cases of *P. cocos* polysaccharides regulating the gut microbiota to promote health and discusses their relationship with bioactive functions. It aims to provide a basis for exploring the new mechanisms of *P. cocos* polysaccharides in promoting intestinal health and offers a new vision for the further development of functional products.

Keywords: *Wolfiporia cocos*; polysaccharides; gut microbiota; pharmacological function; health benefits

1. Introduction

Wolfiporia cocos (F. A. *Wolf*) Ryvarden and Gilb. is a common and famous traditional Chinese medicine, mainly distributed in China, America, Oceania, Japan, and Southeast Asia [1]. *P. cocos* typically parasitizes the roots of pine trees and is classified as the dried mycelium of the fungus *Poria cocos* (Schw.) *Wolf*, belonging to the family Polyporaceae [2]. It is a kind of a large fungal plant, which is popular and has unique medicinal and edible values [3]. As one of the Chinese treasures in the past and present, *P. cocos* has a great demand in the market and has broad development prospects.

P. cocos has been used as a traditional Chinese medicine and dietary supplement for over 2000 years, and it has been described as a "medicine for all seasons". According to TCM, *P. cocos* has the effects of inducing diuresis and seepage of dampness, strengthening the spleen, and tranquilizing the heart [4]. Modern pharmacological studies have indicated that *P. cocos* has a variety of biological activities such as hypoglycemic, hypolipidemic, anti-tumor, anti-inflammatory, antioxidant, and immunomodulatory effects [5,6]. The active ingredients of *P. cocos* include polysaccharides, triterpenes, sterols, amino acids, proteins, nucleotides, and trace elements [7]. Polysaccharides are a class of macromolecular carbohydrates, and polysaccharides are the most important active ingredient in *P. cocos*, accounting for 70–90% of the total mass of the fungus [8]. *P. cocos* triterpenoids are diversified and have significant activities, mainly including *P. cocos* acid, tulmoic acid, and ibruric acid [9]. *P. cocos* polysaccharides and triterpenes are widely used and rich in pharmacological activities, mainly in the fields of anti-tumor, immunity regulation, and hypoglycemia effects [10]. In recent years, isolation technology and pharmacological research on the active ingredients of *P. cocos* have developed rapidly [11]. However, the active ingredients in *P. cocos* have not been fully clarified, and the biological activities of some components are still unknown. In addition, the pharmacological mechanisms and targets of action of *P. cocos* have not been fully elucidated, especially the mechanism of its multicomponent synergistic action. Therefore, the scientific research community needs to adopt more techniques and methods to carry out more in-depth studies and to reveal the mechanism of action of *P. cocos* ingredients to improve diseases, so as to better utilize its edible and medicinal value.

The gut microbiota is a complex ecosystem composed of numerous microorganisms in the gastrointestinal tract, and its composition and diversity play a key role in maintaining the health of the body [12,13]. Imbalances in the gut microbiota contribute to the development and progression of diseases including obesity, diabetes, antibiotic-associated diarrhea (AAD), inflammatory bowel disease (IBD), chronic liver disease, and colorectal cancer [14,15]. Numerous studies have shown that natural products derived from TCM can play a therapeutic role by remodeling the intestinal microecological structure, modulating flora-related metabolites, and influencing intestinal absorption and transport [16,17]. Targeting the gut microbiota for health promotion has great potential, and it is important to explore the specific mechanisms by which natural products modulate the gut microbiota.

Numerous scholars have studied the extraction process, structural identification, and classical pharmacological pathways of polysaccharides, but there are few systematic reviews on *P. cocos* polysaccharides regulating the gut microbiota [18]. Therefore, this paper reviews the bioactive activities and health benefits of *P. cocos* and focuses on the potential relationship between PCPs and the gut microbiota. This review aims to provide a basis for the mechanisms by which *P. cocos* and its active ingredients modulate the gut microbiota to ameliorate diseases, and to provide a new strategy for further research on the potential development of PCP bio-actives in food and drugs.

2. Polysaccharides, the Main Component of *P. cocos*

2.1. *P. cocos Polysaccharides and Other Effective Active Ingredients*

The bioactive ingredients in *P. cocos* include polysaccharides, triterpenes, sterols, volatile oils, proteins, amino acids, nucleotides, and trace elements [19]. Modern pharmacological studies have revealed that polysaccharides are the predominant pharmacologically active ingredients found in *P. cocos*, accounting for about 70% to 90% of the total weight of the whole fungus [20]. Polysaccharides are divided into heteropolysaccharides and homopolysaccharides according to their monosaccharide composition [21]. The polysaccharides in *P. cocos* are mainly divided into a class of branched-chain β-(1–3)-d-glucan containing (1–6) and (1–2) and another class of heteropolysaccharides composed of glucose, arabinose, fucose, mannose, xylose, galactose, and other monosaccharides [22]. Despite continuous advancements in polysaccharide identification techniques, current methods still face limitations in accuracy, consistency, and a comprehensive consideration of dynamic changes in microbial communities, as well as a lack of standardized protocols. These issues may hinder the in-depth understanding of the structure–function relationships of polysaccharides and limit their applications in microbiota research. Triterpenoids are mainly found in *P. cocos* mushroom kernel and skin, containing acid, alcohol, protein, and other components with antioxidant, anti-tumor, anti-inflammatory, and many other pharmacological effects [23]. *P. cocos* polysaccharides show excellent immune response, antioxidant, and anti-tumor activities, and triterpenoids exert their anti-tumor effects by modulating cell signaling and inhibiting tumor cells [24]. It has been shown that lasagna triterpenoids in *P. cocos* extract enhance nonspecific immunity by activating natural killer cells (NK), promoting interferon gamma (IFN-γ) secretion by type 1 helper T cells (Th1), and inhibiting the production of IL-4 and IL-5 [25]. In addition, Poria Acid (PA), another triterpenoid saponin, reduced the invasion and metastasis of gastric cancer cells by inhibiting the EMT process and the expression of MMP proteins [26]. Additionally, other active ingredients in *P. cocos*, such as sterols and ergosterol, have immunomodulatory effects, and alpha-cedrol in volatile oils has anti-inflammatory effects [26].

2.2. Extraction and Structural Characterization of *P. cocos* Polysaccharides

PCPs were mostly extracted by hot water extraction, alkali extraction, enzyme extraction, supercritical fluid extraction, and microwave-assisted and ultrasound-assisted extraction [27]. These methods exhibit distinct trade-offs: hot water and alkali extractions are simple and cost-effective but may degrade polysaccharide structures under harsh thermal or alkaline conditions; enzyme extraction offers mild specificity yet faces limitations in cost and scalability; supercritical fluid extraction is environmentally benign but equipment-intensive; while microwave and ultrasound techniques enhance yield and speed at the risk of localized overheating or radical-induced bioactivity loss. Evidence has demonstrated that deep eutectic solvent (DES) extraction for polysaccharide extraction has the advantages of high efficiency and high yield [28]. A study found that the DES method using a solid–liquid ratio of 1:10 and a ratio of choline chloride to oxalic acid of 1:2 gave a polysaccharide yield of 33.67% after 45 min of extraction [29]. Additionally, Guo et al. also found that the DES method using ternary butylene glycol with a 300 mesh particle size and a solid–liquid ratio of 30 mL/g gave a polysaccharide yield of 55.02% after 30 min of extraction [30]. With the development of instrumentation, as well as extraction, separation, purification, and structure identification techniques, the study of polysaccharides has advanced rapidly [25]. The current methods for polysaccharide extraction and purification are often limited by low yields and insufficient purity, which may introduce contaminants and affect the accuracy of their biological effects on microbiota. To address these issues, there is a need for standardized protocols to improve the yield and purity of polysaccharide preparations, thereby ensuring reliable and reproducible results in microbiota research. The analytical detection of *P. cocos* polysaccharides mainly includes the molecular weight of polysaccharides, monosaccharide composition, and glycosidic bond type [31]. This information can be identified with increasing accuracy by advanced physicochemical methods, chromatographic techniques, and spectroscopic analysis [32]. *P. cocos* polysaccharides can be divided into water-soluble polysaccharides and alkali-soluble polysaccharides according to the different extraction methods [33]. Water-soluble polysaccharides in *P. cocos* have a low content but have significant biological activities, such as anti-tumor and anti-inflammatory effects [34]. Compared with water-soluble polysaccharides, alkali-soluble polysaccharides have a higher content in *P. cocos*, which can reach 93%; however, these polysaccharides have poor water solubility and relatively low bioactivity, and especially almost no anti-tumor activity [35].

2.3. Chemical Modification of P. cocos Polysaccharides

Chemical modification is a widely used modification method employed to change the physicochemical properties and biological activities of polysaccharides by introducing different substituents such as carboxyl, methyl, sulfate, and hydroxyl groups into the polysaccharide molecules [36]. Structural modification of *P. cocos* polysaccharides not only improves the water solubility and stability of polysaccharides but also enhances their biological activities, such as anticancer, antioxidant, anti-inflammatory, and immunomodulatory effects [37]. In addition, chemical modification can help to improve the pharmacokinetic properties and bioavailability of polysaccharides, thus increasing their potential as drugs or functional foods. However, common modification methods, such as acetylation and sulfation, often involve toxic reagents and may generate by-products that could compromise the purity and safety of the modified polysaccharides. Therefore, while chemical modification improves the functionality of polysaccharides, it is essential to optimize the modification processes to minimize the introduction of toxic substances and impurities, ensuring their safe application in food and pharmaceutical industries [38]. It has been shown that by introducing carboxymethyl (-CH_2COOH) into the polysaccharide molecule, the solubility and adsorption capacity of the polysaccharide, as well as its anti-tumor and antioxidant activities, can be increased, [39]. Sulphation is the introduction of sulfate (-SO_4^{2-}) into the polysaccharide molecule, which usually increases the water solubility and anticoagulant activity of the polysaccharide while potentially enhancing its anti-tumor and antiviral activities [40]. Therefore, in order to improve the water solubility and biological activity of *P. cocos* alkali-soluble polysaccharides, they are usually chemically modified by carboxymethylation and sulfate esterification [41]. For example, carboxymethyl porin polysaccharide (CMP) showed good anti-tumor effects, exerting its effects by modulating NF-κB, Nrf2-ARE, and the mitogen-activated protein kinase/P38 protein kinase/c-Jun amino-terminal kinase pathway [42].

Notably, *P. cocos* oligosaccharides (PCOs) are a class of polymers and low-molecular-weight polysaccharides prepared by enzymatic degradation, containing sugar the residues of (1–2)-β-D-Glc_p, (1–2)-α-D-Glc_p, and (1–4)-α-D-Glc_p [43]. PCOs exhibit a wide range of applications in the pharmaceutical and food fields, with a variety of biological activities, including anti-tumor, antiviral, anti-inflammatory, immunomodulatory, and antioxidant effects [24]. Furthermore, they can improve disorders of glycolipid metabolism and protect the structural and functional integrity of the intestinal barrier by regulating intestinal flora [44]. Compared to *P. cocos* polysaccharides, PCOs have better water solubility and bioavailability due to their lower molecular weight, which makes them exhibit stronger antioxidant, immunomodulatory, and anti-tumor properties. To sum up, oligosaccharide degradation and the chemical modification of *P. cocos* polysaccharides, such as carboxymethylation, sulfation, and phosphorylation, can improve their water solubility, increase their molecular flexibility and stretchability, and thus enhance their biological activities, including anti-tumor, immunomodulatory, antioxidant, and anti-inflammatory effects, which makes the modified polysaccharides have a wider range of applications in the field of pharmaceuticals and functional foods (Figure 1).

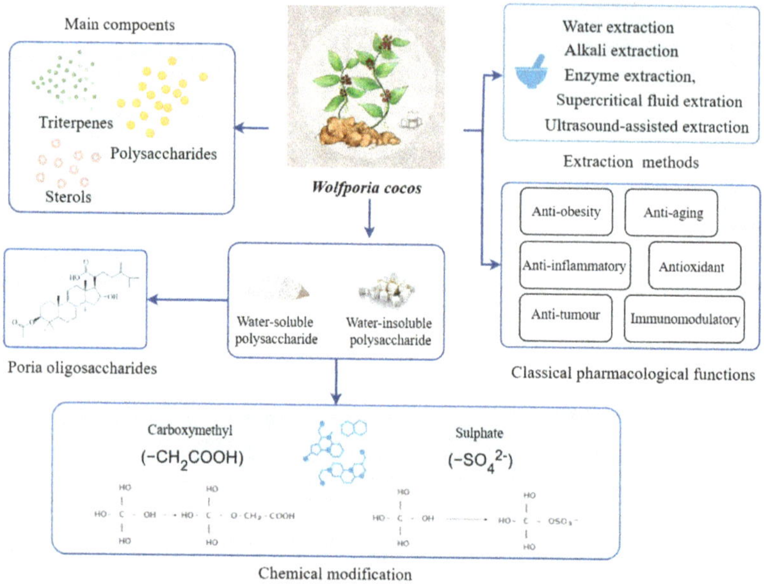

Figure 1. The main active ingredients of *P. cocos* are polysaccharides, triterpenes, and sterols. The extraction and purification methods of PCPs include hot water extraction, alkali extraction, enzyme extraction, supercritical fluid extraction, microwave-assisted and ultrasound-assisted extraction, and deep eutectic solvents (DESs) extraction. The pharmacological functions of polysaccharides include anti-inflammatory, anti-obesity, anticancer, and immunomodulatory functions. PCPs are classified into water-soluble polysaccharides and water-insoluble polysaccharides, and water-insoluble polysaccharides with poor water solubility are β-(1–3)-d-glucan, which are usually modified by sulfate esterification and carboxymethylation.

3. Bioactive Functions of *P. cocos* Polysaccharides

Polysaccharides have great potential to be developed into functional prebiotics and therapeutic drugs due to their wide range of biological activities, making the study of their pharmacological activities and mechanisms a key research area [45]. For the past few years, plenty of studies have revealed the role and mechanism of applying *P. cocos* polysaccharides in the treatment of various diseases, and its pharmacological activities are mainly focused on anti-inflammatory, anti-obesity, anti-tumor, and immunomodulatory functions [46,47] (Table 1).

Table 1. Extensive pharmacological functions of PCPs and their mechanisms.

Name	Structure	Dosage	Model	Pharmacological Function	Molecular Mechanisms and Targets	Symptoms of Improvement	Reference
PCP	PCPs (95% pure) were purchased	100 mg/kg, 200 mg/kg, and 400 mg/kg	Male 8-week C57/BL6 mice and *ApoE*$^{-/-}$ mice	Reduce high-fat diet-induced arteriosclerosis	PCP inhibited the activation of the TLR4/NF-κB pathway in the aorta, serum inflammatory mediators and lipids, and blocked the expression of matrix metalloproteinase 2 and intercellular adhesion molecule 1 proteins.	PCP intervenes in AS by reducing inflammatory factors and blood lipid levels.	[48]
PCP	*N*	225 mg/kg	Male 8-week C57/BL6 mice	Improve lipid metabolism to alleviate NAFLD	PCP affects lipid synthesis, uptake, and oxidation by regulating the expression of genes related to bile acid synthesis (*Cyp7b1* and *Cyp27a1*) and fatty acid metabolism (*Srebp1c*, *Fas*, *Scd1*, *Fatp2*, *Pparα*).	PCP reduced serum and hepatic lipid levels, and improved lipid metabolism by regulating bile acids and fatty acid metabolism.	[49]
PCO	(1 → 2)-β-D-Glcp, (1 → 2)-α-D-Glcp, and (1 → 4)-α-D-Glcp.	200 mg/kg	Male 6-week C57/BL6 mice	Improve HFD-induced dyslipidemia	PCO reversed the expression of bile acid synthesis *genes* (*CYP7A1*, *CYP8B1*, *CYP27A1*, *ABCG1*) to promote lipid metabolism and reduced the mRNA levels of inflammatory cytokines to attenuate inflammatory responses in mouse liver.	PCO inhibits lipid metabolism disorders and reduces lipid accumulation and inflammatory responses in blood and liver tissues.	[50]
PCP	*N*	50, 100, and 200 μg/mL	Vascular smooth muscle cells (VSMCs)	Attenuate ox-LDL-induced inflammation and oxidative stress	PCP activate the ERK/Nrf2/HO-1 signaling pathway in vsmc, decreasing LOX-1 expression, and eliminating intracellular lipid accumulation.	PCP exerts anti-inflammatory effects by inhibiting pro-inflammatory mediators and cytokines and ameliorates oxidative stress.	[51]
PCP	Purity > 98%	0.5–8 μM	RAW264.7 cells	Attenuate RANKL induced osteoclastogenesis	PCP down-regulated the phosphorylation levels of STAT3, P38, ERK, and JNK, and inhibited the expression of NFAcT1 and c-Fos, and TRAcP and CTSK.	PCP inhibits RANKL-induced osteoclast formation and bone resorption.	[52]

Table 1. *Cont.*

Name	Structure	Dosage	Model	Pharmacological Function	Molecular Mechanisms and Targets	Symptoms of Improvement	Reference
PCP	Purity > 90%	200 mg/kg, and 400 mg/kg	Male 6–8-week C57/BL6 mice	Improve fecal-induced peritonitis (FIP)	PCP regulates Treg cells in the spleen and downregulates Annexin-V in the thymus of fp-induced sepsis mice.	PCP reduced inflammatory cytokines and oxidative stress in the plasma and spleen and increased resistance to FIP.	[53]
PCP-1C	*N*	25, 50, and 100 mg/kg	Male C57/BL6 mice	Improve alcohol-induced liver injury	PCP-1C reduced hepatic inflammation by inhibiting the TLR4/NF-κB signaling pathway and ameliorated hepatocyte apoptosis by inhibiting CYP2E1/ROS/MAPKs signaling pathway.	PCP-1C reduces serum biochemical markers, attenuates hepatic steatosis, repairs the intestinal barrier, and reduces lipopolysaccharide (LPS) leakage.	[54]
PCP-1C	Sugar content: 96.97%	50, 100, and 200 μg/mL	RAW264. 7 cells	Regulate the immune response and anti-tumor	PCP-1C activated the Notch signaling pathway in macrophages and up-regulated the expression of Notch1, ligands Jagghd1 and Hes1.	PCP-1C improves M1 macrophage polarization.	[55]
PCP-W1	molecular weight: 18.38 kDa	25, 50, 100, 200 and 400 μg/mL	RAW264. 7 cells	Potential anti-tumor effects	PCP-W1 regulated the TLR4/MD2/NF-κB pathway and activated the release of NO, IL-6, IL-β, TNF-α, CD86, and ROS.	PCP-W1 induced macrophage polarization to m1-type in RAW 264.7 mice, and	[56]
PCP	>90% pure	200 μg/mL for cell and 200 mg/kg for mice	RAW 264.7 cells, female C57BL/10ScNJ, and control C57BL/10J mice	Immunomodulatory effects	PCP elevated the levels of nitric oxide, IL-2, IL-6, IL-17 A, TNF, and IFN-γ and significantly increased the expression of TLR4, MyD88, TRAF-6, p-NF-κB, and p-c-JUN.	PCP led to a significant decrease in tumor volume and an increase in all organ immunoreactivity indices.	[57]
PCAPS1	β-1,3-glucan with 11.5 kDa	500 μg/mL	RAW264. 7 cells	Immunoregulatory capacity	PCAPS1 enhanced the mRNA expression levels of TNF-a and NF-jB, activating RAW264.7 cells by inducing translocation of the NF-jB p65 signaling pathway.	PCAPS1 increased the secretion of TNF-a.	[58]

Table 1. *Cont.*

Name	Structure	Dosage	Model	Pharmacological Function	Molecular Mechanisms and Targets	Symptoms of Improvement	Reference
PCP-2	1,3-β-D-Glc and 1,6-β-D-Glc with 2.35 kDa	2, 10, 50, 200 μg/mL	RAW264. 7 cells	Immunoenhancing effects	PCP-2 promoted the secretion of NO and TNF-α, and increased the levels of IgG, IgA, IgM, and $CD3^+CD4^+$ T cells in the blood.	PCP-2 promoted the development of thymus and spleen immune organs, and improved gut barrier dysfunctions.	[59]
PCP	20.112 kDa	50, 200, 800 μg/mL	BALB/c mice	Inducing immune responses	PCP promotes the activation of dendritic cells and macrophages and binds to Th1 and Th2 immune responses.	PCP markedly induced the cytotoxic T lymphocyte response, and enhanced humoral and cellular immune responses.	[60]

3.1. *Anti-Obesity Effects of P. cocos Polysaccharides*

P. cocos polysaccharides inhibit high-fat-diet-induced metabolic disorders by regulating host metabolic pathways [61]. Polysaccharides can change the synthesis and composition of bile acids, affecting the digestion and absorption of lipids, and then promote the oxidative utilization of fatty acids and reduce the accumulation of fat in the liver, which in turn exerts anti-obesity effects [62]. Meanwhile, *P. cocos* polysaccharides can improve the symptoms of diabetic patients by increasing glucose tolerance, improving abnormal glucose tolerance, and improving glucose metabolism disorder [63]. It was found that 95% pure *P. cocos* polysaccharide (PCP) intervened in atherosclerosis induced by a high-fat diet by inhibiting the activation of the TLR4/NF-κB pathway in the aorta and lowering inflammatory factors and lipid levels [48]. Wang et al. found that PCP reduced serum and liver lipid levels; affected fatty acid metabolism, bile acid metabolism, and metabolic pathways of the tricarboxylic acid cycle; and inhibited lipid synthesis and uptake to improve NAFLD [49]. Zhu et al. showed that PCO can significantly inhibit lipid metabolism disorders and reduce lipid accumulation and inflammation in blood and liver tissues to effectively ameliorate lipid metabolism disorders induced by a high-fat diet [50].

In summary, *P. cocos* polysaccharides exert anti-obesity effects and ameliorate high-fat-diet-induced metabolic disorders by modulating host metabolic pathways, altering bile acid composition to influence lipid digestion and absorption, promoting fatty acid oxidation and utilization, reducing hepatic fat accumulation, increasing glucose tolerance, improving glucose metabolism, inhibiting activation of the TLR4/NF-κB pathway in atherosclerosis, and decreasing inflammation and lipid-level disorders.

3.2. *Anti-Inflammatory Activity of P. cocos Polysaccharides*

P. cocos polysaccharides can reduce inflammatory response and the release of inflammatory factors [43]. Numerous studies have shown that *P. cocos* exerts anti-inflammatory effects by inhibiting the expression of iNOS, COX-2, etc., and the production of inflammatory mediators such as NO, PGE2, IL-1, IL-6, and TNF-α [64]. Zhao et al. found that PCP exerts anti-inflammatory and antioxidant effects by activating the ERK/Nrf2/HO-1 signaling pathway in vsmc, decreasing the expression of LOX-1, and eliminating intracellular lipid accumulation [51]. Song et al. found that PCP inhibited RANKL-induced osteoclast formation and bone resorption by down-regulating the phosphorylation levels of STAT3, P38, ERK, and JNK, inhibiting the expression of NFAcT1 and c-Fos, and impacting the expression of TRAcP and CTSK [52]. A study found that PCP exerts a protective effect against fecal-induced peritonitis (FIP) by decreasing inflammatory cytokines and oxidative stress in the plasma, modulating Treg cells in the spleen, and down-regulating Annexin-V in the thymus of septic mice [53]. Another study showed that PCP reduced alcohol-induced liver inflammation by repairing the intestinal barrier and reducing lipopolysaccharide (LPS) leakage, inhibited the TLR4/NF-κB signaling pathway, and improved hepatocyte apoptosis by inhibiting the CYP2E1/ROS/MAPKs signaling pathway [54].

To sum up, *P. cocos* polysaccharides exert their anti-inflammatory efficacy by inhibiting the production of inflammatory mediators and the release of inflammatory factors, activating the ERK/Nrf2/HO-1 signaling pathway, reducing the accumulation of lipids, attenuating oxidative stress, and protecting the intestinal barrier, as well as by inhibiting the TLR4/NF-κB and CYP2E1/ROS/MAPKs signaling pathways.

3.3. *Anti-Tumor and Immunomodulatory Functions of P. cocos Polysaccharides*

P. cocos polysaccharides have anti-tumor activity, which may play a role by activating the immune system, inhibiting the proliferation of tumor cells, and promoting apoptosis of tumor cells and other mechanisms [65]. Numerous studies have reported that the anti-tumor activity of *P. cocos* polysaccharides is mainly reflected in two aspects: one is to promote the apoptosis of tumor cells through various mechanisms, thus achieving direct tumor suppression effect; the other is to promote the sensitivity of tumor cells to radiotherapy and chemotherapy, thus achieving an indirect tumor suppression effect [66–68]. Polysaccharides can enhance the immune function of the body, activate immune cells such as macrophages and lymphocytes, and promote the production of antibodies, thus improving the body's resistance to pathogens [69]. Current research on the immunomodulatory function of *P. cocos* mainly focuses on polysaccharide and structurally modified polysaccharide derivatives [70]. *P. cocos* polysaccharides (PCPs) regulate the body's immunity by protecting the immune organs, preventing or reducing thymus atrophy and spleen enlargement, activating T and B lymphocytes, enhancing NK cell activity, and regulating inflammatory cytokines such as IL-2, TNF-a, and so on [71]. In a study with RAW264.7 cells, Hu et al. found that the homopolysaccharide PCP-1C further exhibited anti-tumor activity in vivo by activating the Notch signaling pathway in macrophages and upregulating the expression of Notch1, and ligands Jagghd1 and Hes1 [55]. Sun et al. found that PCP-W1 enhanced NO, IL-6, IL-1β, TNF- α, and ROS in macrophages by regulating the TLR4/MD2/NF-κB pathway, suggesting that PCP-W1 may have a potential anti-tumor effect [56]. Tian et al. found that the use of PCP led to a significant reduction in tumor volume and an increase in organ immunoreactivity indexes, and it exerted exogenous and internal immunomodulatory effects by activating the TLR4/TRAF6/NF-κB signaling pathway [57].

Interestingly, water-soluble polysaccharides and water-insoluble polysaccharides derived from *P. cocos* have a large difference in immunomodulatory function and anti-tumor activity [72]. Water-soluble polysaccharides are more easily recognized and processed by the immune system to rapidly stimulate an immune response, which is reflected in the enhancement of the body's immune function through the activation of immune cells [73]. Water-insoluble polysaccharides, on the other hand, exhibit specific anti-tumor activities due to their structural stability and interaction with cell surface receptors, and they can play a role by inhibiting tumor cell proliferation, promoting apoptosis, or affecting the tumor microenvironment [74]. In a study of insoluble polysaccharides, scholars found that PCAPS1 enhanced the mRNA expression levels of TNF-a and nuclear factor jB (NF-jB), while activating RAW264.7 cells by inducing the NF-jB p65 signaling pathway translocation [58]. Lv et al. found that the water-soluble polysaccharide PCP-2 could stimulate the proliferation of RAW264.7 cells, promote the secretion of inflammatory factors such as NO and TNF-α, and increase the levels of IgG, IgA, IgM, and $CD3^+CD4^+$ T cells in the blood [59]. Another study showed that PCP can elicit a strong antibody response in the body by promoting the activation of dendritic cells (DCs) and macrophages in combination with Th1 and Th2 immune responses [60]. In a word, *P. cocos* polysaccharides enhance immune function by activating immune cells and promoting antibody production, and they concurrently exert anti-tumor effects by inhibiting tumor cell proliferation and promoting apoptosis through the activation of signaling pathways such as Notch and TLR4/MD2/NF-κB. Moreover, they can achieve immunomodulation by regulating inflammatory factors and enhancing the function of immune organs, in which water-soluble polysaccharides promote immune responses through rapid activation of the immune system, whereas water-insoluble polysaccharides exert specific anti-tumor activities by affecting the tumor microenvironment and the interaction of cell surface receptors.

In addition to the main pharmacological activities mentioned above, *P. cocos* polysaccharides also have pharmacological effects such as antioxidant, anti-aging, and protection effects on the liver and kidneys [75]. Mechanistic studies have shown that *P. cocos* polysaccharides can elevate superoxide dismutase, which is essential for oxidation and antioxidants in organisms, thus protecting the structure and function of cell membranes from the interference and damage of peroxides and improving the antioxidant capacity of the organism [76,77]. In addition, *P. cocos* polysaccharides inhibited the phosphorylation of mitogen-activated protein kinase p38 antibody (p38MAPK), thereby inhibiting the production of inflammatory factors and thus protecting the kidneys [14]. *P. cocos* polysaccharides protected the liver by down-regulating the expression of TGF01 and PDGF, inhibiting the activation of HSC proliferation, promoting the degradation of the extracellular matrix, and decreasing hepatic fibrous connective tissue deposition [78]. Moreover, *P. cocos* polysaccharides can also be used as prebiotics to widely regulate gut microbiota and improve intestinal barrier function due to their unique activity [79]. Prebiotics are a class of non-digestible macromolecular carbohydrates that produce health benefits for the host by selectively promoting the activity and growth of one or several beneficial bacteria in the gut. A widely used prebiotic are polysaccharides from natural products, which have a variety of positive effects on the health of the host [80,81]. As a powerful prebiotic, *P. cocos* polysaccharides are worth exploring in depth for their multifaceted effects on the maintenance and improvement of intestinal health, helping to improve overall digestive health and the body's immunity.

3.4. P. cocos Polysaccharides Modulate Gut Microbiota to Exert Probiotic Function

With the development of modern biotechnology and pharmacology, polysaccharides have been found to have a wide range of biological functions [82]. The research on the composition, extraction, analysis, and biological activity of *P. cocos* polysaccharides has become a hot spot at home and abroad [83]. Despite extensive reviews on *P. cocos* polysaccharides covering aspects such as extraction processes, structural characterization, anti-tumor activities, anti-inflammatory properties, and immunomodulatory effects, limited attention has been given to summarizing their potential health-promoting effects via modulation of the gut microbiota [84]. Therefore, we will focus on how polysaccharides can ameliorate diseases by modulating the gut microbiota, altering related metabolites, and influencing organismal functions.

Gut microorganisms have a crucial role in human health, and they play a variety of roles in human physiological and pathological processes [85]. The gut microbiota is not only involved in material metabolism and nutrient synthesis but is also closely related to the regulation of the immune system and the development of many diseases [86]. On the one hand, the interaction between gut microbes and the host immune system is crucial for maintaining immune homeostasis [87]. On the other hand, alterations in the composition and function of gut microbes have been associated with a variety of diseases, including diabetes, antibiotic-associated diarrhea, inflammatory bowel disease, and colorectal cancer [88]. Herein, this study of the regulatory effects of *P. cocos* polysaccharides on the gut microbiota is expected to provide new prospects for the effective amelioration of the disease (Figure 2).

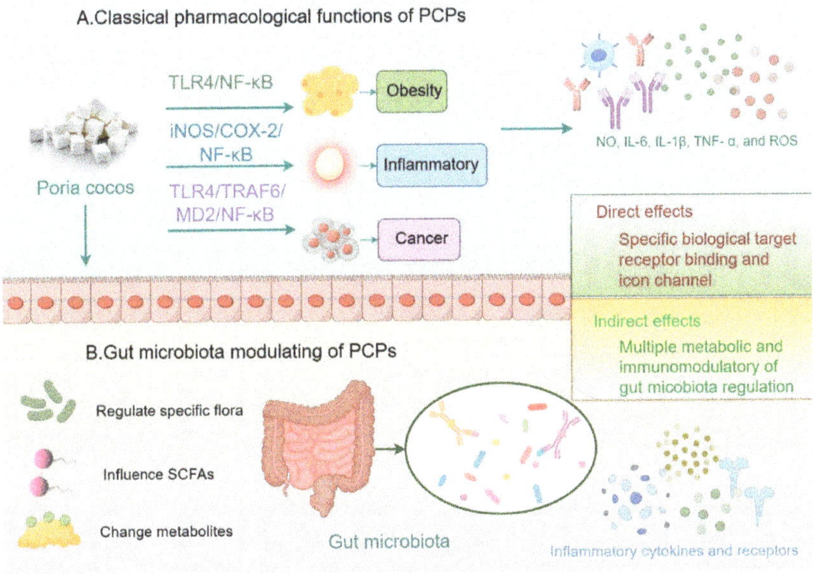

Figure 2. PCPs activate or inhibit the TLR4/NF-κB, CYP2E1/ROS/MAPKs, and TLR4/MD2/NF-κB pathways, releasing cytokines that exert anti-obesity, anti-inflammatory, and anti-tumor effects. In contrast to the above, PCPs affect host metabolic, immune, and inflammatory responses by regulating the gut microbiota, influencing the production of SCFAs, and altering flora-associated metabolites.

3.4.1. Regulate the Composition and Structure of Gut Microbiota

P. cocos polysaccharides can regulate the composition and structure of gut microbiota by promoting the growth of beneficial bacteria (*Muribaculaceae* and *Lachnospiraceae*) and inhibiting the reproduction of harmful bacteria (*Escherichia-Shigella*, *Staphylococcus*, and *Acinetobacter*) [89]. The balance of gut microbiota is crucial to human health, and its diversity and stability are key to maintaining intestinal health [90]. Beneficial bacteria such as *Bifidobacteria* and *Lactobacillus* can enhance the intestinal barrier function and inhibit the invasion of pathogenic bacteria [91]. By regulating the gut microbiota, PCPs can help prevent and treat intestinal-related diseases, such as inflammatory bowel disease (IBD) and irritable bowel syndrome (IBS) [92].

3.4.2. Influence on the Production of Short-Chain Fatty Acids (SCFAs)

SCFAs contain acetate, propionate, and butyrate, and are the main metabolites produced by gut microorganisms fermenting cellulose [93]. PCPs can promote the growth of beneficial intestinal bacteria and increase the production of SCFAs [94]. SCFAs are involved in the regulation of energy metabolism and blood glucose control in the host, which helps to prevent and treat metabolic diseases such as obesity and diabetes [95]. Concomitantly, SCFAs exert anti-tumor effects by enhancing immune cell function, directly acting on tumor cells, regulating the tumor microenvironment, and inhibiting HDAC activity [96]. As ligands for histone deacetylases (HDAC), SCFAs can induce HDAC inhibition to stimulate monocytes and neutrophils, leading to NF-κB inactivation and a reduction in inflammatory cytokines [97]. In addition, SCFAs bind to intestinal GPR43 and GPR41 receptors, which further inhibits MAPK, p-p38/p38, and p-JNK/JNK signaling pathways and increases the expression of immune cytokines (e.g., IL-2, IL-4, IL-6, IL-10, TGF-β, and IFN-γ), thus exerting immune activity [98,99].

3.4.3. Regulation of Flora-Associated Metabolites

Gut flora metabolites are key regulators of host health and disease and are diverse and multifunctional, including short-chain fatty acids (SCFAs), bile acids, tryptophan, and trimethylamine-N-oxide (TMAO). *P. cocos* polysaccharides affect tryptophan and bile acid metabolism by regulating the metabolic activity of the gut microbiota, thus positively affecting host health [100]. Tryptophan is one of the essential amino acids, and gut microbes are able to metabolize tryptophan to produce a variety of metabolites such as 5-hydroxytryptophan (serotonin) and kynurenine [101]. These metabolites play an important role in regulating the host's mood, sleep, and immune response. Bile acids are digestive fluids synthesized by the liver and are involved in the digestion and absorption of fats [102]. Gut microbes metabolize bile acids to produce secondary bile acids, and these metabolites play an important role in regulating the host's metabolic, immune, and cardiovascular health [103]. On the one hand, *P. cocos* polysaccharides can activate immune effector cells and promote the expression of growth factors and cytokines by regulating the intestinal microbiota and metabolic profile, thus enhancing innate and specific immunity. On the other hand, excessive immune responses can damage tissues and organs, aggravate pathological conditions, and induce autoimmune diseases. By regulating metabolites and immune responses, *P. cocos* polysaccharides can both enhance the body's immune defense function and avoid organ damage caused by excessive immune responses [104].

Collectively, *P. cocos* polysaccharides act comprehensively on the intestinal microbiota through a variety of mechanisms, including promoting the growth of beneficial bacteria, increasing the production of SCFAs, regulating the intestinal barrier function, influencing the host metabolism, and altering the structure of the bacterial flora, which work together to maintain the intestinal micro-ecological balance and enhance the body's immune defense ability.

4. *P. cocos* Polysaccharides Improve Disease by Regulating Gut Microbiota

Conventional pharmacology usually relies on direct action on specific molecular targets or signaling pathways [105]. The NF-κB pathway plays a key role in immune, inflammatory, and other processes, and its activation mechanism includes both classical and non-classical pathways involving the IκB kinase complex (IKK) and NF-κB-induced kinase (NIK) [64]. In contrast, the paradigm of targeting the modulation of the gut microbiota for disease amelioration focuses on influencing host health by regulating the composition and metabolic activities of gut microbes [106,107]. Typically, the gut microbiota influences the host's metabolic, immune, and inflammatory responses through the production of metabolites such as SCFAs [18]. Traditional pharmacology focuses on the treatment of specific diseases or symptoms, and the effects of drugs are usually limited to specific organs or systems [108]. In contrast, modulation of the gut microbiota has a broader therapeutic potential, as evidenced by the fact that the gut microbiota is closely related to the function of multiple systems, including metabolism, immunity, and the nervous system [109]. Thus, gut microbiota modulation has a positive impact on a wide range of chronic diseases, and in the next section we will focus on the role of flora modulation in prebiotic function, anti-inflammation, anti-obesity, and immunomodulation (Table 2).

Table 2. The role of PCPs in regulating gut microbiota and its mechanism.

Name	Dosage	Model	Activity	Gut Microbiota Regulation	Metabolites Regulation	Gene and Protein Expression	Reference
PC	750 mg/kg	Male 6-week C57BL/6 mice	Prebiotic functions	*Barnesiella*, *Pseudobutyrivibrio*, and *Dehalobacterium* were decreased.	PC promoted the production of Bacteroides xylanolyticus.	SCFA affects signaling pathways in host intestinal epithelial cells.	[110]
PCP	75 mg/kg, 150 mg/kg, and 300 mg/kg	Male 8-week C57BL/6 mice	Functional food to regulate intestinal mucosal function	PCP treatment increased the abundance of *Muribaculaceae* and *Bacteroides*.	PCP showed significantly higher levels of acetic acid, propionic acid, isobutyric acid, and isovaleric acid.	PCP up-regulates intestinal Occludin and ZO-1 proteins, MUC2, β-defensin and SIgA, and enhances immunity by up-regulating the expression of IL-2, IL-4, IL-6, IL-10, TGF-β and IFN-γ.	[111]
PCPs	12 g/kg	Male 21-day-old Sprague Dawley rats	Functional food to help promote maturation and stability in young rats	The relative abundances of *Bifidobacterium*, *Lactobacillus*, *Allobaculum*, and *Oligella* increased, whereas *Enterococcus* declined.	Improved amino acid, energy, SCFAs and nucleotide metabolism. 35 urinary and 24 feces metabolites was changed.	PCPs could promote the functional maturation of gut microbiota and increase basic metabolism.	[112]
PCX	300 mg/kg	Male 4–6-week Kunming mice	Functional prebiotic	PCX increased *Lachnospiraceae* and decreased *Muribaculaceae*.	The content of short-chain peptides was changed.	PCX significantly elevated IL-10 levels.	[113]
PCY	300 mg/kg	Male 4–6-week Kunming mice	Functional prebiotic	The number of *Lactobacillus* was significantly increased.	The content of short-chain peptides was changed.	PCY significantly decreased IFN-γ levels.	[113]
PCE	20.46 mg/kg, 40.92 mg/kg, 81.84 mg/kg	Male 6–8-week Balb/c mice	Attenuated DSS-induced ulcerative colitis	PCE significantly decreased *Pseudomonas*, and increased *Oscillospira*, *Prevotella*, *Ruminococcus*, and unidentified-*Lachnospiraceae*.	*N*	PCE inhibited the NF-κB pathway, decreased the inflammatory mediators TNF-α, IL-6, and IL-1β, and restored the expression of the colonic tight junction proteins ZO-1 and Claudin-1.	[114]
PCOs	200 mg/kg	Male 6-week BALB/c mice	Attenuated DSS-induced ulcerative colitis	Regulated the relative abundance of *Muribaculum*, *Desulfovibrio*, *Oscillibacter*, *Escherichia–Shigella*, and *Turicibacter*.	Secondary bile acid biosynthesis, the sulfur relay system, and glutathione metabolism were remarkably reversed.	PCOs protect the intestinal barrier from damage by inhibiting TNF-α, IL-1β, and IL-6 cytokines and promoting the expression of tight junction proteins.	[115]

Table 2. *Cont.*

Name	Dosage	Model	Activity	Gut Microbiota Regulation	Metabolites Regulation	Gene and Protein Expression	Reference
PPs	250 mg/kg	Male Sprague Dawley (SD) 7–8-week rats	Alleviated Chronic nonbacterial prostatitis	*Parabacteroides*, *Fusicatenibacter*, and *Parasutterella* were significantly enriched.	PPs increased beneficial metabolites 7-ketodeoxycholic acid and haloperidol glucuronide.	The expression of Alox15 and Pla2g2f increased, and Cyp1a1 and Hsd17b7 reduced in colon epithelium.	[116]
PPs	100 mg/kg, 250 mg/kg, 500 mg/kg	Male Sprague Dawley (SD) 7–8-week rats	Alleviated Chronic non-bacterial prostatitis	*Lachnospiraceae*-NK4A136 group, *Lactobacillus*, and uncultured *bacterium_f_ Erysipelotrichaceae* were decreased, while *Romboutsia* and uncultured *bacterium_f_Desulfovibrionaceae* were increased.	Altered the levels of malondialdehyde (MDA) and superoxide di-uronidase (SOD).	PPs exert anti-CNP effects by decreasing the levels of NF-α and IL-1β and c-reactive protein (CRP) and modulating the production of testosterone (T), dihydrotestosterone (DTH), and estradiol (E2), nitric oxide synthase (iNOS).	[117]
PPs	250 mg/kg	Male Sprague Dawley (SD) 7–8-week rats	Alleviated chronic non-bacterial prostatitis	Restored CNP-induced changes in the bacterial flora, including *Ruminococcaceae NK4A214 group, uncultured bacterium_f_Ruminococcaceae*, *Ruminiclostridium_9*, *Phascolarctobacterium*, *Coriobacteriaceae UCG-002* and *Oribacterium*.	*N*	Inhibited the production of pro-inflammatory cytokines (TNF-α, IL-2 and IL-8) and androgens (dihy_x005f drotestosterone and testosterone).	[118]
WIP	1 g/kg and 0.5 g/kg	Ob/ob 8-week mice	Improved hyperglycemia, hyperlipidemia and hepatic steatosis	WIP promoted an increase in *Lachnospiracea* and *Clostridium*.	WIP treatment ele_x005f vated the level of butyrate in gut.	Improved gut mucosal integrity and activated the intestinal PPAR-γ pathway.	[119]
PCP	100 mg/kg	Male 6-week C57BL/6 mice	Anti-obesity effect	Altered *Eisenbergiella*, *Dorea*, *Proteiniphilum* and *Lachnospira* in response to PCP treatment.	PCP treatment improved vitamin B6 metabolism and ubiquitin system function.	PCP improves fatty acid metabolism and mitigates intestinal barrier disruption induced by HFD in vivo.	[120]
PCO	200 mg/kg	Male 6-week C57BL/6 mice	Improved glycolipid metabolism disturbance	PCO decreased *Ruminococx_0002_caceae* and *Anaeroplasmataceae*, and increased *Lactobacillaceae* and *Rikenellaceae*.	Reverse bile acids (BAs), short-chain fatty acids (SCFAs), and tryptophan metabolites.	PCO inhibited the expression of fatty acid synthesis regulator mRNA and pro-inflammatory cytokines.	[121]

Table 2. *Cont.*

Name	Dosage	Model	Activity	Gut Microbiota Regulation	Metabolites Regulation	Gene and Protein Expression	Reference
PCP	150 mg/kg and 300 mg/kg	Male 9-week C57BL/6 mice	Improved non-alcoholic steatohepatitis	PCP significantly increasing the relative abundance of *Faecalibaculum*.	Decreased the level of endotoxin load derived from gut bacteria.	PCP regulates the expression of the chemokine, Toll-like receptor, and the NF_x0002_kappa B signaling pathway.	[122]
WIP	1.0 g/kg	Male 8-week C57BL/6 mice	Improved gut fungi-induced PGE2 to alcoholic hepatic steatosis	WIP significantly enhanced the ratio of Firmictues to Proteobacteria, and increased *Lachnospiraceae*, *Ruminoclostridum*, and *unidentified_clostridials*	*N*	WIP ameliorates hepatic inflammatory injury and fat accumulation by activating PPAR-γ signaling and reducing colonic inflammation.	[123]
PCWP	100 mg/kg	Male 8-week Wistar rats	Modulated anxiety-like behavior induced by sleep deprivation	Adjusted the abundance of *Rikenellaceae_RC9_ gut_group*, *Ruminococcus*, *Prevotellaceae_UCG-001*, *Prevotellaceae*, and *Fusicatenibacter*.	PCWP intervention moderated sphingolipid, phenyl_x0002_alanine, and taurine and hypotaurine metabolism.	PCWP regulated gastrointestinal peptide levels, reduced inflammatory factors, and inhibited the TNF-α/NF-κB signaling pathway.	[124]
PCP	100 mg/kg	Half male and female BLAB/c mice	Ameliorated CsA-induced immunosuppressive lung injury	PCP intervention significantly reduced the abundance of *Chryseobacterium*, *Lawsonella*, *Paracoccus*, and *Sediminibacterium*, and increased *Alloprevotella*.	The model serum metabolite Americine decreased the expression of PC(O-18:1(4Z)/0:0).	PCP restored organ indices and lung tissue morphology and structure.	[125]
PCP	750 mg/kg	6–8 weeks $Apc^{Min/+}$ mice	Attenuated the adverse effects of 5-FU	PCP stimulated the growth of *Bacteroides acidifaciens*, *Bacteroides intestinihominis*, *Butyricicoccus pullicaecorum*, and the genera *Lactobacillus*, *Bifdobacterium*, and *Eubacterium*.	*N*	Reduced the expressions of pro-inflammatory cytokines and enhanced the tight junction proteins and associated adhesion molecules.	[126]

Table 2. *Cont.*

Name	Dosage	Model	Activity	Gut Microbiota Regulation	Metabolites Regulation	Gene and Protein Expression	Reference
WP	7.6 mg/kg	Male 6–8 weeks C57BL/6 mice	Acted against cisplatin-induced intestinal damage	WP decreased *Proteobacteria*, *Cyanobacteria*, *Ruminococcaceae*, and *Helicobacteraceae*, while promoting *Erysipelotrichaceae* and *Prevotellaceae*.	altered metabolic profiles including xanthine, L-tyrosine, uridine, hypoxanthine, butyrylcarnitine, ribose, plamitic acid, thiamine monophosphate, and indolelactic acid.	WP alleviated weight loss and reversed the elevation of IL-2 and IL-6 in serum.	[127]
PCP	250 mg/kg	Half males and half female 5-week C57BL/6N mice	Ameliorated antibiotic-associated diarrhea	Regulation of seven characteristic species including *Salmonella*, *Parabacteroides*, *Clostridium*, *Ruminoc-occus Lactobacillus*, and *Mucispirillum*.	*N*	PCP increased the expression level of the colonic tight junction protein-occlusion band 1 (ZO-1) and regulated the mRNA expression of FOXP3 and GPR41.	[128]
PCY	300 mg/kg	Male 6-week C57BL/6 mice	Ameliorated antibiotic-associated diarrhea	PCY increased norank_f_*Muribaculaceae* and unclassi-fied_f_*Lachnospiraceae*, and decreased *Escherichia-Shigella*, *Staphylococcus*, and *Acinetobacter*.	The level of acetic and butyric acid in the PCY group was significantly higher.	PCY restored intestinal barrier function and decreased the concentrations of TNF-α, IL-6, and IL-1β.	[129]

4.1. *P. cocos* Polysaccharides as Dietary Supplements for Health Promotion

Previous studies have demonstrated that prebiotics, as dietary supplements, exert significant effects on modulating the gut microbiota by promoting the proliferation of beneficial bacteria such as Bifidobacterium and Lactobacillus, thereby maintaining gut homeostasis, enhancing digestive function, and strengthening the intestinal barrier [130]. Prebiotics are non-digestible food ingredients that selectively promote the growth and activity of beneficial gut microbiota, thereby improving host health [131]. Polysaccharides exhibited prebiotic effects by modulating the composition of the gut microbiota, reducing the abundance of potentially pathogenic bacteria, and promoting the proliferation of SCFA-producing bacteria. A study shows that polysaccharides from *P. cocos* can function as prebiotics by significantly reshaping the composition of the gut microbiome, thereby contributing to health-promoting effects [110]. Duan et al. found that PCP, with a molecular weight of 11.583 kDa, is a functional food that increases the abundance of *Muribaculaceae* and *Bacteroides*, promotes the production of SCFAs, up-regulates the expression of intestinal Occludin and ZO-1, down-regulates serum endotoxin, DAO, d-lactate, and intestinal MPO levels, and enhances the intestinal barrier by increasing the expression of IL-2, IL-4, IL-6, IL-10, TGF-β, and IFN-γ [111]. In male 21-day-old SD young rats, Wang et al. found that supplementation with PCPs favored the development and metabolic activity of the gut microbiota, and that PCPs increased the relative abundance of beneficial bacteria, decreased the relative abundance of detrimental bacteria, and effectively improved energy metabolism and nucleic acid metabolism [112]. A comparative study of *P. cocos* water-soluble polysaccharides (PCX) and water-insoluble polysaccharides (PCY) found that both were effective in modulating the gut microbiota of KM mice and altering short peptide metabolism and inflammatory factors, especially PCY, which has great prebiotic potential [113].

4.2. *P. cocos* Polysaccharides Exert Anti-Inflammatory Effects to Improve Disease

Modern pharmacological studies have demonstrated that *P. cocos* polysaccharides exert their anti-inflammatory effect by affecting the secretion of inflammation-related factors, iNOS and COX-2, and inhibiting the activation of the inflammatory signaling pathway NF-κB [132]. It has been shown that in DSS-induced ulcerative colitis, *P. cocos* oligosaccharides protect the intestinal barrier from damage by regulating the relative abundance of *Muribaculum*, *Desulfovibrio*, *Oscillibacter*, *Escherichia-Shigella*, and *Turicibacter*, inhibiting the expression of TNF-α, IL-1β, and lL-6 cytokines, and promoting the expression of tight junction proteins to protect the intestinal barrier from damage [114]. *P. cocos* aqueous polysaccharides improved IBD by significantly decreasing the number of *Pseudomonas* and increasing the abundance of *Oscillospira*, *Prevotella*, *Ruminococcus*, and unidentified-*Lachnospiraceae*, inhibiting the NF-κB pathway, decreasing inflammatory mediators, and restoring the expression of colonic tight junction proteins ZO-1 and Claudin-1 expression [115]. The gut microbiota affects the immune system, metabolic processes, and intestinal barrier function by influencing the immune system, metabolic processes, and intestinal barrier function in the treatment of chronic nonbacterial prostatitis (CNP). Therefore, natural product polysaccharides modulating the gut microbiota may provide a new strategy for the treatment of CNP [133,134]. *P. cocos* polysaccharides (PPs) reduce CNP symptoms by enriching *Parabacteroides* and *Fusicatenibacter*, increasing beneficial metabolites in the gut microbiome, and upregulating the expression of Alox15 and Pla2g2f in the colonic epithelium to inhibit prostate inflammation [116]. In a study of CNP, Liu et al. found that polysaccharide PPs over-reduced the levels of pro-inflammatory cytokines (TNF-α and IL-1β) and c-reactive protein (CRP), while PPs restored the relative abundance of five genera, reconfigured the DNA methylome of intestinal epithelial cells, and played a key role in alleviating CNP [117]. Furthermore, in their another comparative study of PPs with finasteride in the treatment of CNP, both PPs and finasteride inhibited the production of pro-inflammatory cytokines and androgens, and interfered with CNP by restoring CNP-induced changes in the bacterial flora, including *Ruminococcaceae_NK4A214_group, bacterium_f_Ruminococcaceae, Ruminiclostridium_9, Phascolarctobacterium, Coriobacteriaceae UCG-002,* and *Oribacterium* [118].

4.3. *P. cocos Polysaccharides Effectively Alleviate Metabolic Syndrome*

The metabolic syndrome, typified by obesity, hyperglycaemia and hepatic steatosis, is prevalent worldwide [135]. Metabolites produced by the gut microbiota, such as trimethylamine and secondary bile acids, are involved in the body's glycolipid metabolism and inflammatory response, influencing the development of the metabolic syndrome [45]. Studies have shown that modulating the gut microbiota with prebiotics, probiotics, or fecal mushroom transplantation (FMT) can help improve the symptoms of metabolic syndrome [136]. Sun et al. found that WIP with the repeating unit (1–3)-β-D-glucan modulated the amount of *Lachnospiracea* and *Clostridium,* increased the level of butyrate in the intestine, improved the integrity of the intestinal mucosa, and activated the PPAR-γ pathway [119]. A comprehensive analysis of the Jiang et al. study found that PCP altered the amount of *Eisenbergiella, Dorea, Proteiniphilum,* and *Lachnospira* in the gut, and inhibited inflammatory signaling pathways in adipose tissue induced by a high-fat diet [120]. In addition, Zhu et al. showed that PCO could be used as a new prebiotic, and that PCO inhibited the expression of fatty acid synthesis regulator mRNA and pro-inflammatory cytokines, restored the imbalance of the intestinal microbiota in the HFD mice, and reversed a variety of intestinal metabolites [121]. A study demonstrated that PCP significantly alleviated histological liver injury and impaired liver function in C57BL/6 mice, suggesting that PCP modulates the gut microbiota and downregulates the NF-κB/CCL3/CCR1 axis to ameliorate non-alcoholic steatohepatitis [122]. Another study found that WIP from *P. cocos* treated intestinal fungal-induced PGE2-induced alcoholic hepatic steatosis by activating PPAR-γ signaling, decreasing colonic inflammation, increasing the relative abundance of *Ruminoclostridum* and *unidentified_clostridials,* and inhibiting the overgrowth of fungal and *Proteobacteria* in the intestine [123].

4.4. *P. cocos Polysaccharides Have Superior Immunomodulatory Functions*

P. cocos polysaccharides have a variety of biological activities, especially in immunomodulation, showing great potential to improve a variety of diseases [20]. *P. cocos* polysaccharides can activate macrophages, increase the lymphocyte conversion rate and natural killer cell activity, promote T lymphocyte proliferation, regulate cytokine secretion, and enhance the body's cellular and humoral immune functions [137]. Zhang et al. found that PCWP ameliorated sleep deprivation-induced anxiety by modulating intestinal ecological dysregulation, inhibiting the TNF-α/NF-κB signaling pathway, and alleviating metabolic disturbances [124]. Ye et al. found that PCP exerts an immunomodulatory function and is involved in regulating the composition, function, and metabolism of the gut and lung microbiota to reverse CSA-induced immunosuppressive lung injury [125]. Yin et al. found that PCP attenuated the adverse effects of 5-FU and improved therapeutic efficacy in $Apc^{Min/+}$ mice, and they verified that PCP had a prebiotic effect on enhancing 5-FU by transplanting *Lactobacillus johnsonii* and *Bifdobacterium animalis.* In their study of cisplatin damage to intestinal immunity [126]. Zou et al. found that WP attenuated intestinal injury by modulating the intestinal microbiota and metabolic profile and reversing the elevation of inflammatory mediators [127].

In addition, antibiotic-associated diarrhea is a common and serious problem resulting from the clinical misuse of antibiotics, and its typical diarrhea features are usually accompanied by disturbances in the gut microbiota [138]. Reversing the imbalance in the gut microbiota is one of the most effective treatments for improving AAD, and the intake of polysaccharide prebiotics restores the balance of the flora by increasing the beneficial bacteria and decreasing the pathogenic bacteria [139]. Thus, PCPs ameliorate AAD in mice by modulating the homeostasis of the intestinal microbiota and the intestinal mucosal barrier, showing their potential prebiotic effects and therapeutic efficacy in host immune response and metabolic function [140]. Xu et al. showed that PCP could improve AAD in mice by modulating the homeostasis of the gut microbiota and the intestinal mucosal barrier, by increasing the expression level of the colonic tight junction protein ZO-1, and by regulating the expression of the FOXP3 and GPR41 mRNAs [128]. Interestingly, a study by Lai et al. demonstrated that the PCY originating from *P. cocos* could also alleviate AAD symptoms by increasing the relative abundance of *Muribaculaceae* and *Lachnospiraceae*, decreasing the relative abundance of *Escherichia-Shigella*, *Staphylococcus*, and *Acinetobacter*, promoting the production of SCFAs and decreasing inflammatory response [129].

5. Conclusions and Future Perspective

In this study, we provide information on the bioactivities, extraction methods, structural characterization, and chemical modifications of *P. cocos* and its major ingredients, explore the pharmacological effects of *P. cocos* polysaccharides including anti-obesity, anti-inflammatory, anti-tumor, and immunomodulatory functions, and systematically review the scientific evidence for the modulatory effects of *P. cocos* polysaccharides on the gut microbiota and their health benefits. The conformational relationships of polysaccharides are characterized by their molecular weights, monosaccharide compositions, glycosidic bond types, and high-level structures, which together affect the biological activities, and an in-depth understanding of these conformational relationships is of great significance for the development of natural polysaccharides [141–143]. It is worth noting that *P. cocos* polysaccharides can be categorized into water-soluble polysaccharides and alkali-soluble polysaccharides according to their differences in structure and biological activity. Water-soluble *P. cocos* polysaccharides are more easily absorbed by the body due to their good solubility, and they have excellent biological activities such as anti-tumor, anti-inflammatory, and immunomodulatory effects. The water-insoluble polysaccharides, mainly β-(1 → 3)-D-glucan, are more abundant in *P. cocos*, but have poor water solubility and lower activity than water-soluble polysaccharides [144]. Thus, researchers usually adopt methods, such as degrading polysaccharides into oligosaccharides, or carboxymethylating and sulfating them, to improve water solubility and biological activity [145]. Polysaccharides have been demonstrated to positively impact health on multiple levels by regulating the gut microbiota [146]. As research continues, the relationship between the targets of *P. cocos* polysaccharides acting on the gut microbiota and diseases will be more clearly elucidated [147]. The role of *P. cocos* polysaccharides in improving diseases by targeting the gut microbiota is mainly concentrated on anti-inflammatory, anti-obesity, immune modulation, and prebiotic effects due to the specificity of microbial regulation [148,149]. In this review, we learn that the bioactivities of *P. cocos* polysaccharides targeting the gut microbiota are both related to and different from traditional pharmacological functions. Moreover, the modulatory effects of *P. cocos* polysaccharides on the gut microbiota involve improvement in intestinal barrier function and a reduction in intestinal inflammation via SCFAs, which provides an indirect, yet more integrated and stable, therapeutic approach to treating related diseases. Herein, the main difference between the above two strategies lies in the directness and indirectness of the pathways, as well as the difference in therapeutic focus, with the former indirectly affecting the metabolic and immune status of the host through the modulation of the intestinal microbiota, whereas the latter is usually directly directed to a specific biological target.

In conclusion, this paper reviews the health benefits of *P. cocos* polysaccharides based on the modulation of the gut microbiota, and it emphasizes the relationship between flora modulation and biological functions. Future studies need to combine multidisciplinary knowledge from microbiology, nutrition, immunology, and systems biology to comprehensively understand the regulatory mechanisms of *P. cocos* polysaccharides on the gut microbiota and their integrated effects on human health. This review contributes to the further development of *P. cocos* as a functional product and also provides ideas and insights for developing new therapeutic strategies.

Author Contributions: Y.L. (Yong Lai) and X.L. (Xin Lan): conceptualization, data curation, methodology, visualization, writing—original draft. Z.C., G.L. and C.L.: conceptualization, data curation. Y.L. (Ying Li) and J.F.: data curation, methodology. X.L. (Xi Li) and Y.W.: methodology, supervision, funding acquisition, writing—review and editing. All authors have read and agreed to the published version of the manuscript.

Funding: This work was supported by Sichuan Provincial Department of Science and Technology, project number: 2023JDZH0017; the Basic Research Project of Public Welfare Scientific Research Institutes of Sichuan Province, project number: No. 2024-4-801; and the First Batch of Sichuan Province Qihuang Scholars Capacity Enhancement Project, project number: Chuan Zhong Yi Yao Han [2024]55.

Institutional Review Board Statement: Not applicable.

Informed Consent Statement: Not applicable.

Data Availability Statement: No new data were created or analyzed in this study. Data sharing is not applicable.

Conflicts of Interest: The authors declare that the research was conducted in the absence of any commercial or financial relationships that could be construed as a potential conflict of interest.

References

1. Yang, Z.; Su, C.; Xu, Z.; Liu, Y.; Chen, J.; Wu, X. Mechanistic and Functional Studies on the Microbial Induction of *Wolfiporia cocos* Liquid Fermentation Products. *Foods* **2024**, *13*, 1578. [CrossRef]
2. Liang, D.; Yong, T.; Diao, X.; Chen, S.; Chen, D.; Xiao, C.; Zuo, D.; Xie, Y.; Zhou, X.; Hu, H. Hypouricaemic and nephroprotective effects of *Poria cocos* in hyperuricemic mice by up-regulating ATP-binding cassette super-family G member 2. *Pharm. Biol.* **2021**, *59*, 275–286. [CrossRef] [PubMed]
3. Yuan, J.; Hu, Y.; Yang, D.; Zhou, A.; Luo, S.; Xu, N.; Dong, J.; He, Q.; Zhang, C.; Zhang, X.; et al. The Effects of *Crataegus pinnatifida* and *Wolfiporia extensa* Combination on Diet-Induced Obesity and Gut Microbiota. *Foods* **2024**, *13*, 1633. [CrossRef]
4. Kim, J.H.; Sim, H.A.; Jung, D.Y.; Lim, E.Y.; Kim, Y.T.; Kim, B.J.; Jung, M.H. *Poria cocus* Wolf Extract Ameliorates Hepatic Steatosis through Regulation of Lipid Metabolism, Inhibition of ER Stress, and Activation of Autophagy via AMPK Activation. *Int. J. Mol. Sci.* **2019**, *20*, 4801. [CrossRef]
5. Tong, Q.; Chang, Y.; Shang, G.; Yin, J.; Zhou, X.; Wang, S.; Yan, X.; Zhang, F.; Wang, S.; Yao, W. Integrated chemical characterization, metabolite profiling, and pharmacokinetics analysis of Zhijun Tangshen Decoction by UPLC-Q/TOF-MS. *Front. Pharmacol.* **2024**, *15*, 1363678. [CrossRef] [PubMed]
6. Zong, Y.; Meng, J.; Mao, T.; Han, Q.; Zhang, P.; Shi, L. Repairing the intestinal mucosal barrier of traditional Chinese medicine for ulcerative colitis: A review. *Front. Pharmacol.* **2023**, *14*, 1273407. [CrossRef] [PubMed]
7. Zhu, L.; Wang, X.; Li, S.; Qi, E.R.; Meng, J.; Ching Lam, K.Y.; Dong, X.; Xu, J.; Chen, H.; Zhao, Z. Qualitative and quantitative characterization of carbohydrate profiles in three different parts of *Poria cocos*. *J. Pharm. Biomed. Anal.* **2020**, *179*, 113009. [CrossRef]
8. Park, M.; Yi, J.-M.; Kim, N.S.; Lee, S.-Y.; Lee, H. Effect of *Poria cocos* Terpenes: Verifying Modes of Action Using Molecular Docking, Drug-Induced Transcriptomes, and Diffusion Network Analyses. *Int. J. Mol. Sci.* **2024**, *25*, 4636. [CrossRef]
9. Cheng, Y.; Xie, Y.; Ge, J.C.; Wang, L.; Peng, D.Y.; Yu, N.J.; Zhang, Y.; Jiang, Y.H.; Luo, J.P.; Chen, W.D. Structural characterization and hepatoprotective activity of a galactoglucan from *Poria cocos*. *Carbohydr. Polym.* **2021**, *263*, 117979. [CrossRef]

10. Fang, C.L.; Paul, C.R.; Day, C.H.; Chang, R.L.; Kuo, C.H.; Ho, T.J.; Hsieh, D.J.; Viswanadha, V.P.; Kuo, W.W.; Huang, C.Y. *Poria cocos* (Fuling) targets TGFbeta/Smad7 associated collagen accumulation and enhances Nrf2-antioxidant mechanism to exert anti-skin aging effects in human dermal fibroblasts. *Environ. Toxicol.* **2021**, *36*, 729–736. [CrossRef]
11. Yasuda, S.; Okahashi, N.; Tsugawa, H.; Ogata, Y.; Ikeda, K.; Suda, W.; Arai, H.; Hattori, M.; Arita, M. Elucidation of Gut Microbiota-Associated Lipids Using LC-MS/MS and 16S rRNA Sequence Analyses. *iScience* **2020**, *23*, 101841. [CrossRef]
12. Lai, Y.; Fang, Q.; Guo, X.; Lei, H.; Zhou, Q.; Wu, N.; Song, C. Effect of polysaccharides from Dictyophora indusiata on regulating gut microbiota and short-chain fatty acids in mice. *J. Food Meas. Charact.* **2022**, *17*, 1–11. [CrossRef]
13. Lai, Y.; Deng, H.; Chen, M.; Fan, C.; Chen, Y.; Wang, F.; Zhou, Q.; Song, C. In vitro fermentation properties of grape seed polysaccharides and the effect on regulating gut microbiota in mice. *J. Food Meas. Charact.* **2023**, *17*, 5506–5517. [CrossRef]
14. Liu, C.; Du, P.; Guo, Y.; Xie, Y.; Yu, H.; Yao, W.; Cheng, Y.; Qian, H. Extraction, characterization of aloe polysaccharides and the in-depth analysis of its prebiotic effects on mice gut microbiota. *Carbohydr. Polym.* **2021**, *261*, 117874. [CrossRef] [PubMed]
15. Fang, Q.; Lai, Y.; Zhang, D.; Lei, H.; Wang, F.; Guo, X.; Song, C. Gut microbiota regulation and prebiotic properties of polysaccharides from *Oudemansiella raphanipes* mushroom. *World J. Microbiol. Biotechnol.* **2023**, *39*, 167. [CrossRef]
16. Yin, J.; Ren, W.; Wei, B.; Huang, H.; Li, M.; Wu, X.; Wang, A.; Xiao, Z.; Shen, J.; Zhao, Y.; et al. Characterization of chemical composition and prebiotic effect of a dietary medicinal plant *Penthorum chinense* Pursh. *Food Chem.* **2020**, *319*, 126568. [CrossRef]
17. Cheung, M.K.; Yue, G.G.L.; Chiu, P.W.Y.; Lau, C.B.S. A Review of the Effects of Natural Compounds, Medicinal Plants, and Mushrooms on the Gut Microbiota in Colitis and Cancer. *Front. Pharmacol.* **2020**, *11*, 744. [CrossRef]
18. Feng, Y.L.; Cao, G.; Chen, D.Q.; Vaziri, N.D.; Chen, L.; Zhang, J.; Wang, M.; Guo, Y.; Zhao, Y.Y. Microbiome-metabolomics reveals gut microbiota associated with glycine-conjugated metabolites and polyamine metabolism in chronic kidney disease. *Cell Mol. Life Sci.* **2019**, *76*, 4961–4978. [CrossRef]
19. Ng, C.Y.J.; Lai, N.P.Y.; Ng, W.M.; Siah, K.T.H.; Gan, R.-Y.; Zhong, L.L.D. Chemical structures, extraction and analysis technologies, and bioactivities of edible fungal polysaccharides from *Poria cocos*: An updated review. *Int. J. Biol. Macromol.* **2024**, *261*, 129555. [CrossRef]
20. Jiang, Y.; Fan, L. The effect of *Poria cocos* ethanol extract on the intestinal barrier function and intestinal microbiota in mice with breast cancer. *J. Ethnopharmacol.* **2021**, *266*, 113456. [CrossRef]
21. Li, L.; Zuo, Z.-T.; Wang, Y.-Z. The Traditional Usages, Chemical Components and Pharmacological Activities of *Wolfiporia cocos*: A Review. *Am. J. Chin. Med.* **2022**, *50*, 389–440. [CrossRef] [PubMed]
22. Yang, J.; Dong, X.; Li, B.; Chen, T.; Yu, B.; Wang, X.; Dou, X.; Peng, B.; Hu, Q. *Poria cocos* polysaccharide—Functionalized graphene oxide nanosheet induces efficient cancer immunotherapy in mice. *Front. Bioeng. Biotechnol.* **2023**, *10*, 1050077. [CrossRef]
23. Ríos, J.-L.; Andújar, I.; Recio, M.-C.; Giner, R.-M. Lanostanoids from Fungi: A Group of Potential Anticancer Compounds. *J. Nat. Prod.* **2012**, *75*, 2016–2044. [CrossRef]
24. Wang, D.; Huang, C.; Zhao, Y.; Wang, L.; Yang, Y.; Wang, A.; Zhang, Y.; Hu, G.; Jia, J. Comparative Studies on Polysaccharides, Triterpenoids, and Essential Oil from Fermented Mycelia and Cultivated Sclerotium of a Medicinal and Edible Mushroom, *Poria Cocos*. *Molecules* **2020**, *25*, 1269. [CrossRef] [PubMed]
25. Chao, C.L.; Huang, H.W.; Su, M.H.; Lin, H.C.; Wu, W.M. The Lanostane Triterpenoids in *Poria cocos* Play Beneficial Roles in Immunoregulatory Activity. *Life* **2021**, *11*, 111. [CrossRef]
26. Wang, H.; Luo, Y.; Chu, Z.; Ni, T.; Ou, S.; Dai, X.; Zhang, X.; Liu, Y. Poria Acid, Triterpenoids Extracted from *Poria cocos*, Inhibits the Invasion and Metastasis of Gastric Cancer Cells. *Molecules* **2022**, *27*, 3629. [CrossRef] [PubMed]
27. Meng, Y.; Hu, C.; Cheng, J.; Qiu, W.; Wang, Q.; Chen, X.; Chang, C.; Hu, J.; Qiu, Z.; Zheng, G. The extraction, structure characterization and hydrogel construction of a water-insoluble β-glucan from *Poria cocos*. *Carbohydr. Res.* **2023**, *534*, 108960. [CrossRef]
28. Xu, T.; Zhang, H.; Wang, S.; Xiang, Z.; Kong, H.; Xue, Q.; He, M.; Yu, X.; Li, Y.; Sun, D.; et al. A review on the advances in the extraction methods and structure elucidation of *Poria cocos* polysaccharide and its pharmacological activities and drug carrier applications. *Int. J. Biol. Macromol.* **2022**, *217*, 536–551. [CrossRef]
29. Zhang, W.; Cheng, S.; Zhai, X.; Sun, J.; Hu, X.; Pei, H.; Chen, G. Green and Efficient Extraction of Polysaccharides From *Poria cocos* F. A. Wolf by Deep Eutectic Solvent. *Nat. Prod. Commun.* **2020**, *15*, 1934578X19900708. [CrossRef]
30. Guo, Y.; Li, Y.; Li, Z.; Yan, W.; Chen, P.; Yao, S. Extraction assisted by far infrared radiation and hot air circulation with deep eutectic solvent for bioactive polysaccharides from *Poria cocos* (Schw.) *wolf*. *Green. Chem.* **2021**, *23*, 7170–7192. [CrossRef]
31. Liang, J.; Zhao, M.; Xie, S.; Peng, D.; An, M.; Chen, Y.; Li, P.; Du, B. Effect of steam explosion pretreatment on polysaccharide isolated from *Poria cocos*: Structure and immunostimulatory activity. *J. Food Biochem.* **2022**, *46*, e14355. [CrossRef] [PubMed]
32. Yan, B.; Chen, T.; Tao, Y.; Zhang, N.; Zhao, J.; Zhang, H.; Chen, W.; Fan, D. Fabrication, Functional Properties, and Potential Applications of Mixed Gellan–Polysaccharide Systems: A Review. *Annu. Rev. Food Sci. Technol.* **2024**, *15*, 151–172. [CrossRef]
33. Chen, C.-Y.; Zhang, R.; Zhang, L.-J.; Hu, Z.-Y.; Wang, S.-P.; Mei, X.; Mi, W.; Zhang, J.-Y. Biotransformation and bioaccessibility of active ingredients from Radix Astragali by *Poria cocos* during solid-state fermentation and in vitro digestion and antioxidant activity evaluation. *Sci. Rep.* **2023**, *13*, 6888. [CrossRef] [PubMed]

34. Huang, Q.; Bao, Q.; Wu, C.; Hu, M.; Chen, Y.; Wang, L.; Chen, W. Carbon dots derived from *Poria cocos* polysaccharide as an effective "on-off" fluorescence sensor for chromium (VI) detection. *J. Pharm. Anal.* **2022**, *12*, 104–112. [CrossRef]
35. Nie, A.; Chao, Y.; Zhang, X.; Jia, W.; Zhou, Z.; Zhu, C. Phytochemistry and Pharmacological Activities of *Wolfiporia cocos* (F. A. Wolf) *Ryvarden & Gilb. Front. Pharmacol.* **2020**, *11*, 505249. [CrossRef]
36. Sun, Y. Biological activities and potential health benefits of polysaccharides from *Poria cocos* and their derivatives. *Int. J. Biol. Macromol.* **2014**, *68*, 131–134. [CrossRef]
37. Ríos, J.-L. Chemical Constituents and Pharmacological Properties of *Poria cocos*. *Planta Medica* **2011**, *77*, 681–691. [CrossRef]
38. Zhang, Y.; Huang, J.; Sun, M.; Duan, Y.; Wang, L.; Yu, N.; Peng, D.; Chen, W.; Wang, Y. Preparation, characterization, antioxidant and antianemia activities of *Poria cocos* polysaccharide iron (III) complex. *Heliyon* **2023**, *9*, e12819. [CrossRef]
39. Tan, Z.; Zhang, Q.; Zhao, R.; Huang, T.; Tian, Y.; Lin, Y. A Comparative Study on the Effects of Different Sources of Carboxymethyl Poria Polysaccharides on the Repair of DSS-Induced Colitis in Mice. *Int. J. Mol. Sci.* **2023**, *24*, 9034. [CrossRef]
40. Lu, M.-K.; Chao, C.-H.; Hsu, Y.-C. Advanced culture strategy shows varying bioactivities of sulfated polysaccharides of *Poria cocos*. *Int. J. Biol. Macromol.* **2023**, *253*, 126669. [CrossRef]
41. Liu, F.; Zhang, L.; Feng, X.; Ibrahim, S.A.; Huang, W.; Liu, Y. Immunomodulatory Activity of Carboxymethyl Pachymaran on Immunosuppressed Mice Induced by Cyclophosphamide. *Molecules* **2021**, *26*, 5733. [CrossRef] [PubMed]
42. Liu, X.; Wang, X.; Xu, X.; Zhang, X. Purification, antitumor and anti-inflammation activities of an alkali-soluble and carboxymethyl polysaccharide CMP33 from *Poria cocos*. *Int. J. Biol. Macromol.* **2019**, *127*, 39–47. [CrossRef] [PubMed]
43. Cheng, X.; Cao, L.; Sun, X.; Zhou, S.; Zhu, T.; Zheng, J.; Liu, S.; Liu, H. Metabolomic profile of plasma approach to investigate the mechanism of *Poria cocos* oligosaccharides attenuated LPS-induced acute lung injury in mice. *J. Pharm. Biomed. Anal.* **2024**, *247*, 116262. [CrossRef]
44. Zhang, D.; Li, H.; Luo, X.; Liu, D.; Wei, Q.; Ye, X. Integrated 16S rDNA, metabolomics, and TNF-α/NF-κB signaling pathway analyses to explain the modulatory effect of *Poria cocos* aqueous extract on anxiety-like behavior. *Phytomedicine* **2022**, *104*, 154300. [CrossRef]
45. Cox, A.J.; West, N.P.; Cripps, A.W. Obesity, inflammation, and the gut microbiota. *Lancet Diabetes Endocrinol.* **2015**, *3*, 207–215. [CrossRef] [PubMed]
46. Teame, T.; Wang, A.; Xie, M.; Zhang, Z.; Yang, Y.; Ding, Q.; Gao, C.; Olsen, R.E.; Ran, C.; Zhou, Z. Paraprobiotics and Postbiotics of Probiotic Lactobacilli, Their Positive Effects on the Host and Action Mechanisms: A Review. *Front. Nutr.* **2020**, *7*, 570344. [CrossRef]
47. Moselhy, S.N.; Al-Nashwi, A.A.; Raya-Álvarez, E.; Abu Zaid, F.O.; Shalaby, H.S.T.; El-Khadragy, M.F.; Shahein, M.R.; Hafiz, A.A.; Aljehani, A.A.; Agil, A.; et al. Physicochemical, microbiological, and sensory properties of healthy juices containing aloe vera gel and probiotics and their antidiabetic effects on albino rats. *Front. Nutr.* **2024**, *11*, 1328548. [CrossRef]
48. Li, W.; Yu, J.; Zhao, J.; Xiao, X.; Li, W.; Zang, L.; Yu, J.; Liu, H.; Niu, X. *Poria cocos* polysaccharides reduces high-fat diet-induced arteriosclerosis in ApoE(-/-) mice by inhibiting inflammation. *Phytother. Res.* **2021**, *35*, 2220–2229. [CrossRef]
49. Wang, J.; Zheng, D.; Huang, F.; Zhao, A.; Kuang, J.; Ren, Z.; Chen, T.; Lei, J.; Lin, J.; Wang, X.; et al. Theabrownin and *Poria cocos* Polysaccharide Improve Lipid Metabolism via Modulation of Bile Acid and Fatty Acid Metabolism. *Front. Pharmacol.* **2022**, *13*, 875549. [CrossRef]
50. Zhu, L.; Chen, G.; Guo, Y.; Zheng, J.; Yang, H.; Sun, X.; Liu, Y.; Hu, B.; Liu, H. Structural characterization of *Poria cocos* oligosaccharides and their effects on the hepatic metabolome in high-fat diet-fed mice. *Food Funct.* **2022**, *13*, 6813–6829. [CrossRef]
51. Zhao, J.; Niu, X.; Yu, J.; Xiao, X.; Li, W.; Zang, L.; Hu, Z.; Siu-Po Ip, P.; Li, W. *Poria cocos* polysaccharides attenuated ox-LDL-induced inflammation and oxidative stress via ERK activated Nrf2/HO-1 signaling pathway and inhibited foam cell formation in VSMCs. *Int. Immunopharmacol.* **2020**, *80*, 106173. [CrossRef] [PubMed]
52. Song, D.; Cao, Z.; Tickner, J.; Qiu, H.; Wang, C.; Chen, K.; Wang, Z.; Guo, C.; Dong, S.; Xu, J. *Poria cocos* polysaccharide attenuates RANKL-induced osteoclastogenesis by suppressing NFATc1 activity and phosphorylation of ERK and STAT3. *Arch. Biochem. Biophys.* **2018**, *647*, 76–83. [CrossRef] [PubMed]
53. Wu, Y.; Li, D.; Wang, H.; Wan, X. Protective Effect of *Poria cocos* Polysaccharides on Fecal Peritonitis-Induced Sepsis in Mice Through Inhibition of Oxidative Stress, Inflammation, Apoptosis, and Reduction of Treg Cells. *Front. Microbiol.* **2022**, *13*, 887949. [CrossRef] [PubMed]
54. Jiang, Y.-h.; Wang, L.; Chen, W.-d.; Duan, Y.-t.; Sun, M.-j.; Huang, J.-j.; Peng, D.-y.; Yu, N.-j.; Wang, Y.-y.; Zhang, Y. *Poria cocos* polysaccharide prevents alcohol-induced hepatic injury and inflammation by repressing oxidative stress and gut leakiness. *Front. Nutr.* **2022**, *9*, 963598. [CrossRef]
55. Hu, X.; Hong, B.; Shan, X.; Cheng, Y.; Peng, D.; Hu, R.; Wang, L.; Chen, W. The Effect of *Poria cocos* Polysaccharide PCP-1C on M1 Macrophage Polarization via the Notch Signaling Pathway. *Molecules* **2023**, *28*, 2140. [CrossRef]
56. Sun, M.; Yao, L.; Yu, Q.; Duan, Y.; Huang, J.; Lyu, T.; Yu, N.; Peng, D.; Chen, W.; Wang, Y.; et al. Screening of *Poria cocos* polysaccharide with immunomodulatory activity and its activation effects on TLR4/MD2/NF-κB pathway. *Int. J. Biol. Macromol.* **2024**, *273*, 132931. [CrossRef]

57. Tian, H.; Liu, Z.; Pu, Y.; Bao, Y. Immunomodulatory effects exerted by *Poria cocos* polysaccharides via TLR4/TRAF6/NF-kappaB signaling in vitro and in vivo. *Biomed. Pharmacother.* **2019**, *112*, 108709. [CrossRef]
58. He, J.; Lu, J.; Zhan, L.; Zheng, D.; Wang, Y.; Meng, J.; Li, P.; Zhao, J.; Zhang, W. An Alkali-extracted polysaccharide from *Poria cocos* activates RAW264.7 macrophages via NF-κB signaling pathway. *Arab. J. Chem.* **2023**, *16*, 104592. [CrossRef]
59. Lv, Y.; Yang, Y.; Chen, Y.; Wang, D.; Lei, Y.; Pan, M.; Wang, Z.; Xiao, W.; Dai, Y. Structural characterization and immunomodulatory activity of a water-soluble polysaccharide from *Poria cocos*. *Int. J. Biol. Macromol.* **2024**, *261*, 129878. [CrossRef]
60. Gu, P.; Xu, P.; Zhu, Y.; Zhao, Q.; Zhao, X.; Fan, Y.; Wang, X.; Ma, N.; Bao, Y.; Shi, W. Structural characterization and adjuvant activity of a water soluble polysaccharide from *Poria cocos*. *Int. J. Biol. Macromol.* **2024**, *273*, 133067. [CrossRef]
61. Shao, H.; Zhang, C.; Xiao, N.; Tan, Z. Gut microbiota characteristics in mice with antibiotic-associated diarrhea. *BMC Microbiol.* **2020**, *20*, 313. [CrossRef] [PubMed]
62. Yu, J.; Chen, Z.; Zhou, Q.; Li, P.; Wu, S.; Zhou, T.; Gu, Q. Exopolysaccharide from *Lacticaseibacillus paracasei* alleviates gastritis in Helicobacter pylori-infected mice by regulating gastric microbiota. *Front. Nutr.* **2024**, *11*, 1426358. [CrossRef] [PubMed]
63. Singh, V.K.; Hu, X.-H.; Singh, A.K.; Solanki, M.K.; Vijayaraghavan, P.; Srivastav, R.; Joshi, N.K.; Kumari, M.; Singh, S.K.; Wang, Z.; et al. Precision nutrition-based strategy for management of human diseases and healthy aging: Current progress and challenges forward. *Front. Nutr.* **2024**, *11*, 1427608. [CrossRef] [PubMed]
64. Lu, M.-K.; Chao, C.-H.; Hsu, Y.-C. Effect of carbohydrate-feeding strategy on the production, physiochemical changes, anti-inflammation activities of polysaccharides of *Poria cocos*. *Int. J. Biol. Macromol.* **2021**, *192*, 435–443. [CrossRef]
65. Xu, D.; Yuan, L.; Meng, F.; Lu, D.; Che, M.; Yang, Y.; Liu, W.; Nan, Y. Research progress on antitumor effects of sea buckthorn, a traditional Chinese medicine homologous to food and medicine. *Front. Nutr.* **2024**, *11*, 1430768. [CrossRef]
66. Ma, C.; Lu, J.; Ren, M.; Wang, Q.; Li, C.; Xi, X.; Liu, Z. Rapid identification of α-glucosidase inhibitors from Poria using spectrum-effect, component knock-out, and molecular docking technique. *Front. Nutr.* **2023**, *10*, 1089829. [CrossRef]
67. Mueed, A.; Shibli, S.; Al-Quwaie, D.A.; Ashkan, M.F.; Alharbi, M.; Alanazi, H.; Binothman, N.; Aljadani, M.; Majrashi, K.A.; Huwaikem, M.; et al. Extraction, characterization of polyphenols from certain medicinal plants and evaluation of their antioxidant, antitumor, antidiabetic, antimicrobial properties, and potential use in human nutrition. *Front. Nutr.* **2023**, *10*, 1125106. [CrossRef]
68. Zhao, H.; Liu, G.; Li, Y.; Lu, F.; Yang, N.; Zhao, J. Body fat ratio as a novel predictor of complications and survival after rectal cancer surgery. *Front. Nutr.* **2024**, *11*, 1398807. [CrossRef]
69. Ma, Q.; Ouyang, Y.; Meng, F.; Noolvi, M.N.; Avvaru, S.P.; More, U.A.; Aminabhavi, T.M.; Du, M.; Liu, H.; Zhuang, Y.; et al. A review of pharmacological and clinical studies on the application of Shenling Baizhu San in treatment of Ulcerative colitis. *J. Ethnopharmacol.* **2019**, *244*, 112105. [CrossRef]
70. Qin, L.; Huang, D.; Huang, J.; Qin, F.; Huang, H. Integrated Analysis and Finding Reveal Anti–Liver Cancer Targets and Mechanisms of Pachyman (*Poria cocos* Polysaccharides). *Front. Pharmacol.* **2021**, *12*, 742349. [CrossRef]
71. Zhu, Q.; Zhang, P.; Liu, D.; Tang, L.; Yu, J.; Zhang, C.; Jiang, G. Glucosinolate extract from radish (*Raphanus sativus* L.) seed attenuates high-fat diet-induced obesity: Insights into gut microbiota and fecal metabolites. *Front. Nutr.* **2024**, *11*, 1442535. [CrossRef] [PubMed]
72. Li, Y.-r.; Liu, S.-t.; Gan, Q.; Zhang, J.; Chen, N.; Han, C.-f.; Geng, W.-j.; Wang, B.-x.; Han, N.; Jia, S.-r.; et al. Four polysaccharides isolated from *Poria cocos* mycelium and fermentation broth supernatant possess different activities on regulating immune response. *Int. J. Biol. Macromol.* **2023**, *226*, 935–945. [CrossRef] [PubMed]
73. Yu, Y.; Shen, M.; Song, Q.; Xie, J. Biological activities and pharmaceutical applications of polysaccharide from natural resources: A review. *Carbohydr. Polym.* **2018**, *183*, 91–101. [CrossRef]
74. Nowakowski, P.; Markiewicz-Zukowska, R.; Bielecka, J.; Mielcarek, K.; Grabia, M.; Socha, K. Treasures from the forest: Evaluation of mushroom extracts as anti-cancer agents. *Biomed. Pharmacother.* **2021**, *143*, 112106. [CrossRef]
75. Yang, X.; Lu, S.; Feng, Y.; Cao, C.; Zhang, Y.; Cheng, S. Characteristics and properties of a polysaccharide isolated from *Wolfiporia cocos* as potential dietary supplement for IBS. *Front. Nutr.* **2023**, *10*, 1119583. [CrossRef]
76. Tang, J.; Nie, J.; Li, D.; Zhu, W.; Zhang, S.; Ma, F.; Sun, Q.; Song, J.; Zheng, Y.; Chen, P. Characterization and antioxidant activities of degraded polysaccharides from *Poria cocos* sclerotium. *Carbohydr. Polym.* **2014**, *105*, 121–126. [CrossRef]
77. Koh, A.; De Vadder, F.; Kovatcheva-Datchary, P.; Bäckhed, F. From Dietary Fiber to Host Physiology: Short-Chain Fatty Acids as Key Bacterial Metabolites. *Cell* **2016**, *165*, 1332–1345. [CrossRef] [PubMed]
78. Pi, X.; Du, Z.; Teng, W.; Fu, H.; Hu, L.; Li, J.; Ding, J.; Yang, X.; Zhang, Y. Characteristics of stachyose-induced effects on gut microbiota and microbial metabolites in vitro associated with obesity in children. *Front. Nutr.* **2024**, *11*, 1411374. [CrossRef]
79. Schell, K.R.; Fernandes, K.E.; Shanahan, E.; Wilson, I.; Blair, S.E.; Carter, D.A.; Cokcetin, N.N. The Potential of Honey as a Prebiotic Food to Re-engineer the Gut Microbiome Toward a Healthy State. *Front. Nutr.* **2022**, *9*, 957932. [CrossRef]
80. Zhang, X.-Y.; Chen, J.; Yi, K.; Peng, L.; Xie, J.; Gou, X.; Peng, T.; Tang, L. Phlorizin ameliorates obesity-associated endotoxemia and insulin resistance in high-fat diet-fed mice by targeting the gut microbiota and intestinal barrier integrity. *Gut Microbes* **2020**, *12*, 1842990. [CrossRef]

81. Zhu, Z.; Huang, R.; Huang, A.; Wang, J.; Liu, W.; Wu, S.; Chen, M.; Chen, M.; Xie, Y.; Jiao, C.; et al. Polysaccharide from *Agrocybe cylindracea* prevents diet-induced obesity through inhibiting inflammation mediated by gut microbiota and associated metabolites. *Int. J. Biol. Macromol.* **2022**, *209*, 1430–1438. [CrossRef] [PubMed]
82. Manor, O.; Dai, C.L.; Kornilov, S.A.; Smith, B.; Price, N.D.; Lovejoy, J.C.; Gibbons, S.M.; Magis, A.T. Health and disease markers correlate with gut microbiome composition across thousands of people. *Nat. Commun.* **2020**, *11*, 5206. [CrossRef]
83. Li, M.; Yu, L.; Zhao, J.; Zhang, H.; Chen, W.; Zhai, Q.; Tian, F. Role of dietary edible mushrooms in the modulation of gut microbiota. *J. Funct. Foods* **2021**, *83*, 104538. [CrossRef]
84. Song, C.; Huang, F.; Liu, L.; Zhou, Q.; Zhang, D.; Fang, Q.; Lei, H.; Niu, H. Characterization and prebiotic properties of pectin polysaccharide from *Clausena lansium* (Lour.) Skeels fruit. *Int. J. Biol. Macromol.* **2022**, *194*, 412–421. [CrossRef] [PubMed]
85. Yang, Y.; Ye, H.; Zhao, C.; Ren, L.; Wang, C.; Georgiev, M.I.; Xiao, J.; Zhang, T. Value added immunoregulatory polysaccharides of *Hericium erinaceus* and their effect on the gut microbiota. *Carbohydr. Polym.* **2021**, *262*, 117668. [CrossRef]
86. Liu, Z.; Li, L.; Ma, S.; Ye, J.; Zhang, H.; Li, Y.; Sair, A.T.; Pan, J.; Liu, X.; Li, X.; et al. High-Dietary Fiber Intake Alleviates Antenatal Obesity-Induced Postpartum Depression: Roles of Gut Microbiota and Microbial Metabolite Short-chain Fatty Acid Involved. *J. Agric. Food Chem.* **2020**, *68*, 13697–13710. [CrossRef]
87. Luo, Y.; Fang, Q.; Lai, Y.; Lei, H.; Zhang, D.; Niu, H.; Wang, R.; Song, C. Polysaccharides from the leaves of *Polygonatum sibiricum* Red. regulate the gut microbiota and affect the production of short-chain fatty acids in mice. *AMB Express* **2022**, *12*, 35. [CrossRef] [PubMed]
88. Khinsar, K.H.; Abdul, S.; Hussain, A.; Ud Din, R.; Lei, L.; Cao, J.; Abbasi, M.; Ur Rehman, A.; Farooqui, N.; Yi, X.; et al. Anti-tumor effect of polysaccharide from *Pleurotus ostreatus* on H22 mouse Hepatoma ascites in-vivo and hepatocellular carcinoma in-vitro model. *AMB Express* **2021**, *11*, 160. [CrossRef]
89. Do, M.H.; Lee, H.B.; Oh, M.J.; Jhun, H.; Choi, S.Y.; Park, H.Y. Polysaccharide fraction from greens of *Raphanus sativus* alleviates high fat diet-induced obesity. *Food Chem.* **2021**, *343*, 128395. [CrossRef]
90. Yu, J.; Xiang, H.; Xie, Q. The difference of regulatory effect of two Inonotus obliquus extracts on high-fat diet mice in relation to the fatty acid elongation function of gut microbiota. *Food Sci. Nutr.* **2021**, *9*, 449–458. [CrossRef]
91. Wu, J.; Xu, Y.; Su, J.; Zhu, B.; Wang, S.; Liu, K.; Wang, H.; Shi, S.; Zhang, Q.; Qin, L.; et al. Roles of gut microbiota and metabolites in a homogalacturonan-type pectic polysaccharide from *Ficus pumila* Linn. fruits mediated amelioration of obesity. *Carbohydr. Polym.* **2020**, *248*, 116780. [CrossRef]
92. Yadav, M.K.; Kumari, I.; Singh, B.; Sharma, K.K.; Tiwari, S.K. Probiotics, prebiotics and synbiotics: Safe options for next-generation therapeutics. *Appl. Microbiol. Biotechnol.* **2022**, *106*, 505–521. [CrossRef]
93. Schroeder, B.O.; Backhed, F. Signals from the gut microbiota to distant organs in physiology and disease. *Nat. Med.* **2016**, *22*, 1079–1089. [CrossRef] [PubMed]
94. Yi, Y.; Xu, W.; Wang, H.X.; Huang, F.; Wang, L.M. Natural polysaccharides experience physiochemical and functional changes during preparation: A review. *Carbohydr. Polym.* **2020**, *234*, 115896. [CrossRef] [PubMed]
95. Feng, W.; Ao, H.; Peng, C. Gut Microbiota, Short-Chain Fatty Acids, and Herbal Medicines. *Front. Pharmacol.* **2018**, *9*, 1354. [CrossRef] [PubMed]
96. Xue, H.; Mei, C.F.; Wang, F.Y.; Tang, X.D. Relationship among Chinese herb polysaccharide (CHP), gut microbiota, and chronic diarrhea and impact of CHP on chronic diarrhea. *Food Sci. Nutr.* **2023**, *11*, 5837–5855. [CrossRef]
97. He, Y.; Fu, L.; Li, Y.; Wang, W.; Gong, M.; Zhang, J.; Dong, X.; Huang, J.; Wang, Q.; Mackay, C.R.; et al. Gut microbial metabolites facilitate anticancer therapy efficacy by modulating cytotoxic CD8+ T cell immunity. *Cell Metab.* **2021**, *33*, 988–1000.e7. [CrossRef]
98. Zhang, D.; Jian, Y.-P.; Zhang, Y.-N.; Li, Y.; Gu, L.-T.; Sun, H.-H.; Liu, M.-D.; Zhou, H.-L.; Wang, Y.-S.; Xu, Z.-X. Short-chain fatty acids in diseases. *Cell Commun. Signal.* **2023**, *21*, 212. [CrossRef]
99. Coutzac, C.; Jouniaux, J.-M.; Paci, A.; Schmidt, J.; Mallardo, D.; Seck, A.; Asvatourian, V.; Cassard, L.; Saulnier, P.; Lacroix, L.; et al. Systemic short chain fatty acids limit antitumor effect of CTLA-4 blockade in hosts with cancer. *Nat. Commun.* **2020**, *11*, 2168. [CrossRef]
100. Wang, Z.; Li, Y.; Liao, W.; Huang, J.; Liu, Y.; Li, Z.; Tang, J. Gut microbiota remodeling: A promising therapeutic strategy to confront hyperuricemia and gout. *Front. Cell. Infect. Microbiol.* **2022**, *12*, 935723. [CrossRef]
101. Brown, E.M.; Clardy, J.; Xavier, R.J. Gut microbiome lipid metabolism and its impact on host physiology. *Cell Host Microbe* **2023**, *31*, 173–186. [CrossRef] [PubMed]
102. Kindt, A.; Liebisch, G.; Clavel, T.; Haller, D.; Hormannsperger, G.; Yoon, H.; Kolmeder, D.; Sigruener, A.; Krautbauer, S.; Seeliger, C.; et al. The gut microbiota promotes hepatic fatty acid desaturation and elongation in mice. *Nat. Commun.* **2018**, *9*, 3760. [CrossRef] [PubMed]
103. de Vos, W.M.; Tilg, H.; Van Hul, M.; Cani, P.D. Gut microbiome and health: Mechanistic insights. *Gut* **2022**, *71*, 1020–1032. [CrossRef]
104. Xie, Y.-K.; Pan, X.-Y.; Liang, X.-R.; Zhai, K.-F.; Yu, Q. Research progress on structural characterization and bioactivities of *Poria cocos* and *Ganoderma* polysaccharides. *Food Med. Homol.* **2025**, *2*, 9420040. [CrossRef]

105. Sun, Y.; Liu, Z.; Pi, Z.; Song, F.; Wu, J.; Liu, S. *Poria cocos* could ameliorate cognitive dysfunction in APP/PS1 mice by restoring imbalance of Aβ production and clearance and gut microbiota dysbiosis. *Phytother. Res.* **2021**, *35*, 2678–2690. [CrossRef]
106. Chen, P.; Chen, X.; Hao, L.; Du, P.; Li, C.; Han, H.; Xu, H.; Liu, L. The bioavailability of soybean polysaccharides and their metabolites on gut microbiota in the simulator of the human intestinal microbial ecosystem (SHIME). *Food Chem.* **2021**, *362*, 130233. [CrossRef]
107. Yu, J.; Xiang, J.Y.; Xiang, H.; Xie, Q. Cecal Butyrate (Not Propionate) Was Connected with Metabolism-Related Chemicals of Mice, Based on the Different Effects of the Two Inonotus obliquus Extracts on Obesity and Their Mechanisms. *ACS Omega* **2020**, *5*, 16690–16700. [CrossRef] [PubMed]
108. Wang, Y.-Z.; Zhang, J.; Zhao, Y.-L.; Li, T.; Shen, T.; Li, J.-Q.; Li, W.-Y.; Liu, H.-G. Mycology, cultivation, traditional uses, phytochemistry and pharmacology of *Wolfiporia cocos* (Schwein.) Ryvarden et Gilb.: A review. *J. Ethnopharmacol.* **2013**, *147*, 265–276. [CrossRef]
109. Sun, B.; Huang, B.; Sica, V.P.; Baker, T.R.; Pfuhler, S. A genotoxicity assessment approach for botanical materials demonstrated with *Poria cocos*. *Food Chem. Toxicol.* **2021**, *156*, 112521. [CrossRef]
110. Khan, I.; Huang, G.; Li, X.; Leong, W.; Xia, W.; Hsiao, W.L.W. Mushroom polysaccharides from Ganoderma lucidum and *Poria cocos* reveal prebiotic functions. *J. Funct. Foods* **2018**, *41*, 191–201. [CrossRef]
111. Duan, Y.; Huang, J.; Sun, M.; Jiang, Y.; Wang, S.; Wang, L.; Yu, N.; Peng, D.; Wang, Y.; Chen, W.; et al. *Poria cocos* polysaccharide improves intestinal barrier function and maintains intestinal homeostasis in mice. *Int. J. Biol. Macromol.* **2023**, *249*, 125953. [CrossRef] [PubMed]
112. Wang, M.; Xie, Z.; Li, L.; Chen, Y.; Li, Y.; Wang, Y.; Lu, B.; Zhang, S.; Ma, F.; Ma, C.; et al. Supplementation with compound polysaccharides contributes to the development and metabolic activity of young rat intestinal microbiota. *Food Funct.* **2019**, *10*, 2658–2675. [CrossRef] [PubMed]
113. Lai, Y.; Yu, H.; Deng, H.; Fang, Q.; Lei, H.; Liu, L.; Wu, N.; Guo, X.; Song, C. Three main metabolites from *Wolfiporia cocos* (F. A. *Wolf*) Ryvarden & Gilb regulate the gut microbiota in mice: A comparative study using microbiome-metabolomics. *Front. Pharmacol.* **2022**, *13*, 911140. [CrossRef]
114. Lan, K.; Yang, H.; Zheng, J.; Hu, H.; Zhu, T.; Zou, X.; Hu, B.; Liu, H. *Poria cocos* oligosaccharides ameliorate dextran sodium sulfate-induced colitis mice by regulating gut microbiota dysbiosis. *Food Funct.* **2023**, *14*, 857–873. [CrossRef]
115. Song, X.; Wang, W.; Liu, L.; Zhao, Z.; Shen, X.; Zhou, L.; Zhang, Y.; Peng, D.; Nian, S. *Poria cocos* Attenuated DSS-Induced Ulcerative Colitis via NF-κB Signaling Pathway and Regulating Gut Microbiota. *Molecules* **2024**, *29*, 2154. [CrossRef]
116. Yu, J.; Hu, Q.; Liu, J.; Luo, J.; Liu, L.; Peng, X. Metabolites of gut microbiota fermenting *Poria cocos* polysaccharide alleviates chronic nonbacterial prostatitis in rats. *Int. J. Biol. Macromol.* **2022**, *209*, 1593–1604. [CrossRef]
117. Liu, J.; Yu, J.; Peng, X. *Poria cocos* Polysaccharides Alleviates Chronic Nonbacterial Prostatitis by Preventing Oxidative Stress, Regulating Hormone Production, Modifying Gut Microbiota, and Remodeling the DNA Methylome. *J. Agric. Food Chem.* **2020**, *68*, 12661–12670. [CrossRef]
118. Liu, J.; Liu, L.; Zhang, G.; Peng, X. *Poria cocos* polysaccharides attenuate chronic nonbacterial prostatitis by targeting the gut microbiota: Comparative study of *Poria cocos* polysaccharides and finasteride in treating chronic prostatitis. *Int. J. Biol. Macromol.* **2021**, *189*, 346–355. [CrossRef] [PubMed]
119. Sun, S.-S.; Wang, K.; Ma, K.; Bao, L.; Liu, H.-W. An insoluble polysaccharide from the sclerotium of *Poria cocos* improves hyperglycemia, hyperlipidemia and hepatic steatosis in ob/ob mice via modulation of gut microbiota. *Chin. J. Nat. Med.* **2019**, *17*, 3–14. [CrossRef]
120. Jiang, S.; Liang, C.; Wan, X.; Po Lai, K.; Li, R.; Chen, J.; Liu, J. Integrative analysis reveals the anti-obesity roles of *Poria cocos* polysaccharides through beneficial effects on gut microbiota. *J. Funct. Foods* **2024**, *119*, 106308. [CrossRef]
121. Zhu, L.; Ye, C.; Hu, B.; Xia, H.; Bian, Q.; Liu, Y.; Kong, M.; Zhou, S.; Liu, H. Regulation of gut microbiota and intestinal metabolites by *Poria cocos* oligosaccharides improves glycolipid metabolism disturbance in high-fat diet-fed mice. *J. Nutr. Biochem.* **2022**, *107*, 109019. [CrossRef]
122. Tan, Y.-y.; Yue, S.-r.; Lu, A.-p.; Zhang, L.; Ji, G.; Liu, B.-c.; Wang, R.-r. The improvement of nonalcoholic steatohepatitis by *Poria cocos* polysaccharides associated with gut microbiota and NF-κB/CCL3/CCR1 axis. *Phytomedicine* **2022**, *103*, 154208. [CrossRef]
123. Sun, S.; Wang, K.; Sun, L.; Cheng, B.; Qiao, S.; Dai, H.; Shi, W.; Ma, J.; Liu, H. Therapeutic manipulation of gut microbiota by polysaccharides of *Wolfiporia cocos* reveals the contribution of the gut fungi-induced PGE2 to alcoholic hepatic steatosis. *Gut Microbes* **2020**, *12*, 1830693. [CrossRef] [PubMed]
124. Zhang, D.-d.; Li, H.-j.; Zhang, H.-r.; Ye, X.-c. *Poria cocos* water-soluble polysaccharide modulates anxiety-like behavior induced by sleep deprivation by regulating the gut dysbiosis, metabolic disorders and TNF-α/NF-κB signaling pathway. *Food Funct.* **2022**, *13*, 6648–6664. [CrossRef] [PubMed]

125. Ye, C.; Gao, Z.-H.; Chen, K.-Q.; Lu, F.-G.; Wei, K. Research on Pachymaran to Ameliorate CsA-Induced Immunosuppressive Lung Injury by Regulating Microflora Metabolism. *Microorganisms* **2023**, *11*, 2249. [CrossRef]
126. Yin, L.; Huang, G.; Khan, I.; Su, L.; Xia, W.; Law, B.Y.K.; Wong, V.K.W.; Wu, Q.; Wang, J.; Leong, W.K.; et al. *Poria cocos* polysaccharides exert prebiotic function to attenuate the adverse effects and improve the therapeutic outcome of 5-FU in ApcMin/+ mice. *Chin. Med.* **2022**, *17*, 116. [CrossRef]
127. Zou, Y.T.; Zhou, J.; Wu, C.Y.; Zhang, W.; Shen, H.; Xu, J.D.; Zhang, Y.Q.; Long, F.; Li, S.L. Protective effects of *Poria cocos* and its components against cisplatin-induced intestinal injury. *J. Ethnopharmacol.* **2021**, *269*, 113722. [CrossRef] [PubMed]
128. Xu, H.; Wang, S.; Jiang, Y.; Wu, J.; Chen, L.; Ding, Y.; Zhou, Y.; Deng, L.; Chen, X. *Poria cocos* Polysaccharide Ameliorated Antibiotic-Associated Diarrhea in Mice via Regulating the Homeostasis of the Gut Microbiota and Intestinal Mucosal Barrier. *Int. J. Mol. Sci.* **2023**, *24*, 1423. [CrossRef]
129. Lai, Y.; Deng, H.; Fang, Q.; Ma, L.; Lei, H.; Guo, X.; Chen, Y.; Song, C. Water-Insoluble Polysaccharide Extracted from *Poria cocos* Alleviates Antibiotic-Associated Diarrhea Based on Regulating the Gut Microbiota in Mice. *Foods* **2023**, *12*, 3080. [CrossRef]
130. Mekonnen, S.A.; Merenstein, D.; Fraser, C.M.; Marco, M.L. Molecular mechanisms of probiotic prevention of antibiotic-associated diarrhea. *Curr. Opin. Biotechnol.* **2020**, *61*, 226–234. [CrossRef]
131. Chang, C.J.; Lin, C.S.; Lu, C.C.; Martel, J.; Ko, Y.F.; Ojcius, D.M.; Tseng, S.F.; Wu, T.R.; Chen, Y.Y.; Young, J.D.; et al. Ganoderma lucidum reduces obesity in mice by modulating the composition of the gut microbiota. *Nat. Commun.* **2015**, *6*, 7489. [CrossRef]
132. Zhang, J.; Shu, D.; Cheng, X.; Tian, T.; Xiao, K.; Zhang, D.; Yang, J. Effect of plant polysaccharides (*Poria cocos* and *Astragalus* polysaccharides) on immune responses and intestinal microbiota of Dabry's sturgeons. *Biosci. Microbiota Food Health* **2023**, *42*, 243–253. [CrossRef]
133. Vinolo, M.A.R.; Rodrigues, H.G.; Nachbar, R.T.; Curi, R. Regulation of Inflammation by Short Chain Fatty Acids. *Nutrients* **2011**, *3*, 858–876. [CrossRef]
134. Pickard, J.M.; Zeng, M.Y.; Caruso, R.; Nunez, G. Gut microbiota: Role in pathogen colonization, immune responses, and inflammatory disease. *Immunol. Rev.* **2017**, *279*, 70–89. [CrossRef] [PubMed]
135. Wang, L.; Wang, S.; Zhang, Q.; He, C.; Fu, C.; Wei, Q. The role of the gut microbiota in health and cardiovascular diseases. *Mol. Biomed.* **2022**, *3*, 30. [CrossRef]
136. Wang, Y.; Tang, B.; Long, L.; Luo, P.; Xiang, W.; Li, X.; Wang, H.; Jiang, Q.; Tan, X.; Luo, S.; et al. Improvement of obesity-associated disorders by a small-molecule drug targeting mitochondria of adipose tissue macrophages. *Nat. Commun.* **2021**, *12*, 102. [CrossRef] [PubMed]
137. Peng, X.; Jia, C.; Chi, H.; Wang, P.; Fu, H.; Li, Y.; Wang, Q. Efficacy and Pharmacological Mechanism of *Poria cocos*-Based Formulas Combined with Chemotherapy for Ovarian Cancer: A Integrated Systems Pharmacology Study. *Front. Pharmacol.* **2022**, *13*, 788810. [CrossRef]
138. Willing, B.P.; Russell, S.L.; Finlay, B.B. Shifting the balance: Antibiotic effects on host–microbiota mutualism. *Nat. Rev. Microbiol.* **2011**, *9*, 233–243. [CrossRef] [PubMed]
139. Kopacz, K.; Phadtare, S. Probiotics for the Prevention of Antibiotic-Associated Diarrhea. *Healthcare* **2022**, *10*, 1450. [CrossRef]
140. Tanır Basaranoğlu, S.; Karaaslan, A.; Salı, E.; Çiftçi, E.; Gayretli Aydın, Z.G.; Aldemir Kocabaş, B.; Kaya, C.; Şen Bayturan, S.; Kara, S.S.; Yılmaz Çiftdoğan, D.; et al. Antibiotic associated diarrhea in outpatient pediatric antibiotic therapy. *BMC Pediatr.* **2023**, *23*, 121. [CrossRef]
141. Ji, X.; Guo, J.; Cao, T.; Zhang, T.; Liu, Y.; Yan, Y. Review on mechanisms and structure-activity relationship of hypoglycemic effects of polysaccharides from natural resources. *Food Sci. Hum. Wellness* **2023**, *12*, 1969–1980. [CrossRef]
142. Hou, C.; Yin, M.; Lan, P.; Wang, H.; Nie, H.; Ji, X. Recent progress in the research of *Angelica sinensis* (Oliv.) Diels polysaccharides: Extraction, purification, structure and bioactivities. *Chem. Biol. Technol. Agric.* **2021**, *8*, 13. [CrossRef]
143. Ji, X.; Hou, C.; Gao, Y.; Xue, Y.; Yan, Y.; Guo, X. Metagenomic analysis of gut microbiota modulatory effects of jujube (*Ziziphus jujuba* Mill.) polysaccharides in a colorectal cancer mouse model. *Food Funct.* **2020**, *11*, 163–173. [CrossRef] [PubMed]
144. Wang, Y.; Yu, Y.; Mao, J. Carboxymethylated β-Glucan Derived from *Poria cocos* with Biological Activities. *J. Agric. Food Chem.* **2009**, *57*, 10913–10915. [CrossRef] [PubMed]
145. Zhao, M.; Guan, Z.; Tang, N.; Cheng, Y. The differences between the water- and alkaline-soluble *Poria cocos* polysaccharide: A review. *Int. J. Biol. Macromol.* **2023**, *235*, 123925. [CrossRef]
146. Li, X.; Ma, L.; Zhang, L. Molecular basis for *Poria cocos* mushroom polysaccharide used as an antitumor drug in China. *Prog. Mol. Biol. Transl. Sci.* **2019**, *163*, 263–296. [CrossRef]
147. Yu, C.; Dong, Q.; Chen, M.; Zhao, R.; Zha, L.; Zhao, Y.; Zhang, M.; Zhang, B.; Ma, A. The Effect of Mushroom Dietary Fiber on the Gut Microbiota and Related Health Benefits: A Review. *J. Fungi* **2023**, *9*, 1028. [CrossRef]

148. Qiu, Y.; Lin, G.; Liu, W.; Zhang, F.; Linhardt, R.J.; Wang, X.; Zhang, A. Bioactive compounds in *Hericium erinaceus* and their biological properties: A review. *Food Sci. Hum. Wellness* **2024**, *13*, 1825–1844. [CrossRef]
149. Wu, P.; Tan, H.; Zhan, J.; Wang, W.; Hu, T.; Li, S. Optimization of Bioprocess Extraction of *Poria cocos* Polysaccharide (PCP) with Aspergillus niger β-Glucanase and the Evaluation of PCP Antioxidant Property. *Molecules* **2020**, *25*, 5930. [CrossRef]

molecules

MDPI

Review

Molecular Mechanisms Linking Omega-3 Fatty Acids and the Gut–Brain Axis

Anna Zinkow, Wojciech Grodzicki, Malwina Czerwińska and Katarzyna Dziendzikowska *

Department of Dietetics, Institute of Human Nutrition Sciences, Warsaw University of Life Sciences—SGGW, Nowoursynowska 159C, 02-776 Warsaw, Poland; ania.zinkow@gmail.com (A.Z.); wojciech_grodzicki@sggw.edu.pl (W.G.); malwina_czerwinska@sggw.edu.pl (M.C.)

* Correspondence: katarzyna_dziendzikowska@sggw.edu.pl

Abstract: The gut–brain axis (GBA) is a complex communication network connecting the gastrointestinal tract (GIT) and the central nervous system (CNS) through neuronal, endocrine, metabolic, and immune pathways. Omega-3 (n-3) fatty acids, particularly eicosapentaenoic acid (EPA) and docosahexaenoic acid (DHA), are crucial food components that may modulate the function of this axis through molecular mechanisms. Derived mainly from marine sources, these long-chain polyunsaturated fatty acids are integral to cell membrane structure, enhancing fluidity and influencing neurotransmitter function and signal transduction. Additionally, n-3 fatty acids modulate inflammation by altering eicosanoid production, reducing proinflammatory cytokines, and promoting anti-inflammatory mediators. These actions help preserve the integrity of cellular barriers like the intestinal and blood–brain barriers. In the CNS, EPA and DHA support neurogenesis, synaptic plasticity, and neurotransmission, improving cognitive functions. They also regulate the hypothalamic–pituitary–adrenal (HPA) axis by reducing excessive cortisol production, associated with stress responses and mental health disorders. Furthermore, n-3 fatty acids influence the composition and function of the gut microbiota, promoting beneficial bacterial populations abundance that contribute to gut health and improve systemic immunity. Their multifaceted roles within the GBA underscore their significance in maintaining homeostasis and supporting mental well-being.

Keywords: cognitive function; docosahexaenoic acid (DHA); eicosapentaenoic acid (EPA); gut microbiota; gut–brain axis (GBA); hypothalamic–pituitary–adrenal (HPA) axis; inflammation; omega-3 (n-3) fatty acids

1. Introduction

The gastrointestinal tract (GIT) plays a key physiological role in nutrient digestion and absorption but is also particularly vulnerable, since the alimentary canal is constantly exposed to external and potentially hazardous factors [1]. Given this dual character, GIT has to be closely monitored by the organism's master controller—the brain [2]. The exchange of information between the intestines and the central nervous system (CNS) is mutual. It involves a plethora of neuronal, endocrine, metabolic, and immune factors, known collectively as the gut–brain axis (GBA). The GBA is crucial for maintaining homeostasis and mental health [3]. The pathways that form the axis include interactions with the nervous system as well as molecular signals, like microbial metabolites, tight junction protein expression, and cytokines released during inflammation [4]. Dietary factors, particularly omega-3 polyunsaturated fatty acids (PUFAs), significantly modulate the GBA by influencing gut microbiota composition, enhancing intestinal barrier integrity, and supporting

 https://doi.org/10.3390/molecules30010071

neural function, showing the interplay between nutrition and gut–brain health. Based on the position of the first double bond relative to the terminal end of the carbon chain, PUFAs can be classified into two main groups: omega-3 (n-3) and omega-6 (n-6) fatty acids [5]. n-3 Fatty acids are crucial dietary fats derived from plant sources and marine organisms. α-linolenic acid (ALA, C18:3), an 18-carbon chain fatty acid, is the shortest in the n-3 family and is classified as a short-chain polyunsaturated fatty acid (SC-PUFA). It is also the most abundant n-3 fatty acid found in dietary sources, such as flaxseed, chia seeds, walnuts, and rapeseed oil [6]. ALA plays unique roles supporting cardiovascular health by reducing lipids, blood pressure, and inflammation. Additionally, ALA-derived oxylipins promote vascular health, and emerging evidence highlights its potential in improving cognitive function and supporting brain health [7]. Marine n-3 fatty acids, including eicosapentaenoic acid (EPA, C20:5) and docosahexaenoic acid (DHA, C22:6), are classified as a long-chain PUFAs (LC-PUFA) and exhibit greater biological activity than their plant-derived counterparts [8]. These essential fatty acids cannot be synthesized in the human body and must be supplied through the diet [9]. LCPUFAs, including EPA, DHA, and arachidonic acid (AA, C20:4, n-6 fatty acid), are major components of cellular membrane phospholipids (75–88%, depending on the cell type). Reduced dietary intake of n-3 fatty acids, such as ALA, EPA, and DHA, can lead to decreased content of those fatty acids in brain cells and organelles. DHA, in particular, is the most abundant n-3 fatty acid in the CNS, and is especially concentrated in the membrane lipids of gray matter [8,10]. Therefore, it is to be expected that n-3—and LCPUFAs in particular—would play a crucial role in the GBA, maintaining proper functioning of both the gut and the brain.

2. The Gut–Brain Axis: Definition and Overview

The fundamental part of the GBA is the enteric nervous system (ENS), which entails 100 million nerve cells located in two principal plexuses: the submucosal and the myenteric plexuses [11,12]. ENS forms part of the autonomic nervous system (ANS) and regulates processes related to digestion, nutrient absorption, the release of gastrointestinal hormones, and peristalsis. It serves as an intermediary between the GIT and the CNS by detecting diverse stimuli originating from the intestinal lumen and transferring them to the brain [11–13]. The bidirectional communication network between the CNS and the GIT involves the ENS and parasympathetic innervation, primarily through the vagus nerve fibers that innervate most of the GT. The vagus nerve, also known as the tenth cranial nerve, plays a central role in the complex communication network between the gut and the brain. This nerve is a branch of the ANS that connects the CNS to the ENS through both afferent and efferent nerve fibers [11–13]. Given their multifarious receptors, the constituents of the vagus nerve are sensitive to diverse stimuli, including mechanical tension, hormones, and other chemical incentives. The signals they provide are integrated by the solitary nucleus in the brainstem and elicit a wide array of effects in the brain, stimulating regions related to feeding behavior, anxiety, or emotions [11]. On the other hand, efferent vagal activity has an impact on the gut environment, influencing the immune system and metabolism [11,12].

The CNS also communicates with the GIT through the hypothalamic–pituitary–adrenal (HPA) axis, a key component of the gut–brain communication pathways [11]. The HPA axis activity is initiated by the release of corticotropin-releasing hormone (CRH) from the hypothalamus, which stimulates the anterior pituitary to secrete adrenocorticotropic hormone (ACTH). ACTH, in turn, stimulates the adrenal cortex to release cortisol, a steroid hormone, which plays an important role in regulating metabolism, immune response, and maintaining homeostasis under stress conditions [4,14]. The endocrine factors that influence and regulate the functioning of the GBA include CRH and cortisol. The latter can affect the functioning of immune cells, leading to the production of both proinflammatory cytokines (e.g., tumor necrosis factor-α (TNF-α), interferon-γ (INF-γ), and interleukin 6 (IL-6)) and anti-inflammatory cytokines (e.g., IL-10). Additionally, cortisol increases the permeability of the intestinal barrier, allowing bacterial antigens to pass from the intestinal lumen into the bloodstream, which contributes to the development of systemic inflammation [15].

Gut-associated lymphoid tissue (GALT), which consists of immune cells, is another component of the GBA, positioned at the interface between gut contents and the internal environment of the body [16]. It constitutes 70–80% of the human immune system, highlighting the crucial and sensitive role the intestines play in the body's defense mechanisms [17]. M cells and dendritic cells interact with luminal antigens, activating T and B lymphocytes in Peyer's patches [1]. Cytokine release from immune cells and enterocytes triggers an immune response that can extend beyond the GI tract, reaching the CNS via the bloodstream and affecting vagus nerve signaling. The immune cells' defense is complemented by the protective function of the intestinal barrier [1,11]. The intestinal mucosa functions as a physical and immunological defense barrier, consisting of key components, such as the outer mucus layer with commensal microbiota, antimicrobial peptides, and secretory immunoglobulin A. It also includes a central single layer of epithelial cells and an inner lamina propria containing innate and adaptive immune cells like T cells, B cells, macrophages, and dendritic cells [18].

GALT is also a very important site of interaction with microbial agents and their metabolites [11,16]. Collectively known as the gut microbiota, these microorganisms significantly influence the host's physiology [19]. Interestingly, the number of microbes within the digestive tract exceeds the number of human cells by a factor of 1.3, which highlights their essential role in both health and disease [20,21]. Intestinal microorganisms produce a number of neurotransmitters and neuromodulators—including serotonin, melatonin, γ-aminobutyric acid (GABA), catecholamines, and histamine—which contribute significantly to the proper functioning of brain areas involved in emotion processing, motor activity, and cognitive skills [21,22]. Intestinal microorganisms synthesize and metabolize tryptophan, producing about 95% of systemic serotonin in the gut, which also participates in gut–brain communication [23,24]. Current research demonstrates that the microbiota not only interacts with the CNS but also shapes its development by influencing growth and maturation of brain cells [11,16,25]. Additionally, alterations in microbiota composition have been associated with the onset of various CNS-related disorders, such as Alzheimer's disease, Parkinson's disease, autism, and depression [12].

GALT and gut microbiota collaboratively reinforce the intestinal barrier, contributing to immune protection and maintaining gut homeostasis. Epithelial cells are the primary physical components of the intestinal barrier [26]. Due to the impermeability of cell membranes to hydrophilic solutes without specific transporters, the passage of such molecules through intestinal epithelial cells (IECs) is highly restricted. Lipophilic or larger molecules are primarily absorbed via diffusion and endocytosis that is controlled by junctional complexes, with the most crucial being tight junctions (TJs), adherens junctions (AJs), and desmosomes. TJs, located at the apical region, seal the intercellular space and include proteins such as claudins, occludin, and zonula occludens (ZO)-1 and ZO-2. AJs are positioned below TJs and, together with desmosomes, maintain the epithelial integrity through strong adhesive bonds [27]. The proper functioning of the intestinal barrier is ensured by the tight adhesion of these cells, allowing for transcellular transport and enabling selective absorption.

The GBA also includes the physical barrier that protects the CNS. The blood–brain barrier (BBB) is formed by endothelial cells that are connected by protein junctions [28]. These specialized squamous epithelial cells create a single layer of polarized lining on the inner side of the capillary wall [29]. The intercellular spaces of the capillary endothelium are covered by a dense network of high-resistance junctions, with TJs being the most significant ones. The main components of these TJs are the proteins occludin and claudin [30]. Another set of proteins found in the barrier junctions of the brain are cell adhesion molecules—junctional adhesion molecules (JAM)-A, -B, -C, and -D—with JAM-A believed to influence TJs formation. Along with membrane proteins, the barrier connections also include cytosolic proteins such as ZO-1, -2, and -3 [31]. Additionally, astrocytes contribute to the neurovascular cell complex by forming an extra barrier that circulating blood compounds must cross to reach the brain, enhancing the selectivity of the BBB during periods of increased neuronal activity. Transport of substrates and metabolites is carefully regulated by membrane systems, including the sodium–potassium pump. The BBB serves as a protective barrier against neuroactive substances (e.g., catecholamines) and blood-borne toxins, while also supplying neurons with essential nutrients like glucose and amino acids. Moreover, this barrier protects also against the entry of immune system cells [30].

In summary, multiple communication pathways link the gut and the brain, encompassing systems like the ANS, HPA axis, ENS, intestinal barrier, GALT, microbiota, and the BBB. These systems engage in continuous interaction and information exchange within the GBA (Figure 1) [13].

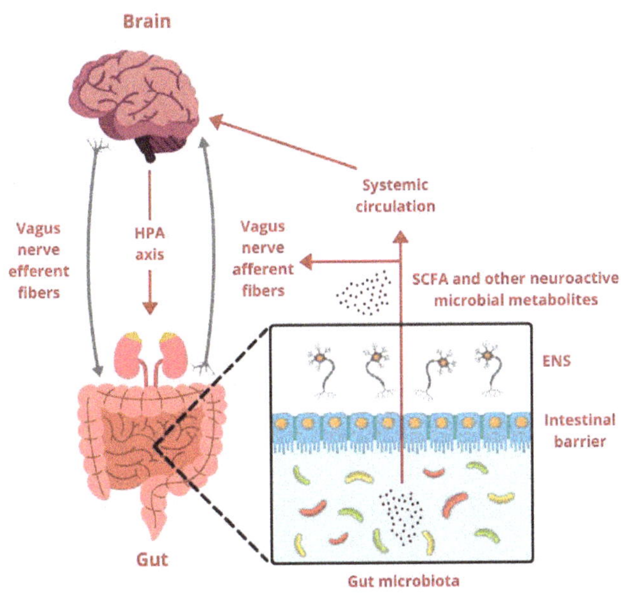

Figure 1. Interaction Between the gut and the brain through the gut–brain axis. HPA axis, hypothalamic-pituitary-adrenal axis; ENS, enteric nervous system; SCFA, short-chain fatty acids. Designed using elements by ©Canva, sparklestroke, Pixeden, iconsy, OpenClipart-Vectors via Canva.com (access date: 18 November 2024).

3. Molecular Mechanisms Linking n-3 Fatty Acids, Microbiota, and Brain Function

3.1. Omega-3 Fatty Acids as Components of Cell Membranes

The multifaceted roles of n-3 fatty acids within biological systems include complex interactions with the GBA. They are integral components of phospholipids in the nerve cell membranes, which enhance their structure and are crucial for their optimal fluidity [32]. This fluidity influences neuronal information transfer by affecting neurotransmitter binding and the speed and integrity of cell signaling [33–35]. DHA represents approximately 15% of all fatty acids in the gray matter of the prefrontal cortex, while EPA and n-3 docosapentaenoic acid (DPA) account for only ~1% of brain fatty acids [36–38]. However, the hydroxy derivative of DHA (2-hydroxydocosahexaenoic acid, OHDHA) has demonstrated therapeutic potential in treating Alzheimer's disease in a mouse model. Administration of this DHA derivative increased brain DHA levels and reduced Aβ (amyloid-β) levels as well as Aβ-induced tau phosphorylation—key factors in the progression of the disease. These effects supported neuronal cell membranes, preserving proper synaptic function, which is essential for signaling and membrane stability in the CNS [39]. The mechanism through which neuronal fluidity changes is based on the displacement of cholesterol from the membrane as well as the induction of non-lamellar structure formation in the membrane [40–42]. Different lipid concentrations in the cell membrane can alter its fluidity as well as the structure and functioning of embedded proteins, such as enzymes, receptors, and ion channels. It is believed that the incorporation of fatty acids into cell membranes also affects the inflammatory cellular responses [43–45]. EPA and DHA compete with dihomogammalinolenic acid and AA for incorporation into the phospholipid membrane, sharing enzymes involved in the eicosanoid production process [46,47]. Metabolic transformations of DHA and EPA carried out by cyclooxygenases (COX), lipoxygenases (LOX), and cytochrome P450 enzymes result in the production of numerous eicosanoids and docosanoids [48,49]. These metabolites influence the brain-derived neurotrophic factor (BDNF), increasing synaptic plasticity and enhancing neurotransmission, thus providing neuroprotective effects, as demonstrated in studies conducted on the multipotent human hippocampal progenitor cell line HPC0A07/03C and the human bone marrow neuroblastoma SH-SY5Y cell line (multipotent human hippocampal progenitor cell line) [48–50]. Both animal and human studies indicate that the incorporation of EPA and DHA into cell phospholipids during inflammatory processes is dose-dependent and occurs at the expense of AA content [47,51–56]. The role of n-3 fatty acids as components of CNS cellular membranes is summarized in Figure 2.

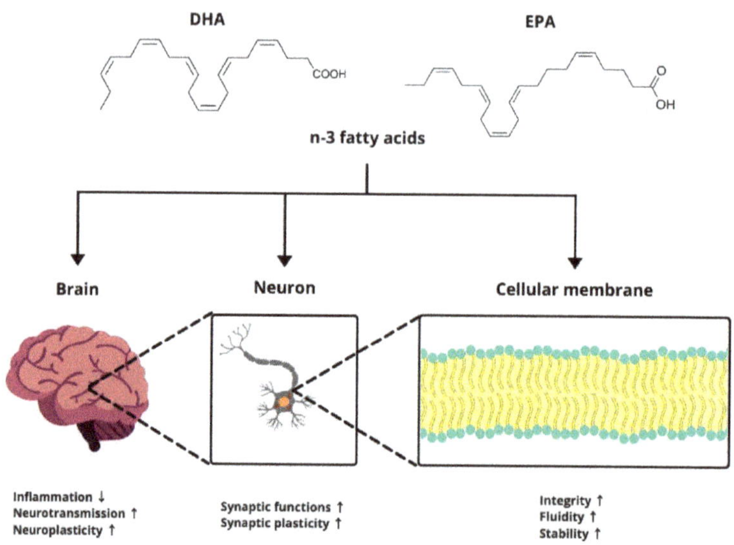

Figure 2. The role of omega-3 fatty acids as components of cell membranes. ↑ indicates an increase, ↓ indicates a decrease. Designed using elements by ©Canva, sparklestroke, Pixeden, iconsy, OpenClipart-Vectors via Canva.com (access date: 18 November 2024).

3.2. Impact of Omega-3 Fatty Acids on Inflammation

The modulation of inflammation by n-3 fatty acids, mainly through their effects on eicosanoid production, illustrates a critical mechanism by which dietary fats influence both neurological health and systemic inflammatory responses [57,58]. Prostaglandins, thromboxanes, leukotrienes, and hydroxyl and hydroxy fatty acids are enzymatic metabolic products of PUFA, known as eicosanoids. These compounds play a pivotal role in the inflammatory processes and neurological pathways within the GBA [59,60]. The structural differences in eicosanoids derived from EPA and AA affect the biological activity of EPA derivatives, as eicosanoid receptors have a lower affinity for the mediators derived from EPA than ARA [61]. An in vitro study on HEK293 cell lines demonstrated 50–80% lower activity of prostaglandin E3 (PGE3) compared to prostaglandin E2 (PGE2) on prostaglandin E2 receptors 1, 2, 3, and 4 (EP1, EP2, EP3, and EP4), indicating nuanced influence of dietary fats on neuroinflammatory responses [62]. Eicosanoids derived from EPA and DHA have anti-inflammatory properties [47,55,58,63]. EPA competes with AA for the cyclooxygenase enzyme system, effectively inhibiting the production of proinflammatory eicosanoids from AA. Both DHA and EPA reduce the release of proinflammatory cytokines, such as interleukin-1β (IL-1β), -2 (IL-2), and -6 (IL-6), along with IFN-γ and TNF-α [57,63–65]. These cytokines can affect the CNS both indirectly and directly by reducing the availability of neurotransmitter precursors, influencing their metabolism, transport, and regulation, as well as impacting the HPA axis and mRNA-encoding proteins involved in neurotransmitter metabolism [66–69]. Flaxseed oil inhibits the synthesis of proinflammatory cytokines, thereby regulating neurotransmitter production and the HPA axis [70]. Marine-derived n-3 fatty acids lead to the production of pro-resolving lipid mediators, such as EPA-derived resolvins (E series), DHA-derived resolvins (D series), and resolvins derived from DPA n-3 (RvDn-3 DPA), along with protectins (also known as neuroprotectins when produced in the nervous tissue) and maresins derived from DHA. Their synthesis occurs through COX and LOX pathways, acting intercellularly [57,71–74]. The anti-inflammatory actions of n-3 fatty acids involve binding to peroxisome proliferator-activated receptors (PPARs), G-protein–coupled receptor 40 (GPR40), and free fatty acid receptor 4 (FFA4), also known as GPR120, which promote the production of anti-inflammatory lipids—resolvins and protectins. These lipids play a crucial role in inhibiting the activation of key inflammatory regulators, including transcription factor nuclear factor kappa B (NF-kB), IL-1 β, and TNF-α release [75–79]. Supplementation with EPA and DHA in mice has been shown to increase the number of T lymphocytes [80]. Additionally, DHA and EPA are able to inhibit IL-6 and interleukin 8 (IL-8) production stimulated by lipopolysaccharide (LPS) in human endothelial cells. Moreover, EPA has been observed to inhibit TNF-α production by cultured monocytes [81,82]. LC-PUFAs also reduce LPS-induced proinflammatory cytokine production in human blood monocytes and in murine fetal liver-derived macrophages, leading to a decrease in TNF-α level in serum, NF-kB activation, and IL-1 β production by monocytes [82–84]. This reduction can trigger the release of substantial amounts of anti-inflammatory factors, such as interleukin-10 (IL-10), from resident macrophages. LC-PUFAs play a critical role in directly modulating cytokine production and immune cell regulation. They also exert broader anti-inflammatory effects through key intracellular signaling pathways, such as NFκB, that influence overall immune response and inflammatory status mainly due to the increased level of inflammatory cytokines, adhesion molecules, and cyclooxygenase-2 (COX-2) [82,85,86]. NFκB is activated by the signaling cascade triggered by external inflammatory stimuli, including endotoxin binding to toll-like receptor (TLR) 4. Upon activation, the NFκB dimer is translocated to the nucleus, where it upregulates gene expression [87–90].

The documented anti-inflammatory and regulatory capabilities of EPA and DHA on cytokine dynamics and cellular mediator pathways also help preserve the integrity of cellular barriers, such as the BBB, by reducing inflammation-induced disruption and enhancing barrier functions. Transmembrane proteins, including claudin-5 and occludin, along with scaffold proteins, like ZO-1 and ZO-2, participate in the tight junction complex of endothelial cells in the CNS [91,92]. LC-PUFAs indirectly enhance the integrity of the BBB and reduce its permeability by modulating levels of inflammatory cytokines [93, 94]. Systemic administration of IL-1β has been demonstrated to cause prolonged BBB disruption, activate matrix metalloproteinase-9, and induce rearrangement of claudin-5 in cerebral vessels following transient middle cerebral artery occlusion in mice [95]. Therefore, it is suggested that n-3 fatty acids may strengthen the integrity of the BBB by downregulating the expression of proinflammatory cytokines. Interestingly, research indicates that certain anti-inflammatory cytokines, including IL-4, IL-10, and IL-13, can also contribute to damaging the BBB, but the precise mechanisms behind these effects are not yet well understood [96]. However, the disruption kinetics of the barrier via IL-4 seems to be similar to that of n-6 PUFAs, such as di-homo-gamma-linolenic acid (DGLA, C20:3 n-6) and AA. In comparison n-3 PUFAs, including EPA and DHA, support epithelial barrier integrity by enhancing trans-epithelial electrical resistance (TER) and significantly reducing IL-4-induced permeability. This suggests that LC-PUFAs play a crucial role in maintaining barrier function, as demonstrated by Willemsen Le et al. [97]. Tight junction complexes actively control paracellular permeability and are sensitive to soluble barrier-disrupting mediators [98,99]. Proteins such as occludin, ZO-1, and claudins play critical roles in regulating the intestinal barrier, controlled by the perijunctional actomyosin ring and myosin light chain kinase [100–102]. LC-PUFAs improve trans-epithelial resistance, but the exact mechanism of its impact on this process is not fully understood. Several mechanisms have been proposed to explain the effects of n-3 LC-PUFAs on BBB integrity, particularly their roles in modulating inflammatory pathways and enhancing antioxidant defense systems. Notably, n-3 PUFAs suppress IFN-γ-induced expression of TNF-α, IL-6, nitric oxide synthase (NOS), and COX-2, while promoting the upregulation of heme oxygenase-1 (HO-1) in BV-2 microglia cells. BBB disruption and "leaky gut" phenomenon increase the transfer of neurotoxins into the brain, leading to elevated production of proinflammatory molecules, reactive oxygen species, and increased bacterial adhesion through receptors, thereby disrupting endothelial connections [103]. n-3 Fatty acids, specifically EPA and DHA, have been shown to enhance basal trans-epithelial resistance (TER), thereby reducing the permeability of the gut barrier in human intestinal epithelial cells (T84) in vitro, indirectly through mechanisms involving IL-4. LCPUFAs, such as dihomo-γ-linolenic acid (DGLA), AA, EPA, and DHA, stimulate basal resistance and mitigate IL-4-induced permeability changes [97,104,105]. Supplementation with EPA in rats has been shown to increase the expression of occludin, a protein playing an important role in the intestinal barrier integrity [106–108]. These protective effects are associated with support and protection of the tight junction structure and function. Additionally, n-3 fatty acids have been shown to increase the number of goblet cells, promote the growth of beneficial bacteria, and elevate the expression of mucin 2, all of which contribute to improved intestinal barrier integrity [104,109]. Summarized anti-inflammatory effects of n-3 fatty acids in the gut and the brain are shown in Figure 3.

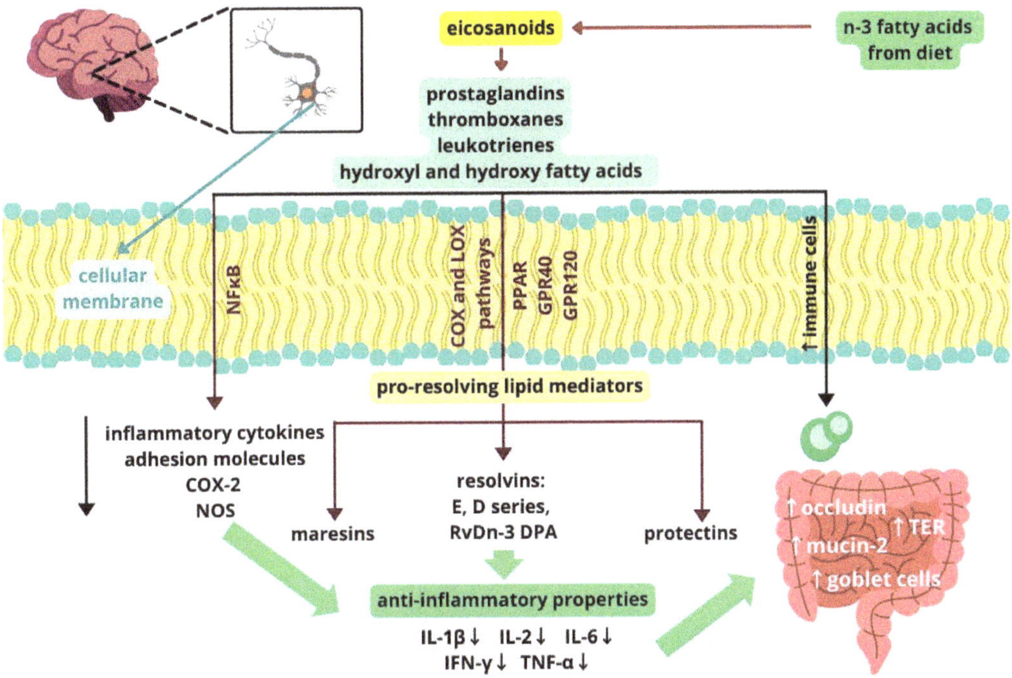

Figure 3. Anti-inflammatory role of n-3 fatty acids. NF-kB—nuclear factor kappa B; COX-2—cyclooxygenase-2, prostaglandin-endoperoxide synthase 2; LOX—lipoxygenase; NOS—nitric oxide synthase; PPAR—peroxisome proliferator-activated receptors; GPR40—G-protein–coupled receptor 40; GPR120—G-protein–coupled receptor 120; RvDn DPA—resolvins derived from DPA n-3; Il-1β—interleukin 1β; IL-2—interleukin 2; IL-6—interleukin 6; INF-γ—interferon-γ; TNF-α—tumor necrosis factor α; TER—trans-epithelial electrical resistance. ↑ indicates an increase, ↓ indicates a decrease. Designed using elements by ©Canva, sparklestroke, Pixeden, iconsy, OpenClipart-Vectors via Canva.com (access date: 18 November 2024).

3.3. *Impact of Omega-3 Fatty Acids on the Nervous System and Cognitive Functions*

Omega-3 fatty acids, mainly DHA and EPA, are essential for maintaining neural integrity and improving cognitive functions, as they serve as integral components of neuron membrane structure and play a critical role in neurogenesis, neural signaling, and neuroprotection. DHA also promotes neuron growth by enhancing protein kinase B signaling [110]. This process requires the accumulation of lipids in newly formed membranes and DHA facilitates the incorporation of cholesterol into structures important for myelination and neurite extension, thereby assisting in the organization of the lipid raft domain of the membrane [111–113]. Summarized data presenting the effects of n-3 fatty acids on cognitive functions are presented in Table 1.

Neurogenesis is essential for cognitive function, as it supports brain plasticity and adaptability, fundamental for learning and memory retention. This process is most apparent during prenatal development, but it persists in certain parts of the adult brain, most notably in the hippocampus, a structure crucial for learning and memory formation [114,115]. BDNF is a protein that belongs to the neurotrophin family of growth factors, which are vital for the growth, survival, and differentiation of neuron cells. It plays a key role in neuroplasticity, and it is a critical mediator that links neurogenesis to broader brain functions, particularly those related to learning, memory, and overall cognitive health [116–

118]. n-3 Fatty acids—especially DHA—increase BDNF levels, thereby influencing the growth, differentiation, and viability of neurons in the hippocampus, playing a significant role in the regulation of various neurotransmitter systems [119–122]. Direct administration of BDNF to the dorsal hippocampus in rats significantly increased the granule cell layer of the hilar region [123]. Deuterated polyunsaturated fatty acids (D-PUFAs) supplementation has been shown to alleviate cognitive decline through its antioxidant activity and reduction in lipid peroxidation in a Huntington's disease mouse model [124]. In an animal model of spinal cord injury, DHA treatment following injury led to comprehensive functional improvements, evidenced by enhanced fore and hindlimb locomotion and better motor control in the grid exploration and staircase tests. This was accompanied by structural neural adaptations, including increased synaptophysin density around motor neurons, enhanced cortical synaptogenesis, amplified serotonergic innervation, and increased sprouting of corticospinal axons in both rostral and caudal regions of the injured area [125]. DHA also promotes hippocampal neuron development in vitro by supporting neurite growth and branching and also synaptogenesis. Moreover, in vivo DHA depletion in the fetal hippocampus resulted in inhibition of hippocampal neuron development in culture, which can be reversed with DHA supplementation [126].

n-3 Fatty acids increase synaptic plasticity in hippocampal neurons and improve its glutaminergic activity, which is crucial for cognitive function as it mediates synaptic plasticity and neurotransmission, fundamental for learning, memory formation, and overall brain cell connectivity [127–129]. A 6-month randomized controlled trial showed that supplementation at a dose of almost 2 g of EPA and DHA decreases depression symptoms in the Geriatric Depression Scale in geriatric patients and DHA improves cognitive function, i.e., verbal fluency tested with Initial Letter Fluency [130]. In a model of accelerated aging with prediabetic status, dietary enrichment with flaxseed and fish oils enhanced spatial learning and working memory performance in the Morris water maze test through reduction in inflammatory markers and toxic metabolites in the CNS of male rats. Elevated n-3 fatty acids levels in the frontal cortex following supplementation were associated with protective effects against cognitive impairment and reduced depressive-like behaviors linked to gray matter atrophy, suggesting a crucial role of EPA in preventing cognitive decline [131].

The cognitive enhancements provided by n-3 fatty acids primarily stem from their profound impact on cellular structures, which leads to the modulation of the physical aspects of brain health, particularly the stabilization of neuronal membranes and ion channels [132–134]. In a randomized, double-blind, controlled trial, healthy older adults who consumed 3.7 g per day of flaxseed oil containing 2.2 g of ALA over 12 weeks demonstrated improved verbal fluency. This improvement is believed to result from changes in neuronal cell membrane structure across broad anatomical regions, enhanced membrane fluidity, and improved intercellular connectivity, which typically decline with age [135]. LC-PUFAs influence the integrity of membrane proteins, including enzymes, receptors, and ion channels. They regulate membrane protein integrity, affecting enzymatic activity, receptor function, and ion channel conductance. Administration of DHA demonstrated neuromodulatory effects via ion channel regulation, subsequently reducing the amplitude of epileptiform discharges in experimental rodent models of seizure activity [134,136]. These changes occurred through sodium channel blockade and neuronal membrane stabilization by suppressing calcium-gated membrane tension, thereby blocking synaptic transmission [132–134,136–138]. Research indicates that n-3 LC-PUFAs play a crucial role in promoting brain health. They enhance neuroprotective capabilities, support neuroplasticity, and reduce neuroinflammation, all of which are essential for sustaining cognitive functions. Short-term exposure to EPA and DHA reversed spatial working memory deficits in older mice by reducing IL-1β expression in inflammation-associated hippocampi [139]. Similarly, a high-fat diet enriched with flaxseed oil improved spatial learning and working memory in male mice during the Morris water maze test by reducing levels of inflammatory markers and toxic metabolites in the CNS [140].

n-3 Fatty acids contribute to brain health by modulating membrane structures and reducing neuronal damage. Additionally, they directly impact cellular mechanisms that eliminate harmful proteins and facilitate cellular repair, highlighting their potential therapeutic roles in neurodegenerative diseases [141]. DHA and EPA stimulate and increase the expression of insulin-degrading enzyme (IDE) genes, which raises the levels of IDE, the main enzyme responsible for degrading amyloid-beta (Aβ) peptide secreted into the extracellular space of neuronal and microglial cells [142]. The accumulation of Aβ peptides is linked to the development of AD, and the effect of n-3 fatty acids may assist in removing these peptides from the brain and modulating inflammation, thereby supporting brain glial cells [143,144]. Additionally, DHA exhibits a protective effect on dopaminergic neurons in a Parkinson's disease animal model induced by the neurotoxin 1-methyl-4-phenyl-1,2,3,6-tetrahydropyridine (MPTP) [142]. Moreover, another study demonstrated that DHA administration significantly increased TH-positive neurons compared to the control group when exposed to MPTP, suggesting changes in dopaminergic activity [145]. It has been suggested that the DHA may delay or slow the progression of Parkinson disease development by blocking the conversion of MPTP to MPP+ (methylpyridinium ion) or by preventing the uptake of MPP+ into dopaminergic terminals. Furthermore, DHA has been shown to influence synaptic plasticity and cognitive functions by activating syntaxin 3, a plasma membrane protein that plays a significant role in membrane expansion [146,147].

Table 1. Effects of n-3 fatty acids on the CNS and cognitive functions.

Models	Type of Study	Source and Dose	Exposure	Effect Related to Nervous System and Cognitive Functions	Reference
			In vitro model studies		
Embryonic neurons from E18 mouse hippocampi pregnant C57/BL6 mice	in vitro	Diet with 2.5 wt% of linolenic acid plus 0.9 wt% DHA	16 days	- Increased neurite growth and synaptogenesis - Enhance glutamatergic synaptic activity	[126]
Hippocampus of Sprague Dawley rats	in vitro	50 µM of DHA	Single dose	- Attenuation of epileptic activity	[136]
			In vivo model studies		
Q140 mouse model of Huntington's disease	in vivo	Deuterium-reinforced D_2-Lin (KI D-PUFA)	5 months	- Alleviation of cognitive decline	[124]
Female Sprague Dawley rats	in vivo	5 mL/kg of DHA (i.v. injection) post-injury	Single bolus	- Improve locomotion and BBB score - Enhanced synaptogenesis in cortical neurons	[125]
Male Sprague Dawley rats with prediabetic status	in vivo	2% fish oil (EPA + DHA) or 2% flaxseed oil	3 months	- Improved spatial memory	[131]
Adult male Sprague Dawley rats	in vivo	Diet with n-6/n-3 PUFA ratio at 6:1 (1.25% DHA, 0.25% EPA)	12 days	- Enhanced synaptic function underlying learning and memory - Improved spatial learning	[146]
C57Bl6/J mice 22 months old (aged)	in vivo	EPA and DHA from tuna oil	2 months	- Inhibition proinflammatory cytokine expression - Prevention of morphological alterations in hippocampal tissue - Amelioration of spatial memory impairments	[139]
Obese male C57BL/6 mice 8 weeks old	in vivo	n-3 PUFA from linseed oil	16 weeks	- Improved spatial memory - Reduced inflammatory markers (TNF-α) - Decreased toxic metabolite levels in the CNS	[140]
Male C57BL/6 mice model of Parkinson's disease (3 months old)	in vivo	36 mg/kg/d of DHA (in corn oil)	30 days	- Decrease levels and activity of heme oxygenase (HO) in substantia nigra- Decrease in levels of Nuclear Factor E2-related factor 2, HO-1 and HO-2 in substantia nigra	[148]

Table 1. *Cont.*

Models	Type of Study	Source and Dose	Exposure	Effect Related to Nervous System and Cognitive Functions	Reference
Male C57BL/6 mice model of Parkinson's disease (10 months old)	in vivo	36 mg/kg/d of DHA (in corn oil)	30 days	- Protection against oxidative stress - Significant increase in TH-positive neurons	[145]
Human subject studies					
Healthy older adults 65–80 years old	human subjects	3.7 g/day of flaxseed oil with 2.2 g of alpha-linolenic acid	12 weeks	- Improve lexical fluency	[135]
Elderly people (over 65 years old)	human subjects	1.67 g EPA + 0.16 g DHA/d or 1.55 g DHA + 0.40 g EPA/d	6 months	- Decrease in depression symptoms	[130]

3.4. Impact of Omega-3 Fatty Acids on the HPA Axis

As a neuroendocrine factor, cortisol is essential in the stress response and plays a critical role in regulating GBA functions. As a primary stress hormone released by the adrenal glands in response to stress, cortisol forms part of the body's HPA axis, which is closely connected to the GBA. Dysregulation of this system, particularly HPA axis hyperactivity, has been implicated in the pathophysiology of anxiety, depression, and other stress-related conditions [149,150]. n-3 fatty acids, particularly EPA and DHA, have been shown to regulate the HPA axis by reducing excessive cortisol production. Research has shown a reduced cortisol response to acute mental stress in healthy men who were given 7.2 g/day of fish oil for 3 weeks [151]. Preclinical and clinical data indicate that low plasma levels of n-3 fatty acids are correlated with higher CRH [149] and plasma concentration of cortisol [152,153], while n-3 fatty acid supplementation may decrease CRH expression and corticosterone secretion [154,155]. CRH, crucial in regulating the HPA axis, is produced in neurons within the hypothalamic paraventricular nucleus (PVN), which receives input from the limbic system and the brainstem. This connectivity enables these neurons to respond to both psychological and physical stressors [156]. In vitro studies confirmed that n-3 fatty acid-deficient rats had exaggerated distress behaviours in comparison with rats with the appropriate n-3 fatty acid levels during administration of CRH and were normalized upon restoration of n-3 fatty acid levels [157]. Studies conducted on male Finnish psychiatric patients (with diagnosed depression, alcoholism, or both) and healthy patients without psychiatric disorders have also shown that excessive stress response and HPA hyperactivity may be related to concentrations of brain and plasma neuroactive steroids (NASs) [158]. NASs are produced in the CNS from cholesterol and have the ability to alter neuronal excitability rapidly. In a study carried out on male psychiatric patients from Finland, the authors observed that lower plasma levels of n-3 fatty acids were linked to higher plasma levels of neurosteroids. Specifically, reduced concentrations of DHA and EPA were correlated with increased levels of NASs in healthy control subjects [158]. DHA supplementation reduced stress-related increases in aggression and hostility among Japanese students [159]. The research conducted by Oravcova et al. [160] on patients aged 11–18 confirmed the hypothesis that long-term (12 weeks) supplementation of n-3 fatty acids from fish oil emulsion reduces morning cortisol levels in saliva. These findings are in line with the current understanding of the connection between HPA axis activity and fatty acid metabolism in adults with recurrent depressive disorder [155]. Adults with lower levels of n-3 fatty acids demonstrated HPA axis dysregulation, suggesting that supplementation with these fatty acids could potentially improve both physical and mental health [161]. Notably, dietary supplementation with LC-PUFAs from marine oils has been shown to lower corticosterone levels in rats and to reduce cortisol secretion in both healthy individuals and adults experiencing depression [151,162,163]. Results from a randomized, placebo-controlled trial in midlife adults demonstrated that EPA and DHA supplementation significantly reduced cortisol levels during stress in a dose–response manner. Patients receiving the higher doses of n-3 fatty acids had the lowest overall cortisol levels, while those in the placebo group exhibited the highest levels [164]. Additionally, supplementation with n-3 fatty acids (2400 mg of total omega-3 fatty acids; 1000 mg of EPA and 750 mg of DHA; EPA:DHA ratio of 1.33:1) over a 12-week period was shown to significantly reduce clinical symptoms of depression in older children and adolescents [165]. In adolescent patients, the positive treatment effects from n-3 fatty acid supplementation were also associated with a decrease in various oxidative stress markers, such as 8-isoprostane, advanced oxidation protein products, and nitrotyrosine blood levels, as well as increased Trolox equivalent antioxidant capacity and superoxide dismutase activity [166].

Chronic stress or inflammation can result in the overactivation of the HPA axis. Previous studies have demonstrated increased levels of inflammatory markers, including IL-6 and TNF-α, in numerous chronic diseases such as cardiovascular diseases, obesity, and depression, contributing to their development and progression [167–169]. Additionally, HPA axis hyperactivity has been observed in obesity, and increased morning cortisol levels have been reported in individuals with depression [170,171]. Given their anti-inflammatory and immunomodulatory effects, n-3 PUFAs may help mitigate these detrimental processes and thereby potentially alleviate conditions characterized by HPA axis dysregulation [172,173]. n-3 fatty acids can lower HPA axis hyperactivity by decreasing proinflammatory cytokines levels, such as IL-6 and TNF-α, which influence the stress response. By downregulating the proinflammatory cytokine pathways and modulating the stress response, n-3 fatty acids reduce the sensitivity of the HPA axis. This means that the axis is less likely to become overactive in response to minor stressors, potentially lowering the risk of stress-related disorders. In a randomized, double blind, placebo-controlled trial conduced on healthy man, n-3 supplementation in combination with phosphatidylserine significantly improved the functioning of the HPA axis by lowering chronic and acute stress [174]. The authors concluded that individuals experiencing high levels of chronic stress and/or having a dysfunctional HPA axis response could benefit from n-3 phosphatidylserine supplementation. The impact of n-3 fatty acids on regulating the activity of the HPA axis may be related to their anti-inflammatory properties, coupled with the increase in the HPA axis sensitivity to negative feedback [175,176].

3.5. Modulation of the Gut Microbiota by Omega-3 Fatty Acids

The beneficial physiological effects of LC-PUFAs encompass their influence on the composition and function of the gut microbiota, as demonstrated in various studies linking fatty acid intake to microbial diversity and health outcomes. n-3 fatty acids can influence the modulation and abundance of gut bacteria types. At the same time, gut microbiota can affect the absorption and metabolism of these fatty acids. Fish oil, for instance, reduces the growth of *Enterobacteria*, while increasing that of *Bifidobacteria*. EPA and DHA are partially metabolized by anaerobic bacteria, such as *Bifidobacteria* and *Lactobacilli*, in the distal gut [177]. In a study conducted on gnotobiotic piglets fed with PUFA from seal oil, a significant increase in the number of *Lactobacillus paracasei* adhering to the jejunal mucosa was shown [178]. Similarly, n-3 fatty acids administered to male transgenic fat-1 mice significantly increased the number and percentage of *Bifidobacterium*, *Akkermansia muciniphila*, *Lactobacillus*, *Clostridium clusters IV* and *XIVa*, and *Enterococcus faecium* in the intestines [179]. The modulatory functions of n-3 fatty acids are also attributed to increased levels of SCFAs. It has been shown that dietary supplementation with DHA and EPA in mice infected with *Salmonella* increased SCFA fecal content, enhancing resistance against the pathogen [180]. Consuming 3 g per day of DHA and EPA from sardines significantly altered the gut microbiota composition in patients with untreated type 2 diabetes. Specifically, the proportions of *Bacteroides/Prevotella* increased, while the *Firmicutes/Bacteroidetes* ratio decreased [181]. In a study of birds, a diet rich in omega-3 PUFA significantly increased the presence of *Firmicutes* (e.g., *Faecalibacterium*, *Clostridium*, and *Ruminococcus*, all of which are butyrate producers), in the gut microbiota [182]. Additionally, serum levels of omega-3 fatty acids, particularly DHA, were positively correlated with gut microbiome diversity and the abundance of specific bacterial taxa, such as *Lachnospiraceae*, in a cohort of 876 elderly women, suggesting a potential role for LC-PUFA intake in modulating microbiome composition [183]. A 6-week intervention study further demonstrated that omega-3 supplementation alters gut microbiome composition, increasing the abundance of butyrate-associated *Coprococcus* spp. and beneficial fermentation products, suggesting a potential prebiotic-like role for omega-3 fatty acids [184].

On the other hand, gut microbiota can both indirectly and directly modulate the absorption, bioavailability, and biotransformation of n-3 fatty acids [185–187]. Certain bacterial species, such as *Bacillus proteus* or *Lactobacillus plantarum*, convert ALA and linoleic acid (LA) into conjugated linoleic acid (CLA) and conjugated alpha-linolenic acid (CALA), which are then hydrogenated to stearic acid, changing the PUFA content in the brain and heart [188]. A study of mice demonstrated that high tissue levels of n-3 fatty acids were associated with variations in the amounts of *Bifidobacterium* and *Lactobacillus* [189]. Conversely, mice fed a diet low in n-3 fatty acids for two generations showed a significant decrease in lactic acid bacteria and an increase in *Bifidobacteria* in the oral cavity compared to those fed a diet adequate in n-3 fatty acids [190]. While studies suggest that *Bifidobacterium* can significantly modulate fatty acid metabolism and its absorption by the intestinal epithelium, specific mechanisms underlying this relationship remain unexplained [191–193].

n-3 Fatty acids can modulate gut microbiota by either inhibiting the production of proinflammatory mediators or promoting the production of anti-inflammatory mediators. For instance, DHA reduces its activation by lowering IkappaB kinase (IκB) phosphorylation in response to LPS in cultured macrophages and dendritic cells, thereby decreasing NFκB activation [194,195]. Similarly, EPA reduced NFκB activation induced by LPS in human monocytes due to reduced IκB phosphorylation [196]. Furthermore, peroxisome proliferator-activated receptor gamma (PPAR-γ), which functions by inhibiting NFκB translocation to the nucleus, is regulated by the binding of EPA and DHA [197]. This binding interaction significantly influences inflammatory processes [198]. Supplementation with these acids significantly influences changes in the gut microbiota by altering the content of immune cell membranes and influencing proinflammatory signaling pathways. n-3 Fatty acids increase the number of regulatory T lymphocytes (Tregs), thereby reducing inflammatory reactions [199]. n-3 Fatty acids are mainly absorbed in the intestine, where their metabolites can be directly utilized by certain microorganisms. Their protective action on the intestinal mucosa includes increasing its thickness and improving barrier functions [200]. Summarized data presenting the mechanistic effects of LC-PUFAs on gut microbiota, immune function, and intestinal barrier integrity are presented in Table 2.

Table 2. Summarized effects of LC-PUFAs on the gut microbiota, immune function, and intestinal barrier integrity.

Models	Type of Study	Source and Dose of n-3 PUFA	Exposure	Effect	Reference
		In vitro model studies			
RAW 264.7 murine macrophage-like cell line	in vitro	100 µM DHA	24 h	- DHA reduced NFκB-DNA binding activity - Reduced inflammation	[194]
Murine bone marrow-derived DC	in vitro	100 µM DHA	24 h	- Reduction NFκB translocation mediated by inhibition of IκB degradation - Reduced inflammation	[195]
RAW 264.7 murine MØ cell line	in vitro	12 mg%, ω-3 FA emulsion	4 h	- Reduction in endotoxin-induced NFκB activation through decreased IκB phosphorylation - Reduced inflammation	[198]
Human Jurkat T cell lines E6-1	in vitro	50 µm EPA	48 h	- Promotion of regulatory T lymphocyte (Treg) induction and prevention of excessive development of T helper 17 (Th17) cells increase the number of regulatory T lymphocytes (Tregs) - Reduced inflammation	[199]
		In vivo model and human subject studies			
Male BALB/c mice with chronic stress	in vivo	Squid egg and sea cucumber (9% EPA and 38.9% DHA or 36% EPA and 5% DHA or 79% EPA and 10% DHA)	21 days	- Increase *Lactobacillus*, *Prevotella* spp., *Bacteroides fragilis*, and *Roseburia* spp. - Decrease *Enterobacteriaceae* and *Enterococcus* spp. - Protection against intestinal dysfunction - Attenuation of proinflammatory processes - Amelioration of LPS increase	[177]
Poultry	in vivo	0.2% and 0.6% of total n-3 PUFA in the diet (marine algal biomass or flaxseed oil)	8 weeks	- Increased population of *Firmicutes* (e.g., *Faecalibacterium*, *Clostridium* and *Ruminococcus*	[182]
C57BL/6J female mice were and their male offspring	in vivo	~1 g EPADHA/100 g of the diet	12 weeks	- Increased fecal *Bifidobacterium* and *Lactobacillus* abundance in offspring	[189]

Table 2. *Cont.*

Models	Type of Study	Source and Dose of n-3 PUFA	Exposure	Effect	Reference
Male Sprague Dawley rats with intestinal damage	in vivo	300 µg/kg per day (EPA 180 µg + DHA 120 µg)	Once per day 48 h before and 72 h after MTX injection	- Increased mass of the colon and ileum - Greater mass of the ileal mucosa—increased villus height and crypt depth in the ileum	[200]
Drug-naïve patients with type 2 diabetes	human subjects	3.0 ± 0.2 g EPA + DHA/d (sardines)	5 days a week for 6 months	- Increased ratio of *Bacteroides*/*Prevotella* - Decreased ratio of *Firmicutes*/*Bacteroidetes*	[181]

4. Conclusions

n-3 Fatty acids, particularly EPA and DHA, play a pivotal role in the intricate communication network of the GBA. Their incorporation into cell membranes enhances membrane fluidity, which is essential for optimal neurotransmitter function and efficient signal transduction. By modulating inflammatory responses—reducing proinflammatory cytokines and promoting anti-inflammatory mediators—n-3 fatty acids help preserve the integrity of critical barriers, like the intestinal barrier and the BBB. This not only supports gut health but also protects the CNS from potential neurotoxins and inflammatory agents. In the CNS, EPA and DHA contribute to neurogenesis and synaptic plasticity, thereby enhancing cognitive functions such as learning and memory. They also regulate the HPA axis by mitigating excessive cortisol production, which is often associated with stress responses and mental health disorders, like depression and anxiety. Furthermore, n-3 fatty acids positively influence gut microbiota composition, promoting growth of beneficial bacterial populations that contribute to gut health and systemic immunity. The effects of n-3 fatty acids on the GBA are summarized in Figure 4.

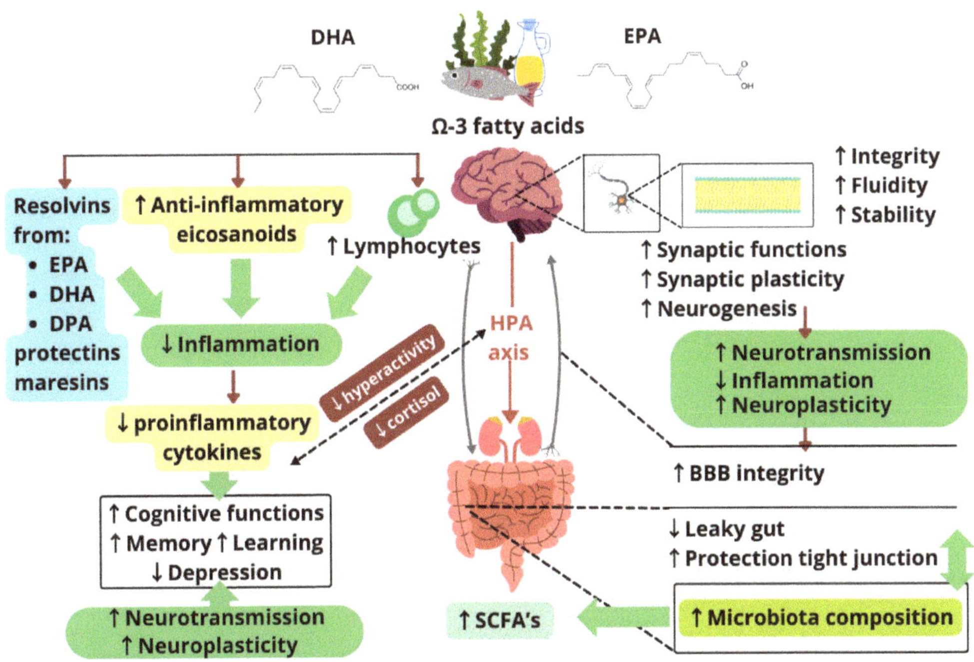

Figure 4. Summary of n-3 PUFAs' mechanisms of action: a schematic representation of the possible mechanisms through which n-3 PUFAs influence the gut–brain axis. DHA—docosahexaenoic acid; EPA—eicosapentaenoic acid; DPA—n-3 docosapentaenoic acid; HPA—hypothalamic-pituitary-adrenal; BBB—blood–brain barrier; SCFAs—short-chain fatty acids. ↑ indicates an increase, ↓ indicates a decrease. Designed using elements by ©Canva, sparklestroke, Pixeden, iconsy, OpenClipart-Vectors via Canva.com (access date: 18 November 2024).

Given the multifaceted benefits of n-3 fatty acids on the GBA, it is recommended to incorporate adequate amounts of EPA and DHA into the diet by consuming marine foods, like fatty fish, or through supplementation. Additionally, based on the significant benefits of n-3 fatty acids on the GBA and overall health, the following nutritional recommendations are proposed:

1. Incorporate fish rich in n-3 fatty acids, such as salmon, mackerel, sardines, trout, and herring, into the diet at least twice a week to boost EPA and DHA intake according to recommendation to achieve essentiality and cardiovascular benefits [201].
2. Consider n-3 fatty acid supplements based on fish oil or algae, especially for individuals with limited access to n-3-rich foods or with dietary restrictions [202].
3. Consume fiber-rich foods, like whole grains, fruits, and vegetables, along with fermented foods like yogurt, kefir, and sauerkraut, to support beneficial gut microbiota that synergizes with n-3 fatty acids [203].
4. Use cooking methods that preserve n-3 content, such as baking, steaming, or grilling, and avoid high-temperature frying, which can oxidize these delicate fats [204].
5. To ensure adequate intake of omega-3 fatty acids, individuals are encouraged to follow national or international dietary guidelines, such as those provided by the World Health Organization, the Institute of Medicine, or the European Food Safety Authority, which offer evidence-based recommendations for maintaining optimal health.

5. Limitations and Current Knowledge Gaps

Despite the existing research on the influence of LC-PUFAs on the GBA, critical gaps in our understanding of the precise mechanisms underlying this interaction persist. For instance, the exact processes by which n-3 PUFAs stabilize physiological barriers—such as the BBB and the intestinal barrier—and how they modulate the activity of both immune and neuronal cells, remain incompletely elucidated. Furthermore, the complex relationships between gut microbiota composition, n-3 fatty acid metabolism, and the regulation of inflammatory states require more investigations to fully clarify their interconnected roles. Despite substantial evidence demonstrating the beneficial effects of LC-PUFAs on the GBA, the major limitation is the difficulty of extrapolating doses and outcomes from in vitro and animal models to human populations. The concentrations of fatty acids used in cell culture studies and the dietary interventions used in animal experiments often exceed physiologically achievable levels in human.

Author Contributions: Conceptualization, K.D.; writing—original draft preparation, A.Z., W.G., M.C. and K.D.; writing—review and editing, W.G. and K.D.; visualization, A.Z. and W.G.; supervision, K.D. All authors have read and agreed to the published version of the manuscript.

Funding: This research received no external funding.

Institutional Review Board Statement: Not applicable.

Informed Consent Statement: Not applicable.

Data Availability Statement: Not applicable.

Conflicts of Interest: The authors declare no conflicts of interest.

References

1. Shen, L. Functional Morphology of the Gastrointestinal Tract. *Mol. Mech. Bact. Infect. Gut* **2009**, *337*, 1–35.
2. Deisseroth, K. A Look Inside the Brain. *Sci. Am.* **2016**, *315*, 30. [CrossRef] [PubMed]
3. Lu, S.; Zhao, Q.; Guan, Y.; Sun, Z.; Li, W.; Guo, S.; Zhang, A. The Communication Mechanism of the Gut-Brain Axis and Its Effect on Central Nervous System Diseases: A Systematic Review. *Biomed. Pharmacother.* **2024**, *178*, 117207. [CrossRef] [PubMed]
4. Morys, J.; Małecki, A.; Nowacka-Chmielewska, M. Stress and the Gut-Brain Axis: An Inflammatory Perspective. *Front. Mol. Neurosci.* **2024**, *17*, 1415567. [CrossRef] [PubMed]
5. Shahidi, F.; Ambigaipalan, P. Omega-3 Polyunsaturated Fatty Acids and Their Health Benefits. *Annu. Rev. Food Sci. Technol.* **2018**, *9*, 345–381. [CrossRef]

6. Liput, K.P.; Lepczyński, A.; Ogłuszka, M.; Nawrocka, A.; Poławska, E.; Grzesiak, A.; Ślaska, B.; Pareek, C.S.; Czarnik, U.; Pierzchała, M. Effects of Dietary n–3 and n–6 Polyunsaturated Fatty Acids in Inflammation and Cancerogenesis. *Int. J. Mol. Sci.* **2021**, *22*, 6965. [CrossRef] [PubMed]
7. Sala-Vila, A.; Fleming, J.; Kris-Etherton, P.; Ros, E. Impact of α-Linolenic Acid, the Vegetable ω-3 Fatty Acid, on Cardiovascular Disease and Cognition. *Adv. Nutr.* **2022**, *13*, 1584–1602. [CrossRef] [PubMed]
8. Chandola, H.M.; Tanna, I. Role of Omega-3 Fatty Acids in Brain and Neurological Health with Special Reference to Clinical Depression. In *Omega-3 Fatty Acids in Brain and Neurological Health*; Academic Press: Cambridge, MA, USA, 2014; pp. 163–179, ISBN 9780124105270. [CrossRef]
9. Drobner, T.; Braun, T.S.; Kiehntopf, M.; Schlattmann, P.; Lorkowski, S.; Dawczynski, C. Evaluation of Influencing Factors on Metabolism of Land-Based n-3 Poly Unsaturated Fatty Acids—The KoALA Study. *Nutrients* **2023**, *15*, 4461. [CrossRef] [PubMed]
10. Yu, H.; Bi, Y.; Ma, W.; He, L.; Yuan, L.; Feng, J.; Xiao, R. Long-Term Effects of High Lipid and High Energy Diet on Serum Lipid, Brain Fatty Acid Composition, and Memory and Learning Ability in Mice. *Int. J. Dev. Neurosci.* **2010**, *28*, 271–276. [CrossRef]
11. Cryan, J.F.; O'Riordan, K.J.; Cowan, C.S.; Sandhu, K.V.; Bastiaanssen, T.F.; Boehme, M.; Codagnone, M.G.; Cussotto, S.; Fulling, C.; Golubeva, A.V.; et al. The Microbiota-Gut-Brain Axis. *Physiol. Rev.* **2019**, *99*, 1877–2013. [CrossRef] [PubMed]
12. Morais, L.H.; Schreiber, H.L.; Mazmanian, S.K. The Gut Microbiota–Brain Axis in Behaviour and Brain Disorders. *Nat. Rev. Microbiol.* **2021**, *19*, 241–255. [CrossRef]
13. Carabotti, M.; Scirocco, A.; Antonietta Maselli, M.; Severi, C. The Gut-Brain Axis: Interactions between Enteric Microbiota, Central and Enteric Nervous Systems. *Ann. Gastroenterol.* **2015**, *28*, 203. [PubMed]
14. Gjerstad, J.K.; Lightman, S.L.; Spiga, F. Role of Glucocorticoid Negative Feedback in the Regulation of HPA Axis Pulsatility. *Stress* **2018**, *21*, 403–416. [CrossRef] [PubMed]
15. Gareau, M.G.; Jury, J.; MacQueen, G.; Sherman, P.M.; Perdue, M.H. Probiotic Treatment of Rat Pups Normalises Corticosterone Release and Ameliorates Colonic Dysfunction Induced by Maternal Separation. *Gut* **2007**, *56*, 1522–1528. [CrossRef] [PubMed]
16. Liang, S.; Wu, X.; Jin, F. Gut-Brain Psychology: Rethinking Psychology from the Microbiota–Gut–Brain Axis. *Front. Integr. Neurosci.* **2018**, *12*, 33. [CrossRef] [PubMed]
17. Kumar, S.; Kumar, A. Microbial Pathogenesis in Inflammatory Bowel Diseases. *Microb. Pathog.* **2022**, *163*, 105383. [CrossRef] [PubMed]
18. Vancamelbeke, M.; Vermeire, S. The Intestinal Barrier: A Fundamental Role in Health and Disease. *Expert Rev. Gastroenterol. Hepatol.* **2017**, *11*, 821–834. [CrossRef] [PubMed]
19. Ma, Q.; Xing, C.; Long, W.; Wang, H.Y.; Liu, Q.; Wang, R.-F. Impact of Microbiota on Central Nervous System and Neurological Diseases: The Gut-Brain Axis. *J. Neuroinflamm.* **2019**, *16*, 53. [CrossRef]
20. Sender, R.; Fuchs, S.; Milo, R. Are We Really Vastly Outnumbered? Revisiting the Ratio of Bacterial to Host Cells in Humans. *Cell* **2016**, *164*, 337–340. [CrossRef]
21. Bruce-Keller, A.J.; Salbaum, J.M.; Luo, M.; Blanchard, E.; Taylor, C.M.; Welsh, D.A.; Berthoud, H.R. Obese-Type Gut Microbiota Induce Neurobehavioral Changes in the Absence of Obesity. *Biol. Psychiatry* **2015**, *77*, 607–615. [CrossRef] [PubMed]
22. Chen, Y.; Xu, J.; Chen, Y. Regulation of Neurotransmitters by the Gut Microbiota and Effects on Cognition in Neurological Disorders. *Nutrients* **2021**, *13*, 2099. [CrossRef] [PubMed]
23. Eisenstein, M. Microbiome: Bacterial Broadband. *Nature* **2016**, *533*, S104–S106. [CrossRef] [PubMed]
24. Nichols, E.; Szoeke, C.E.I.; Vollset, S.E.; Abbasi, N.; Abd-Allah, F.; Abdela, J.; Aichour, M.T.E.; Akinyemi, R.O.; Alahdab, F.; Asgedom, S.W.; et al. Global, Regional, and National Burden of Alzheimer's Disease and Other Dementias, 1990–2016: A Systematic Analysis for the Global Burden of Disease Study 2016. *Lancet Neurol.* **2019**, *18*, 88–106. [CrossRef] [PubMed]
25. Erny, D.; De Angelis, A.L.H.; Jaitin, D.; Wieghofer, P.; Staszewski, O.; David, E.; Keren-Shaul, H.; Mahlakoiv, T.; Jakobshagen, K.; Buch, T.; et al. Host Microbiota Constantly Control Maturation and Function of Microglia in the CNS. *Nat. Neurosci.* **2015**, *18*, 965–977. [CrossRef] [PubMed]
26. Di Tommaso, N.; Gasbarrini, A.; Ponziani, F.R. Intestinal Barrier in Human Health and Disease. *Int. J. Environ. Res. Public Health* **2021**, *18*, 12836. [CrossRef]
27. Ghosh, S.; Whitley, C.S.; Haribabu, B.; Jala, V.R. Regulation of Intestinal Barrier Function by Microbial Metabolites. *Cell. Mol. Gastroenterol. Hepatol.* **2021**, *11*, 1463–1482. [CrossRef]
28. Ballabh, P.; Braun, A.; Nedergaard, M. The Blood-Brain Barrier: An Overview: Structure, Regulation, and Clinical Implications. *Neurobiol. Dis.* **2004**, *16*, 1–13. [CrossRef]
29. Adil, M.S.; Narayanan, S.P.; Somanath, P.R. Cell-Cell Junctions: Structure and Regulation in Physiology and Pathology. *Tissue Barriers* **2021**, *9*, 1848212. [CrossRef] [PubMed]
30. Petty, M.A.; Lo, E.H. Junctional Complexes of the Blood-Brain Barrier: Permeability Changes in Neuroinflammation. *Prog. Neurobiol.* **2002**, *68*, 311–323. [CrossRef] [PubMed]
31. Serlin, Y.; Shelef, I.; Knyazer, B.; Friedman, A. Anatomy and Physiology of the Blood-Brain Barrier. *Semin. Cell Dev. Biol.* **2015**, *38*, 2–6. [CrossRef]

32. Guixà-González, R.; Javanainen, M.; Gómez-Soler, M.; Cordobilla, B.; Domingo, J.C.; Sanz, F.; Pastor, M.; Ciruela, F.; Martinez-Seara, H.; Selent, J. Membrane Omega-3 Fatty Acids Modulate the Oligomerisation Kinetics of Adenosine A2A and Dopamine D2 Receptors. *Sci. Rep.* **2016**, *6*, 19839. [CrossRef]
33. Bazan, N.G.; Musto, A.E.; Knott, E.J. Endogenous Signaling by Omega-3 Docosahexaenoic Acid-Derived Mediators Sustains Homeostatic Synaptic and Circuitry Integrity. *Mol. Neurobiol.* **2011**, *44*, 216–222. [CrossRef] [PubMed]
34. Heinrichs, S.C. Dietary ω-3 Fatty Acid Supplementation for Optimizing Neuronal Structure and Function. *Mol. Nutr. Food Res.* **2010**, *54*, 447–456. [CrossRef]
35. Hennebelle, M.; Champeil-Potokar, G.; Lavialle, M.; Vancassel, S.; Denis, I. Omega-3 Polyunsaturated Fatty Acids and Chronic Stress-Induced Modulations of Glutamatergic Neurotransmission in the Hippocampus. *Nutr. Rev.* **2014**, *72*, 99–112. [CrossRef]
36. McNamara, R.K.; Able, J.; Jandacek, R.; Rider, T.; Tso, P.; Eliassen, J.C.; Alfieri, D.; Weber, W.; Jarvis, K.; Delbello, M.P.; et al. Docosahexaenoic Acid Supplementation Increases Prefrontal Cortex Activation during Sustained Attention in Healthy Boys: A Placebo-Controlled, Dose-Ranging, Functional Magnetic Resonance Imaging Study. *Am. J. Clin. Nutr.* **2010**, *91*, 1060–1067. [CrossRef] [PubMed]
37. Dyall, S.C. Long-Chain Omega-3 Fatty Acids and the Brain: A Review of the Independent and Shared Effects of EPA, DPA and DHA. *Front. Aging Neurosci.* **2015**, *7*, 52. [CrossRef] [PubMed]
38. Carver, J.D.; Benford, V.J.; Han, B.; Cantor, A.B. The Relationship between Age and the Fatty Acid Composition of Cerebral Cortex and Erythrocytes in Human Subjects. *Brain Res. Bull.* **2001**, *56*, 79–85. [CrossRef] [PubMed]
39. Torres, M.; Price, S.L.; Fiol-Deroque, M.A.; Marcilla-Etxenike, A.; Ahyayauch, H.; Barceló-Coblijn, G.; Terés, S.; Katsouri, L.; Ordinas, M.; López, D.J.; et al. Membrane Lipid Modifications and Therapeutic Effects Mediated by Hydroxydocosahexaenoic Acid on Alzheimer's Disease. *Biochim. Biophys. Acta Biomembr.* **2014**, *1838*, 1680–1692. [CrossRef] [PubMed]
40. de Santis, A.; Scoppola, E.; Ottaviani, M.F.; Koutsioubas, A.; Barnsley, L.C.; Paduano, L.; D'Errico, G.; Krauss, I.R. Order vs. Disorder: Cholesterol and Omega-3 Phospholipids Determine Biomembrane Organization. *Int. J. Mol. Sci.* **2022**, *2*, 5322. [CrossRef] [PubMed]
41. De Santis, A.; Vitiello, G.; Appavou, M.S.; Scoppola, E.; Fragneto, G.; Barnsley, L.C.; Clifton, L.A.; Ottaviani, M.F.; Paduano, L.; Russo Krauss, I.; et al. Not Just a Fluidifying Effect: Omega-3 Phospholipids Induce Formation of Non-Lamellar Structures in Biomembranes. *Soft Matter* **2020**, *16*, 10425–10438. [CrossRef]
42. Rubin, D.; Laposata, M. Cellular Interactions between N-6 and n-3 Fatty Acids: A Mass Analysis of Fatty Acid Elongation/Desaturation, Distribution among Complex Lipids, and Conversion to Eicosanoids. *J. Lipid Res.* **1992**, *33*, 1431–1440. [CrossRef]
43. Sunshine, H.; Iruela-Arispe, M.L. Membrane Lipids and Cell Signaling. *Curr. Opin. Lipidol.* **2017**, *28*, 408–413. [CrossRef] [PubMed]
44. Zhang, X.; Hurng, J.; Rateri, D.L.; Daugherty, A.; Schmid-Schönbein, G.W.; Shin, H.Y. Membrane Cholesterol Modulates the Fluid Shear Stress Response of Polymorphonuclear Leukocytes via Its Effects on Membrane Fluidity. *Am. J. Physiol. Cell Physiol.* **2011**, *301*, 451–460. [CrossRef] [PubMed]
45. Cammarota, E.; Soriani, C.; Taub, R.; Morgan, F.; Sakai, J.; Veatch, S.L.; Bryant, C.E.; Cicuta, P. Criticality of Plasma Membrane Lipids Reflects Activation State of Macrophage Cells. *J. R. Soc. Interface* **2020**, *17*, 163. [CrossRef]
46. Whelan, J. Antagonistic Effects of Dietary Arachidonic Acid and N-3 Polyunsaturated Fatty Acids. *J. Nutr.* **1996**, *126*, 1086S–1091S. [CrossRef] [PubMed]
47. Calder, P.C. Polyunsaturated Fatty Acids and Inflammatory Processes: New Twists in an Old Tale. *Biochimie* **2009**, *91*, 791–795. [CrossRef] [PubMed]
48. Borsini, A.; Nicolaou, A.; Camacho-Muñoz, D.; Kendall, A.C.; Di Benedetto, M.G.; Giacobbe, J.; Su, K.P.; Pariante, C.M. Omega-3 Polyunsaturated Fatty Acids Protect against Inflammation through Production of LOX and CYP450 Lipid Mediators: Relevance for Major Depression and for Human Hippocampal Neurogenesis. *Mol. Psychiatry* **2021**, *26*, 6773–6788. [CrossRef] [PubMed]
49. Fischer, R.; Konkel, A.; Mehling, H.; Blossey, K.; Gapelyuk, A.; Wessel, N.; Von Schacky, C.; Dechend, R.; Muller, D.N.; Rothe, M.; et al. Dietary Omega-3 Fatty Acids Modulate the Eicosanoid Profile in Man Primarily via the CYP-Epoxygenase Pathway. *J. Lipid Res.* **2014**, *55*, 1150–1164. [CrossRef]
50. Ceccarini, M.R.; Ceccarelli, V.; Codini, M.; Fettucciari, K.; Calvitti, M.; Cataldi, S.; Albi, E.; Vecchini, A.; Beccari, T. The Polyunsaturated Fatty Acid EPA, but Not DHA, Enhances Neurotrophic Factor Expression through Epigenetic Mechanisms and Protects against Parkinsonian Neuronal Cell Death. *Int. J. Mol. Sci.* **2022**, *23*, 16176. [CrossRef] [PubMed]
51. Norris, P.C.; Dennis, E.A. Omega-3 Fatty Acids Cause Dramatic Changes in TLR4 and Purinergic Eicosanoid Signaling. *Proc. Natl. Acad. Sci. USA* **2012**, *109*, 8517–8522. [CrossRef] [PubMed]
52. Palombo, J.D.; Demichele, S.J.; Lydon, E.E.; Gregory, T.J.; Banks, P.L.; Forse, R.A.; Bistrian, B.R. Rapid Modulation of Lung and Liver Macrophage Phospholipid Fatty Acids in Endotoxemic Rats by Continuous Enteral Feeding with N-3 and y-Linolenic Fatty Acids. *Am. J. Clin. Nutr.* **1996**, *63*, 208–219. [CrossRef] [PubMed]

53. Hayashi, D.; Mouchlis, V.D.; Dennis, E.A. Omega-3 versus Omega-6 Fatty Acid Availability Is Controlled by Hydrophobic Site Geometries of Phospholipase A2s. *J. Lipid Res.* **2021**, *62*, 100113. [CrossRef]
54. Nieves, D.; Moreno, J.J. Effect of Arachidonic and Eicosapentaenoic Acid Metabolism on RAW 264.7 Macrophage Proliferation. *J. Cell Physiol.* **2006**, *208*, 428–434. [CrossRef]
55. So, J.; Wu, D.; Lichtenstein, A.H.; Tai, A.K.; Matthan, N.R.; Maddipati, K.R.; Lamon-Fava, S. EPA and DHA Differentially Modulate Monocyte Inflammatory Response in Subjects with Chronic Inflammation in Part via Plasma Specialized Pro-Resolving Lipid Mediators: A Randomized, Double-Blind, Crossover Study. *Atherosclerosis* **2021**, *316*, 90–98. [CrossRef]
56. Rees, D.; Miles, E.A.; Banerjee, T.; Wells, S.J.; Roynette, C.E.; Wahle, K.W.; Calder, P.C. Dose-Related Effects of Eicosapentaenoic Acid on Innate Immune Function in Healthy Humans: A Comparison of Young and Older Men. *Am. J. Clin. Nutr.* **2006**, *83*, 331–342. [CrossRef]
57. Calder, P.C. Omega-3 Fatty Acids and Inflammatory Processes. *Nutrients* **2010**, *2*, 355–374. [CrossRef]
58. Wall, R.; Ross, R.P.; Fitzgerald, G.F.; Stanton, C. Fatty Acids from Fish: The Anti-Inflammatory Potential of Long-Chain Omega-3 Fatty Acids. *Nutr. Rev.* **2010**, *68*, 280–289. [CrossRef]
59. Calder, P.C. Eicosapentaenoic and Docosahexaenoic Acid Derived Specialised Pro-Resolving Mediators: Concentrations in Humans and the Effects of Age, Sex, Disease and Increased Omega-3 Fatty Acid Intake. *Biochimie* **2020**, *178*, 105–123. [CrossRef] [PubMed]
60. Calder, P.C. Dietary Fatty Acids, Lipid Mediators, Immunity, and Inflammation. In *Functional Dietary Lipids: Food Formulation, Consumer Issues, and Innovation for Health*, 2nd ed.; Woodhead Publishing: Sawston, UK, 2024; pp. 187–214. [CrossRef]
61. Larsen, L.N.; Bremer, J.; Flock, S.; Skattebø, L. α- and β- Alkyl-Substituted Eicosapentaenoic Acids: Incorporation into Phospholipids and Effets on Prostaglandin H Synthase and 5-Lipoxygenase. *Biochem. Pharmacol.* **1998**, *55*, 405–411. [CrossRef]
62. Wada, M.; DeLong, C.J.; Hong, Y.H.; Rieke, C.J.; Song, I.; Sidhu, R.S.; Yuan, C.; Warnock, M.; Schmaier, A.H.; Yokoyama, C.; et al. Enzymes and Receptors of Prostaglandin Pathways with Arachidonic Acid-Derived versus Eicosapentaenoic Acid-Derived Substrates and Products. *J. Biol. Chem.* **2007**, *282*, 22254–22266. [CrossRef]
63. Allaire, J.; Couture, P.; Leclerc, M.; Charest, A.; Marin, J.; Lépine, M.C.; Talbot, D.; Tchernof, A.; Lamarche, B. A Randomized, Crossover, Head-to-Head Comparison of Eicosapentaenoic Acid and Docosahexaenoic Acid Supplementation to Reduce Inflammation Markers in Men and Women: The Comparing EPA to DHA (ComparED) Study. *Am. J. Clin. Nutr.* **2016**, *104*, 280–287. [CrossRef] [PubMed]
64. Liu, J.-Y. Editorial: Eicosanoids and Cytokines: Resolution of Inflammation. *Front. Pharmacol.* **2022**, *13*, 978331. [CrossRef] [PubMed]
65. Sierra, S.; Lara-Villoslada, F.; Comalada, M.; Olivares, M.; Xaus, J. Dietary Eicosapentaenoic Acid and Docosahexaenoic Acid Equally Incorporate as Decosahexaenoic Acid but Differ in Inflammatory Effects. *Nutrition* **2008**, *24*, 245–254. [CrossRef] [PubMed]
66. Skelly, D.T.; Hennessy, E.; Dansereau, M.A.; Cunningham, C. A Systematic Analysis of the Peripheral and CNS Effects of Systemic LPS, IL-1B, TNF-α and IL-6 Challenges in C57BL/6 Mice. *PLoS ONE* **2013**, *8*, 10. [CrossRef]
67. Vezzani, A.; Viviani, B. Neuromodulatory Properties of Inflammatory Cytokines and Their Impact on Neuronal Excitability. *Neuropharmacology* **2015**, *96*, 70–82. [CrossRef] [PubMed]
68. Brebner, K.; Hayley, S.; Zacharko, R.; Merali, Z.; Anisman, H. Synergistic Effects of Interleukin-1, Interleukin-6, and Tumor Necrosis Factor-: Central Monoamine, Corticosterone, and Behavioral Variations. *Neuropsychopharmacology* **2000**, *22*, 566–580. [CrossRef]
69. Wang, J.; Chen, Z.; Walston, J.D.; Gao, P.; Gao, M.; Leng, S.X. Interferon-γ Potentiates α-Synuclein-Induced Neurotoxicity Linked to Toll-like Receptors 2 and 3 and Tumor Necrosis Factor-α in Murine Astrocytes. *Mol. Neurobiol.* **2019**, *56*, 7664–7679. [CrossRef] [PubMed]
70. Caroprese, M.; Ciliberti, M.G.; Annicchiarico, G.; Albenzio, M.; Muscio, A.; Sevi, A. Hypothalamic-Pituitary-Adrenal Axis Activation and Immune Regulation in Heat-Stressed Sheep after Supplementation with Polyunsaturated Fatty Acids. *J. Dairy Sci.* **2014**, *97*, 4247–4258. [CrossRef]
71. Kwon, Y. Immuno-Resolving Ability of Resolvins, Protectins, and Maresins Derived from Omega-Fatty Acids in Metabolic Syndrome. *Mol. Nutr. Food Res.* **2020**, *64*, 1900824. [CrossRef] [PubMed]
72. Pilkington, S.M.; Rhodes, L.E.; Al-Aasswad, N.M.I.; Massey, K.A.; Nicolaou, A. Impact of EPA Ingestion on COX- and LOX-Mediated Eicosanoid Synthesis in Skin with and without a pro-Inflammatory UVR Challenge—Report of a Randomised Controlled Study in Humans. *Mol. Nutr. Food Res.* **2014**, *58*, 580–590. [CrossRef]
73. Ferreira, I.; Falcato, F.; Bandarra, N.; Rauter, A.P. Resolvins, Protectins, and Maresins: DHA-Derived Specialized Pro-Resolving Mediators, Biosynthetic Pathways, Synthetic Approaches, and Their Role in Inflammation. *Molecules* **2022**, *27*, 1677. [CrossRef] [PubMed]
74. Singer, P.; Shapiro, H.; Theilla, M.; Anbar, R.; Singer, J.; Cohen, J. Anti-Inflammatory Properties of Omega-3 Fatty Acids in Critical Illness: Novel Mechanisms and an Integrative Perspective. *Intensive Care Med.* **2008**, *34*, 1580–1592. [CrossRef] [PubMed]

75. Zúñiga, J.; Cancino, M.; Medina, F.; Varela, P.; Vargas, R.; Tapia, G.; Videla, L.A.; Fernández, V. N-3 PUFA Supplementation Triggers PPAR-α Activation and PPAR-α/NF-KB Interaction: Anti-Inflammatory Implications in Liver Ischemia-Reperfusion Injury. *PLoS ONE* **2011**, *6*, e28502. [CrossRef] [PubMed]
76. Tapia, G.; Valenzuela, R.; Espinosa, A.; Romanque, P.; Dossi, C.; Gonzalez-Mañán, D.; Videla, L.A.; D'Espessailles, A. N-3 Long-Chain PUFA Supplementation Prevents High Fat Diet Induced Mouse Liver Steatosis and Inflammation in Relation to PPAR-α Upregulation and NF-KB DNA Binding Abrogation. *Mol. Nutr. Food Res.* **2014**, *58*, 1333–1341. [CrossRef]
77. Bosviel, R.; Joumard-Cubizolles, L.; Chinetti-Gbaguidi, G.; Bayle, D.; Copin, C.; Hennuyer, N.; Duplan, I.; Staels, B.; Zanoni, G.; Porta, A.; et al. DHA-Derived Oxylipins, Neuroprostanes and Protectins, Differentially and Dose-Dependently Modulate the Inflammatory Response in Human Macrophages: Putative Mechanisms through PPAR Activation. *Free Radic. Biol. Med.* **2017**, *103*, 146–154. [CrossRef] [PubMed]
78. El-Ashmawy, N.E.; Khedr, N.F.; El-Bahrawy, H.A.; Helal, S.A. Upregulation of PPAR-γ Mediates the Renoprotective Effect of Omega-3 PUFA and Ferulic Acid in Gentamicin-Intoxicated Rats. *Biomed. Pharmacother.* **2018**, *99*, 504–510. [CrossRef] [PubMed]
79. Magee, P.; Pearson, S.; Whittingham-Dowd, J.; Allen, J. PPARγ as a Molecular Target of EPA Anti-Inflammatory Activity during TNF-α-Impaired Skeletal Muscle Cell Differentiation. *J. Nutr. Biochem.* **2012**, *23*, 1440–1448. [CrossRef]
80. Campanari, D.D.; Cipriano, U.G.; Fraga-Silva, T.F.D.C.; Ramalho, L.N.Z.; Ovidio, P.P.; Jordão Júnior, A.A.; Bonato, V.L.D.; Ferriolli, E. Effect of Dietary Supplementation with Omega-3 Fatty Acid on the Generation of Regulatory T Lymphocytes and on Antioxidant Parameters and Markers of Oxidative Stress in the Liver Tissue of IL−10 Knockout Mice. *Nutrients* **2024**, *16*, 634. [CrossRef]
81. Khalfoun, B.; Thibault, F.; Watier, H.; Bardos, P.; Lebranchu, Y. Docosahexaenoic and Eicosapentaenoic Acids Inhibit In vitro Human Endothelial Cell Production of Interleukin-6. *Adv. Exp. Med. Biol.* **1997**, *400*, 589–597.
82. Mullen, A.; Loscher, C.E.; Roche, H.M. Anti-Inflammatory Effects of EPA and DHA Are Dependent upon Time and Dose-Response Elements Associated with LPS Stimulation in THP-1-Derived Macrophages. *J. Nutr. Biochem.* **2010**, *21*, 444–450. [CrossRef] [PubMed]
83. Wierenga, K.A.; Riemers, F.M.; Westendorp, B.; Harkema, J.R.; Pestka, J.J. Single Cell Analysis of Docosahexaenoic Acid Suppression of Sequential LPS-Induced Proinflammatory and Interferon-Regulated Gene Expression in the Macrophage. *Front. Immunol.* **2022**, *13*, 993614. [CrossRef] [PubMed]
84. Weldon, S.M.; Mullen, A.C.; Loscher, C.E.; Hurley, L.A.; Roche, H.M. Docosahexaenoic Acid Induces an Anti-Inflammatory Profile in Lipopolysaccharide-Stimulated Human THP-1 Macrophages More Effectively than Eicosapentaenoic Acid. *J. Nutr. Biochem.* **2007**, *18*, 250–258. [CrossRef] [PubMed]
85. Dennis, E.A.; Norris, P.C. Eicosanoid Storm in Infection and Inflammation. *Nat. Rev. Immunol.* **2015**, *15*, 511–523. [CrossRef] [PubMed]
86. Draper, E.; Reynolds, C.M.; Canavan, M.; Mills, K.H.; Loscher, C.E.; Roche, H.M. Omega-3 Fatty Acids Attenuate Dendritic Cell Function via NF-KB Independent of PPARγ. *J. Nutr. Biochem.* **2011**, *22*, 784–790. [CrossRef]
87. Perkins, N.D. Integrating Cell-Signalling Pathways with NF-KB and IKK Function. *Nat. Rev. Mol. Cell Biol.* **2007**, *8*, 49–62. [CrossRef]
88. Downton, P.; Bagnall, J.S.; England, H.; Spiller, D.G.; Humphreys, N.E.; Jackson, D.A.; Paszek, P.; White, M.R.H.; Adamson, A.D. Overexpression of IκBα Modulates NF-KB Activation of Inflammatory Target Gene Expression. *Front. Mol. Biosci.* **2023**, *10*, 1187187. [CrossRef]
89. Adelaja, A.; Hoffmann, A. Signaling Crosstalk Mechanisms That May Fine-Tune Pathogen-Responsive NFκB. *Front. Immunol.* **2019**, *10*, 433. [CrossRef]
90. Liu, T.; Zhang, L.; Joo, D.; Sun, S.-C. NF-KB Signaling in Inflammation. *Signal Transduct. Target. Ther.* **2017**, *2*, 17023. [CrossRef] [PubMed]
91. Jiao, H.; Wang, Z.; Liu, Y.; Wang, P.; Xue, Y. Specific Role of Tight Junction Proteins Claudin-5, Occludin, and ZO-1 of the Blood-Brain Barrier in a Focal Cerebral Ischemic Insult. *J. Mol. Neurosci.* **2011**, *44*, 130–139. [CrossRef] [PubMed]
92. Balbuena, P.; Li, W.; Ehrich, M. Assessments of Tight Junction Proteins Occludin, Claudin 5 and Scaffold Proteins ZO1 and ZO2 in Endothelial Cells of the Rat Blood-Brain Barrier: Cellular Responses to Neurotoxicants Malathion and Lead Acetate. *Neurotoxicology* **2011**, *32*, 58–67. [CrossRef]
93. Wang, X.; Pan, L.; Lu, J.; Li, N.; Li, J. N-3 PUFAs Attenuate Ischemia/Reperfusion Induced Intestinal Barrier Injury by Activating I-FABP-PPARγ Pathway. *Clin. Nutr.* **2012**, *31*, 951–957. [CrossRef] [PubMed]
94. Zhang, W.; Zhang, H.; Mu, H.; Zhu, W.; Jiang, X.; Hu, X.; Shi, Y.; Leak, R.K.; Dong, Q.; Chen, J.; et al. Omega-3 Polyunsaturated Fatty Acids Mitigate Blood-Brain Barrier Disruption after Hypoxic-Ischemic Brain Injury. *Neurobiol. Dis.* **2016**, *91*, 37–46. [CrossRef] [PubMed]
95. McColl, B.W.; Rothwell, N.J.; Allan, S.M. Systemic Inflammation Alters the Kinetics of Cerebrovascular Tight Junction Disruption After Experimental Stroke in Mice. *J. Neurosci.* **2008**, *28*, 9451–9462. [CrossRef] [PubMed]

96. Smyth, L.C.D.; Rustenhoven, J.; Park, T.I.H.; Schweder, P.; Jansson, D.; Heppner, P.A.; O'Carroll, S.J.; Mee, E.W.; Faull, R.L.M.; Curtis, M.; et al. Unique and Shared Inflammatory Profiles of Human Brain Endothelia and Pericytes. *J. Neuroinflamm.* **2018**, *15*, 138. [CrossRef]
97. Willemsen, L.E.M.; Koetsier, M.A.; Balvers, M.; Beermann, C.; Stahl, B.; Van Tol, E.A.F. Polyunsaturated Fatty Acids Support Epithelial Barrier Integrity and Reduce IL-4 Mediated Permeability In Vitro. *Eur. J. Nutr.* **2008**, *47*, 183–191. [CrossRef] [PubMed]
98. Naser, A.N.; Lu, Q.; Chen, Y.-H. Trans-Compartmental Regulation of Tight Junction Barrier Function. *Tissue Barriers* **2023**, *11*, 2133880. [CrossRef]
99. Krug, S.M.; Schulzke, J.D.; Fromm, M. Tight Junction, Selective Permeability, and Related Diseases. *Semin. Cell Dev. Biol.* **2014**, *36*, 166–176. [CrossRef] [PubMed]
100. Cunningham, K.E.; Turner, J.R. Myosin Light Chain Kinase: Pulling the Strings of Epithelial Tight Junction Function. *Ann. N. Y. Acad. Sci.* **2012**, *1258*, 34–42. [CrossRef]
101. Musch, M.W.; Mary Walsh-Reitz, M.; Chang, E.B.; Chang Roles, E.B. Roles of ZO-1, Occludin, and Actin in Oxidant-Induced Barrier Disruption. *Am. J. Physiol. Gastrointest. Liver Physiol.* **2006**, *290*, 222–231. [CrossRef]
102. Yu, D.; Marchiando, A.M.; Weber, C.R.; Raleigh, D.R.; Wang, Y.; Shen, L.; Turner, J.R. MLCK-Dependent Exchange and Actin Binding Region-Dependent Anchoring of ZO-1 Regulate Tight Junction Barrier Function. *Proc. Natl. Acad. Sci. USA* **2010**, *107*, 8237–8241. [CrossRef] [PubMed]
103. Lukiw, W.J. Gastrointestinal (GI) Tract Microbiome-Derived Neurotoxins—Potent Neuro-Inflammatory Signals from the GI Tract via the Systemic Circulation into the Brain. *Front. Cell Infect. Microbiol.* **2020**, *10*, 22. [CrossRef] [PubMed]
104. Xiao, G.; Tang, L.; Yuan, F.; Zhu, W.; Zhang, S.; Liu, Z.; Geng, Y.; Qiu, X.; Zhang, Y.; Su, L. Eicosapentaenoic Acid Enhances Heat Stress-Impaired Intestinal Epithelial Barrier Function in Caco-2 Cells. *PLoS ONE* **2013**, *8*, e73571. [CrossRef] [PubMed]
105. Usami, M.; Muraki, K.; Iwamoto, M.; Ohata, A.; Matsushita, E.; Miki, A. Effect of Eicosapentaenoic Acid (EPA) on Tight Junction Permeability in Intestinal Monolayer Cells. *Clin. Nutr.* **2001**, *20*, 351–359. [CrossRef]
106. Xiao, G.; Yuan, F.; Geng, Y.; Qiu, X.; Liu, Z.; Lu, J.; Tang, L.; Zhang, Y.; Su, L. Eicosapentaenoic Acid Enhances Heatstroke-Impaired Intestinal Epithelial Barrier Function in Rats. *Shock* **2015**, *44*, 348–356. [CrossRef] [PubMed]
107. Yu, T.-X.; Wang, P.-Y.; Rao, J.N.; Zou, T.; Liu, L.; Xiao, L.; Gorospe, M.; Wang, J.-Y. Chk2-Dependent HuR Phosphorylation Regulates Occludin MRNA Translation and Epithelial Barrier Function. *Nucleic Acids Res.* **2011**, *39*, 8472–8487. [CrossRef] [PubMed]
108. Chelakkot, C.; Ghim, J.; Ryu, S.H. Mechanisms Regulating Intestinal Barrier Integrity and Its Pathological Implications. *Exp. Mol. Med.* **2018**, *50*, 1–9. [CrossRef] [PubMed]
109. Tian, F.; Gao, X.; Zhang, L.; Wang, X.; Wan, X.; Jiang, T.; Wu, C.; Bi, J.; Lei, Q. Effects of N-3 PUFAs on Intestinal Mucosa Innate Immunity and Intestinal Microbiota in Mice after Hemorrhagic Shock Resuscitation. *Nutrients* **2016**, *8*, 609. [CrossRef] [PubMed]
110. Kim, H.-Y.; Akbar, M.; Kim, Y.-S. Phosphatidylserine-Dependent Neuroprotective Signaling Promoted by Docosahexaenoic Acid. *Prostaglandins Leukot. Essent. Fat. Acids* **2010**, *82*, 165–172. [CrossRef] [PubMed]
111. Xie, Q.; Zhang, Y.; Zhang, J.; Cui, D.; Zhou, Q.; Guo, M. Promotion Effect of the Blend Containing 2′-FL, OPN and DHA on Oligodendrocyte Progenitor Cells Myelination In Vitro. *Front. Nutr.* **2022**, *9*, 1054431. [CrossRef] [PubMed]
112. Dagai, L.; Peri-Naor, R.; Birk, R.Z. Docosahexaenoic Acid Significantly Stimulates Immediate Early Response Genes and Neurite Outgrowth. *Neurochem. Res.* **2009**, *34*, 867–875. [CrossRef] [PubMed]
113. Chen, S.; Zhang, H.; Pu, H.; Wang, G.; Li, W.; Leak, R.K.; Chen, J.; Liou, A.K.; Hu, X. N-3 PUFA Supplementation Benefits Microglial Responses to Myelin Pathology. *Sci. Rep.* **2014**, *4*, 7458. [CrossRef]
114. Götz, M.; Barde, Y.A. Radial Glial Cells: Defined and Major Intermediates between Embryonicstem Cells and CNS Neurons. *Neuron* **2005**, *46*, 369–372. [CrossRef] [PubMed]
115. Ming, G.L.; Song, H. Adult Neurogenesis in the Mammalian Brain: Significant Answers and Significant Questions. *Neuron* **2011**, *70*, 687–702. [CrossRef]
116. Kowiański, P.; Lietzau, G.; Czuba, E.; Waśkow, M.; Steliga, A.; Moryś, J. BDNF: A Key Factor with Multipotent Impact on Brain Signaling and Synaptic Plasticity. *Cell. Mol. Neurobiol.* **2018**, *38*, 579–593. [CrossRef] [PubMed]
117. Miranda, M.; Morici, J.F.; Zanoni, M.B.; Bekinschtein, P. Brain-Derived Neurotrophic Factor: A Key Molecule for Memory in the Healthy and the Pathological Brain. *Front. Cell. Neurosci.* **2019**, *13*, 363. [CrossRef] [PubMed]
118. Müller, P.; Duderstadt, Y.; Lessmann, V.; Müller, N.G. Lactate and BDNF: Key Mediators of Exercise Induced Neuroplasticity? *J. Clin. Med.* **2020**, *9*, 1136. [CrossRef]
119. Cysneiros, R.M.; Ferrari, D.; Arida, R.M.; Terra, V.C.; de Almeida, A.C.G.; Cavalheiro, E.A.; Scorza, F.A. Qualitative Analysis of Hippocampal Plastic Changes in Rats with Epilepsy Supplemented with Oral Omega-3 Fatty Acids. *Epilepsy Behav.* **2010**, *17*, 33–38. [CrossRef]
120. Kolarow, R.; Kuhlmann, C.R.W.; Munsch, T.; Zehendner, C.; Brigadski, T.; Luhmann, H.J.; Lessmann, V. BDNF-Induced Nitric Oxide Signals in Cultured Rat Hippocampal Neurons: Time Course, Mechanism of Generation, and Effect on Neurotrophin Secretion. *Front. Cell. Neurosci.* **2014**, *8*, 323. [CrossRef] [PubMed]

121. Sugasini, D.; Yalagala, P.C.R.; Subbaiah, P.V. Plasma BDNF Is a More Reliable Biomarker than Erythrocyte Omega-3 Index for the Omega-3 Fatty Acid Enrichment of Brain. *Sci. Rep.* **2020**, *10*, 10809. [CrossRef] [PubMed]
122. Mita, T.; Mayanagi, T.; Ichijo, H.; Fukumoto, K.; Otsuka, K.; Sakai, A.; Sobue, K. Docosahexaenoic Acid Promotes Axon Outgrowth by Translational Regulation of Tau and Collapsin Response Mediator Protein 2 Expression. *J. Biol. Chem.* **2016**, *291*, 4955–4965. [CrossRef] [PubMed]
123. Scharfman, H.; Goodman, J.; Macleod, A.; Phani, S.; Antonelli, C.; Croll, S. Increased Neurogenesis and the Ectopic Granule Cells after Intrahippocampal BDNF Infusion in Adult Rats. *Exp. Neurol.* **2005**, *192*, 348–356. [CrossRef] [PubMed]
124. Hatami, A.; Zhu, C.; Relaño-Gines, A.; Elias, C.; Galstyan, A.; Jun, M.; Milne, G.; Cantor, C.R.; Chesselet, M.F.; Shchepinov, M.S. Deuterium-Reinforced Linoleic Acid Lowers Lipid Peroxidation and Mitigates Cognitive Impairment in the Q140 Knock in Mouse Model of Huntington's Disease. *FEBS J.* **2018**, *285*, 3002–3012. [CrossRef] [PubMed]
125. Liu, Z.-H.; Yip, P.K.; Adams, L.; Davies, M.; Lee, J.W.; Michael, G.J.; Priestley, J.V.; Michael-Titus, A.T. A Single Bolus of Docosahexaenoic Acid Promotes Neuroplastic Changes in the Innervation of Spinal Cord Interneurons and Motor Neurons and Improves Functional Recovery after Spinal Cord Injury. *J. Neurosci.* **2015**, *35*, 12733–12752. [CrossRef]
126. Cao, D.; Kevala, K.; Kim, J.; Moon, H.S.; Jun, S.B.; Lovinger, D.; Kim, H.Y. Docosahexaenoic Acid Promotes Hippocampal Neuronal Development and Synaptic Function. *J. Neurochem.* **2009**, *111*, 510–521. [CrossRef] [PubMed]
127. González, L.M.; Bourissai, A.; Lessard-Beaudoin, M.; Lebel, R.; Tremblay, L.; Lepage, M.; Graham, R.K. Amelioration of Cognitive and Olfactory System Deficits in APOE4 Transgenic Mice with DHA Treatment. *Mol. Neurobiol.* **2023**, *60*, 5624–5641. [CrossRef] [PubMed]
128. Liu, J.H.; Wang, Q.; You, Q.L.; Li, Z.L.; Hu, N.Y.; Wang, Y.; Jin, Z.L.; Li, S.J.; Li, X.W.; Yang, J.M.; et al. Acute EPA-Induced Learning and Memory Impairment in Mice Is Prevented by DHA. *Nat. Commun.* **2020**, *11*, 5465. [CrossRef] [PubMed]
129. Xiao, M.; Xiang, W.; Chen, Y.; Peng, N.; Du, X.; Lu, S.; Zuo, Y.; Li, B.; Hu, Y.; Li, X. DHA Ameliorates Cognitive Ability, Reduces Amyloid Deposition, and Nerve Fiber Production in Alzheimer's Disease. *Front. Nutr.* **2022**, *9*, 852433. [CrossRef]
130. Sinn, N.; Milte, C.M.; Street, S.J.; Buckley, J.D.; Coates, A.M.; Petkov, J.; Howe, P.R.C. Effects of N-3 Fatty Acids, EPA v. DHA, on Depressive Symptoms, Quality of Life, Memory and Executive Function in Older Adults with Mild Cognitive Impairment: A 6-Month Randomised Controlled Trial. *Br. J. Nutr.* **2012**, *107*, 1682–1693. [CrossRef]
131. Guo, Y.-R.; Lee, H.-C.; Lo, Y.-C.; Yu, S.-C.; Huang, S.-Y. N-3 Polyunsaturated Fatty Acids Prevent d-Galactose-Induced Cognitive Deficits in Prediabetic Rats. *Food Funct.* **2018**, *9*, 2228–2239. [CrossRef] [PubMed]
132. Javanainen, M.; Enkavi, G.; Guixà-Gonzaléz, R.; Kulig, W.; Martinez-Seara, H.; Levental, I.; Vattulainen, I. Reduced Level of Docosahexaenoic Acid Shifts GPCR Neuroreceptors to Less Ordered Membrane Regions. *PLoS Comput. Biol.* **2019**, *15*, e1007033. [CrossRef] [PubMed]
133. Moreno, C.; de la Cruz, A.; Valenzuela, C. In-Depth Study of the Interaction, Sensitivity, and Gating Modulation by PUFAs on K+ Channels; Interaction and New Targets. *Front. Physiol.* **2016**, *7*, 578. [CrossRef]
134. Elinder, F.; Liin, S.I. Actions and Mechanisms of Polyunsaturated Fatty Acids on Voltage-Gated Ion Channels. *Front. Physiol.* **2017**, *8*, 43. [CrossRef]
135. Ogawa, T.; Sawane, K.; Ookoshi, K.; Kawashima, R. Supplementation with Flaxseed Oil Rich in Alpha-Linolenic Acid Improves Verbal Fluency in Healthy Older Adults. *Nutrients* **2023**, *15*, 1499. [CrossRef]
136. Young, C.; Gean, P.-W.; Chiou, L.-C.; Shen, Y.-Z. Docosahexaenoic Acid Inhibits Synaptic Transmission and Epileptiform Activity in the Rat Hippocampus. *Synapse* **2000**, *37*, 90–94. [CrossRef]
137. Cordero-Morales, J.F.; Vásquez, V. How Lipids Contribute to Ion Channel Function, a Fat Perspective on Direct and Indirect Interactions. *Curr. Opin. Struct. Biol.* **2018**, *51*, 92–98. [CrossRef] [PubMed]
138. Leaf, A.; Xiao, Y.-F.; Kang, J.X. Interactions of N-3 Fatty Acids with Ion Channels in Excitable Tissues. *Prostaglandins Leukot. Essent. Fat. Acids* **2002**, *67*, 113–120. [CrossRef] [PubMed]
139. Labrousse, V.F.; Nadjar, A.; Joffre, C.; Costes, L.; Aubert, A.; Grégoire, S.; Bretillon, L.; Layé, S. Short-Term Long Chain Omega3 Diet Protects from Neuroinflammatory Processes and Memory Impairment in Aged Mice. *PLoS ONE* **2012**, *7*, e36861. [CrossRef] [PubMed]
140. Fan, R.; Hua, Y.; Shen, J.; Xiao, R.; Ma, W. Dietary Fatty Acids Affect Learning and Memory Ability via Regulating Inflammatory Factors in Obese Mice. *J. Nutr. Biochem.* **2022**, *103*, 108959. [CrossRef] [PubMed]
141. Luchtman, D.W.; Song, C. Cognitive Enhancement by Omega-3 Fatty Acids from Child-Hood to Old Age: Findings from Animal and Clinical Studies. *Neuropharmacology* **2013**, *64*, 550–565. [CrossRef]
142. Grimm, M.O.W.; Mett, J.; Stahlmann, C.P.; Haupenthal, V.J.; Blümel, T.; Stötzel, H.; Grimm, H.S.; Hartmann, T. Eicosapentaenoic Acid and Docosahexaenoic Acid Increase the Degradation of Amyloid-β by Affecting Insulin-Degrading Enzyme1. *Biochem. Cell Biol.* **2016**, *94*, 534–542. [CrossRef] [PubMed]
143. Yan, L.; Xie, Y.; Satyanarayanan, S.K.; Zeng, H.; Liu, Q.; Huang, M.; Ma, Y.; Wan, J.-B.; Yao, X.; Su, K.-P.; et al. Omega-3 Polyunsaturated Fatty Acids Promote Brain-to-Blood Clearance of β-Amyloid in a Mouse Model with Alzheimer's Disease. *Brain Behav. Immun.* **2020**, *85*, 35–45. [CrossRef] [PubMed]

144. Ren, H.; Luo, C.; Feng, Y.; Yao, X.; Shi, Z.; Liang, F.; Kang, J.X.; Wan, J.-B.; Pei, Z.; Su, H. Omega-3 Polyunsaturated Fatty Acids Promote Amyloid-b Clearance from the Brain through Mediating the Function of the Glymphatic System. *FASEB J.* **2017**, *31*, 282–293. [CrossRef]
145. Ozsoy, O.; Seval-Celik, Y.; Hacioglu, G.; Yargicoglu, P.; Demir, R.; Agar, A.; Aslan, M. The Influence and the Mechanism of Docosahexaenoic Acid on a Mouse Model of Parkinson's Disease. *Neurochem. Int.* **2011**, *59*, 664–670. [CrossRef]
146. Chytrova, G.; Ying, Z.; Gomez-Pinilla, F. Exercise Contributes to the Effects of DHA Dietary Supplementation by Acting on Membrane-Related Synaptic Systems. *Brain Res.* **2010**, *1341*, 32–40. [CrossRef] [PubMed]
147. Wu, A.; Ying, Z.; Gomez-Pinilla, F. The Salutary Effects of DHA Dietary Supplementation on Cognition, Neuroplasticity, and Membrane Homeostasis after Brain Trauma. *J. Neurotrauma* **2011**, *28*, 2113–2122. [CrossRef] [PubMed]
148. Ozkan, A.; Parlak, H.; Tanriover, G.; Dilmac, S.; Ulker, S.N.; Birsen, L.; Agar, A. The Protective Mechanism of Docosahexaenoic Acid in Mouse Model of Parkinson: The Role of Heme Oxygenase. *Neurochem. Int.* **2016**, *101*, 110–119. [CrossRef]
149. Jezova, D.; Hlavacova, N. Endocrine Factors in Stress and Psychiatric Disorders: Focus on Anxiety and Salivary Steroids. *Ann. N. Y. Acad. Sci.* **2008**, *1148*, 495–503. [CrossRef] [PubMed]
150. Chrousos, G.P. Stress and Disorders of the Stress System. *Nat. Rev. Endocrinol.* **2009**, *5*, 374–381. [CrossRef]
151. Delarue, J.; Matzinger, O.; Binnert, C.; Schneiter, P.; Chioléro, R.; Tappy, L. Fish Oil Prevents the Adrenal Activation Elicited by Mental Stress in Healthy Men. *Diabetes Metab.* **2003**, *29*, 289–295. [CrossRef]
152. Song, C.; Xiang, Y.Z.; Manku, M. Increased Phospholipase A2 Activity and Inflammatory Response but Decreased Nerve Growth Factor Expression in the Olfactory Bulbectomized Rat Model of Depression: Effects of Chronic Ethyl-Eicosapentaenoate Treatment. *J. Neurosci.* **2009**, *29*, 14–22. [CrossRef] [PubMed]
153. Levant, B.; Ozias, M.K.; Davis, P.F.; Winter, M.; Russell, K.L.; Carlson, S.E.; Reed, G.A.; McCarson, K.E. Decreased Brain Docosahexaenoic Acid Content Produces Neurobiological Effects Associated with Depression: Interactions with Reproductive Status in Female Rats. *Psychoneuroendocrinology* **2008**, *33*, 1279–1292. [CrossRef] [PubMed]
154. Morgese, M.G.; Tucci, P.; Mhillaj, E.; Bove, M.; Schiavone, S.; Trabace, L.; Cuomo, V. Lifelong Nutritional Omega-3 Deficiency Evokes Depressive-Like State Through Soluble Beta Amyloid. *Mol. Neurobiol.* **2017**, *54*, 2079–2089. [CrossRef] [PubMed]
155. Mocking, R.J.T.; Ruhé, H.G.; Assies, J.; Lok, A.; Koeter, M.W.J.; Visser, I.; Bockting, C.L.H.; Schene, A.H. Relationship between the Hypothalamic-Pituitary-Adrenal-Axis and Fatty Acid Metabolism in Recurrent Depression. *Psychoneuroendocrinology* **2013**, *38*, 1607–1617. [CrossRef]
156. Lightman, S.L. The Neuroendocrinology of Stress: A Never Ending Story. *J. Neuroendocrinol.* **2008**, *20*, 880–884. [CrossRef] [PubMed]
157. Takeuchi, T.; Iwanaga, M.; Harada, E. Possible Regulatory Mechanism of DHA-Induced Anti-Stress Reaction in Rats. *Brain Res.* **2003**, *964*, 136–143. [CrossRef]
158. Nieminen, L.R.G.; Makino, K.K.; Mehta, N.; Virkkunen, M.; Kim, H.Y.; Hibbeln, J.R. Relationship between Omega-3 Fatty Acids and Plasma Neuroactive Steroids in Alcoholism, Depression and Controls. *Prostaglandins Leukot. Essent. Fat. Acids* **2006**, *75*, 309–314. [CrossRef] [PubMed]
159. Hamazaki, T.; Sawazaki, S.; Itomura, M.; Asaoka, E.; Nagao, Y.; Nishimura, N.; Yazawa, K.; Kuwamori, T.; Kobayashi, M. Effect of Docosahexaenoic Acid on Aggression Rapid Publication The Effect of Docosahexaenoic Acid on Aggression in Young Adults A Placebo-Controlled Double-Blind Study. *J. Clin. Investig.* **1996**, *97*, 1129–1133. [CrossRef] [PubMed]
160. Oravcova, H.; Katrencikova, B.; Garaiova, I.; Durackova, Z.; Trebaticka, J.; Jezova, D. Stress Hormones Cortisol and Aldosterone, and Selected Markers of Oxidative Stress in Response to Long-Term Supplementation with Omega-3 Fatty Acids in Adolescent Children with Depression. *Antioxidants* **2022**, *11*, 1546. [CrossRef]
161. Thesing, C.S.; Bot, M.; Milaneschi, Y.; Giltay, E.J.; Penninx, B.W.J.H. Omega-3 Polyunsaturated Fatty Acid Levels and Dysregulations in Biological Stress Systems. *Psychoneuroendocrinology* **2018**, *97*, 206–215. [CrossRef] [PubMed]
162. Jazayeri, S.; Keshavarz, S.A.; Tehrani-Doost, M.; Djalali, M.; Hosseini, M.; Amini, H.; Chamari, M.; Djazayery, A. Effects of Eicosapentaenoic Acid and Fluoxetine on Plasma Cortisol, Serum Interleukin-1beta and Interleukin-6 Concentrations in Patients with Major Depressive Disorder. *Psychiatry Res.* **2010**, *178*, 112–115. [CrossRef]
163. Song, C.; Phillips, A.G.; Leonard, B.E.; Horrobin, D.F. Ethyl-Eicosapentaenoic Acid Ingestion Prevents Corticosterone-Mediated Memory Impairment Induced by Central Administration of Interleukin-1β in Rats. *Mol. Psychiatry* **2004**, *9*, 630–638. [CrossRef]
164. Madison, A.A.; Belury, M.A.; Andridge, R.; Renna, M.E.; Rosie Shrout, M.; Malarkey, W.B.; Lin, J.; Epel, E.S.; Kiecolt-Glaser, J.K. Omega-3 Supplementation and Stress Reactivity of Cellular Aging Biomarkers: An Ancillary Substudy of a Randomized, Controlled Trial in Midlife Adults. *Mol. Psychiatry* **2021**, *26*, 3034–3042. [CrossRef]
165. Trebatická, J.; Hradečná, Z.; Surovcová, A.; Katrenčíková, B.; Gushina, I.; Waczulíková, I.; Sušienková, K.; Garaiova, I.; Šuba, J.; Ďuračková, Z. Omega-3 Fatty-Acids Modulate Symptoms of Depressive Disorder, Serum Levels of Omega-3 Fatty Acids and Omega-6/Omega-3 Ratio in Children. A Randomized, Double-Blind and Controlled Trial. *Psychiatry Res.* **2020**, *287*, 112911. [CrossRef]

166. Katrenčíková, B.; Vaváková, M.; Paduchová, Z.; Nagyová, Z.; Garaiova, I.; Muchová, J.; Ďuračková, Z.; Trebatická, J. Oxidative Stress Markers and Antioxidant Enzymes in Children and Adolescents with Depressive Disorder and Impact of Omega-3 Fatty Acids in Randomised Clinical Trial. *Antioxidants* **2021**, *10*, 1256. [CrossRef] [PubMed]
167. Lasselin, J.; Magne, E.; Beau, C.; Ledaguenel, P.; Dexpert, S.; Aubert, A.; Layé, S.; Capuron, L. Adipose Inflammation in Obesity: Relationship with Circulating Levels of Inflammatory Markers and Association with Surgery-Induced Weight Loss. *J. Clin. Endocrinol. Metab.* **2014**, *99*, E53–E61. [CrossRef] [PubMed]
168. Kiecolt-Glaser, J.K.; Derry, H.M.; Fagundes, C.P. Inflammation: Depression Fans the Flames and Feasts on the Heat. *Am. J. Psychiatry* **2015**, *172*, 1075–1091. [CrossRef]
169. Gupta, S.; Gupta, I.; Gupta, R.; Gupta, P. Role of C-Reactive Protein in Periodontal Disease—A Review. *Int. J. Contemp. Med. Res.* **2017**, *4*, 980–985.
170. Incollingo Rodriguez, A.C.; Epel, E.S.; White, M.L.; Standen, E.C.; Seckl, J.R.; Tomiyama, A.J. Hypothalamic-Pituitary-Adrenal Axis Dysregulation and Cortisol Activity in Obesity: A Systematic Review. *Psychoneuroendocrinology* **2015**, *62*, 301–318. [CrossRef] [PubMed]
171. Vreeburg, S.A.; Hoogendijk, W.J.; van Pelt, J.; DeRijk, R.H.; Verhagen, J.C.; van Dyck, R.; Smit, J.H.; Zitman, F.G.; Penninx, B.W. Major Depressive Disorder and Hypothalamic-Pituitary-Adrenal Axis Activity Results from a Large Cohort Study. *Arch. Gen. Psychiatry* **2009**, *66*, 617–626. [CrossRef] [PubMed]
172. Bowden, R.G.; Wilson, R.L.; Deike, E.; Gentile, M. Fish Oil Supplementation Lowers C-Reactive Protein Levels Independent of Triglyceride Reduction in Patients with End-Stage Renal Disease. *Nutr. Clin. Pract.* **2009**, *24*, 508–512. [CrossRef] [PubMed]
173. Zhao, Y.T.; Shao, L.; Teng, L.L.; Hu, B.; Luo, Y.; Yu, X.; Zhang, D.F.; Zhang, H. Effects of N-3 Polyunsaturated Fatty Acid Therapy on Plasma Inflammatory Markers and N-Terminal Pro-Brain Natriuretic Peptide in Elderly Patients with Chronic Heart Failure. *J. Int. Med. Res.* **2009**, *37*, 1831–1841. [CrossRef] [PubMed]
174. Hellhammer, J.; Hero, T.; Franz, N.; Contreras, C.; Schubert, M. Omega-3 Fatty Acids Administered in Phosphatidylserine Improved Certain Aspects of High Chronic Stress in Men. *Nutr. Res.* **2012**, *32*, 241–250. [CrossRef] [PubMed]
175. Pace, T.W.; Hu, F.; Miller, A.H. Cytokine-Effects on Glucocorticoid Receptor Function: Relevance to Glucocorticoid Resistance and the Pathophysiology and Treatment of Major Depression. *Brain Behav. Immun.* **2007**, *21*, 9–19. [CrossRef] [PubMed]
176. Escoll, P.; Ranz, I.; Muñoz-Antón, N.; Van-Den-Rym, A.; Alvarez-Mon, M.; Martínez-Alonso, C.; Sanz, E.; De-La-Hera, A. Sustained Interleukin-1β Exposure Modulates Multiple Steps in Glucocorticoid Receptor Signaling, Promoting Split-Resistance to the Transactivation of Prominent Anti-Inflammatory Genes by Glucocorticoids. *Mediat. Inflamm.* **2015**, *2015*, 347965. [CrossRef] [PubMed]
177. Cao, W.; Wang, C.; Chin, Y.; Chen, X.; Gao, Y.; Yuan, S.; Xue, C.; Wang, Y.; Tang, Q. DHA-Phospholipids (DHA-PL) and EPA-Phospholipids (EPA-PL) Prevent Intestinal Dysfunction Induced by Chronic Stress. *Food Funct.* **2019**, *10*, 277–288. [CrossRef]
178. Bomba, A.; Nemcová, R.; Gancarcíková, S.; Herich, R.; Guba, P.; Mudronová, D. Improvement of the Probiotic Effect of Micro-Organisms by Their Combination with Maltodextrins, Fructo-Oligosaccharides and Polyunsaturated Fatty Acids. *Br. J. Nutr.* **2002**, *88*, S95–S99. [CrossRef] [PubMed]
179. Kaliannan, K.; Wang, B.; Li, X.-Y.; Kim, K.-J.; Kang, J.X. A Host-Microbiome Interaction Mediates the Opposing Effects of Omega-6 and Omega-3 Fatty Acids on Metabolic Endotoxemia. *Sci. Rep.* **2015**, *5*, 11276. [CrossRef]
180. Liu, J.; Huang, H.; Yang, Q.; Zhao, J.; Zhang, H.; Chen, W.; Peng, X.; Gu, Z. Dietary Supplementation of N-3 LCPUFAs Prevents Salmonellosis in a Murine Model. *J. Agric. Food Chem.* **2020**, *68*, 128–137. [CrossRef] [PubMed]
181. Balfegò, M.; Canivell, S.; Hanzu, F.A.; Sala-Vila, A.; Martínez-Medina, M.; Murillo, S.; Mur, T.; Ruano, E.G.; Linares, F.; Porras, N.; et al. Effects of Sardine-Enriched Diet on Metabolic Control, Inflammation and Gut Microbiota in Drug-Naïve Patients with Type 2 Diabetes: A Pilot Randomized Trial. *Lipids Health Dis.* **2016**, *15*, 78. [CrossRef] [PubMed]
182. Neijat, M.; Habtewold, J.; Li, S.; Jing, M.; House, J.D. Effect of Dietary N-3 Polyunsaturated Fatty Acids on the Composition of Cecal Microbiome of Lohmann Hens. *Prostaglandins Leukot. Essent. Fat. Acids* **2020**, *162*, 102182. [CrossRef]
183. Menni, C.; Zierer, J.; Pallister, T.; Jackson, M.A.; Long, T.; Mohney, R.P.; Steves, C.J.; Spector, T.D.; Valdes, A.M. Omega-3 Fatty Acids Correlate with Gut Microbiome Diversity and Production of N-Carbamylglutamate in Middle Aged and Elderly Women. *Sci. Rep.* **2017**, *7*, 11079. [CrossRef] [PubMed]
184. Vijay, A.; Astbury, S.; Le Roy, C.; Spector, T.D.; Valdes, A.M. The Prebiotic Effects of Omega-3 Fatty Acid Supplementation: A Six-Week Randomised Intervention Trial. *Gut Microbes* **2021**, *13*, 1863133. [CrossRef]
185. Jayapala, H.P.S.; Lim, S.Y. N-3 Polyunsaturated Fatty Acids and Gut Microbiota. *Comb. Chem. High Throughput Screen.* **2022**, *26*, 892–905. [CrossRef]
186. Tao, F.; Xing, X.; Wu, J.; Jiang, R. Enteral Nutrition Modulation with N-3 PUFAs Directs Microbiome and Lipid Metabolism in Mice. *PLoS ONE* **2021**, *16*, e0248482. [CrossRef]
187. Robertson, R.C.; Oriach, C.S.; Murphy, K.; Moloney, G.M.; Cryan, J.F.; Dinan, T.G.; Ross, R.P.; Stanton, C. Deficiency of Essential Dietary N-3 PUFA Disrupts the Caecal Microbiome and Metabolome in Mice. *Br. J. Nutr.* **2017**, *118*, 959–970. [CrossRef]

188. Blanchard, H.; Pédrono, F.; Boulier-Monthéan, N.; Catheline, D.; Rioux, V.; Legrand, P. Comparative Effects of Well-Balanced Diets Enriched in α-Linolenic or Linoleic Acids on LC-PUFA Metabolism in Rat Tissues. *Prostaglandins Leukot. Essent. Fat. Acids* **2013**, *88*, 383–389. [CrossRef] [PubMed]
189. Robertson, R.C.; Seira Oriach, C.; Murphy, K.; Moloney, G.M.; Cryan, J.F.; Dinan, T.G.; Paul Ross, R.; Stanton, C. Omega-3 Polyunsaturated Fatty Acids Critically Regulate Behaviour and Gut Microbiota Development in Adolescence and Adulthood. *Brain Behav. Immun.* **2017**, *59*, 21–37. [CrossRef]
190. Pachikian, B.D.; Neyrinck, A.M.; Portois, L.; De Backer, F.C.; Sohet, F.M.; Hacquebard, M.; Carpentier, Y.A.; Cani, P.D.; Delzenne, N.M. Involvement of Gut Microbial Fermentation in the Metabolic Alterations Occurring in N-3 Polyunsaturated Fatty Acids-Depleted Mice. *Nutr. Metab.* **2011**, *8*, 44. [CrossRef]
191. Horiuchi, H.; Kamikado, K.; Aoki, R.; Suganuma, N.; Nishijima, T.; Nakatani, A.; Kimura, I. Bifidobacterium Animalis Subsp. Lactis GCL2505 Modulates Host Energy Metabolism via the Short-Chain Fatty Acid Receptor GPR43. *Sci. Rep.* **2020**, *10*, 4158. [CrossRef]
192. Patterson, E.; Wall, R.; Lisai, S.; Ross, R.P.; Dinan, T.G.; Cryan, J.F.; Fitzgerald, G.F.; Banni, S.; Quigley, E.M.; Shanahan, F.; et al. Bifidobacterium Breve with α-Linolenic Acid Alters the Composition, Distribution and Transcription Factor Activity Associated with Metabolism and Absorption of Fat. *Sci. Rep.* **2017**, *7*, 43300. [CrossRef]
193. Lu, J.; Shataer, D.; Yan, H.; Dong, X.; Zhang, M.; Qin, Y.; Cui, J.; Wang, L. Probiotics and Non-Alcoholic Fatty Liver Disease: Unveiling the Mechanisms of Lactobacillus Plantarum and Bifidobacterium Bifidum in Modulating Lipid Metabolism, Inflammation, and Intestinal Barrier Integrity. *Foods* **2024**, *13*, 2992. [CrossRef] [PubMed]
194. Honda, K.L.; Lamon-Fava, S.; Matthan, N.R.; Wu, D.; Lichtenstein, A.H. Docosahexaenoic Acid Differentially Affects TNFα and IL-6 Expression in LPS-Stimulated RAW 264.7 Murine Macrophages. *Prostaglandins Leukot. Essent. Fat. Acids* **2015**, *97*, 27–34. [CrossRef] [PubMed]
195. Kong, W.; Yen, J.-H.; Vassiliou, E.; Adhikary, S.; Toscano, M.G.; Ganea, D. Docosahexaenoic Acid Prevents Dendritic Cell Maturation and In Vitro and In Vivo Expression of the IL-12 Cytokine Family. *Lipids Health Dis.* **2010**, *9*, 12. [CrossRef] [PubMed]
196. Zhao, Y.; Joshi-Barve, S.; Barve, S.; Chen, L.H. Eicosapentaenoic Acid Prevents LPS-Induced TNF-α Expression by Preventing NF-KB Activation. *J. Am. Coll. Nutr.* **2004**, *23*, 71–78. [CrossRef] [PubMed]
197. Vanden Berghe, W.; Vermeulen, L.; Delerive, P.; De Bosscher, K.; Staels, B.; Haegeman, G. A Paradigm for Gene Regulation: Inflammation, NF-KB and PPAR. In *Peroxisomal Disorders and Regulation of Genes*; Springer: Boston, MA, USA, 2003.
198. Novak, T.E.; Babcock, T.A.; Jho, D.H.; Helton, W.S.; Espat, N.J.; Joseph, N. NF-B Inhibition by-3 Fatty Acids Modulates LPS-Stimulated Macrophage TNF-Transcription. *Am. J. Physiol. Lung Cell. Mol. Physiol.* **2003**, *284*, 84–89. [CrossRef] [PubMed]
199. Zeyda, M.; Staffler, G.; Hořejší, V.; Waldhäusl, W.; Stulnig, T.M. LAT Displacement from Lipid Rafts as a Molecular Mechanism for the Inhibition of T Cell Signaling by Polyunsaturated Fatty Acids. *J. Biol. Chem.* **2002**, *277*, 28418–28423. [CrossRef] [PubMed]
200. Koppelmann, T.; Pollak, Y.; Mogilner, J.; Bejar, J.; Coran, A.G.; Sukhotnik, I. Reversal of Severe Methotrexate-Induced Intestinal Damage Using Enteral n-3 Fatty Acids. *Br. J. Nutr.* **2013**, *109*, 89–98. [CrossRef] [PubMed]
201. Gebauer, S.K.; Psota, T.L.; Harris, W.S.; Kris-Etherton, P.M. N−3 Fatty Acid Dietary Recommendations and Food Sources to Achieve Essentiality and Cardiovascular Benefits. *Am. J. Clin. Nutr.* **2006**, *83*, 1526S–1535S. [CrossRef] [PubMed]
202. Van Dael, P. Role of N-3 Long-Chain Polyunsaturated Fatty Acids in Human Nutrition and Health: Review of Recent Studies and Recommendations. *Nutr. Res. Pract.* **2021**, *15*, 137–159. [CrossRef]
203. Schneider, E.; Balasubramanian, R.; Ferri, A.; Cotter, P.D.; Clarke, G.; Cryan, J.F. Fibre & fermented foods: Differential effects on the microbiota-gut-brain axis. *Proc Nutr Soc.*. [CrossRef]
204. de Oliveira, V.S.; Viana, D.S.B.; Keller, L.M.; de Melo, M.T.T.; Mulandeza, O.F.; Barbosa, M.I.M.J.; Barbosa Júnior, J.L.; Saldanha, T. Impact of Air Frying on Food Lipids: Oxidative Evidence, Current Research, and Insights into Domestic Mitigation by Natural Antioxidants. *Trends Food Sci. Technol.* **2024**, *147*, 104465. [CrossRef]

molecules

MDPI

Article

Influence of Ovophospholipids on Lymphocyte Subsets and Humoral Immune Response in Mice

Magdalena Lis [1,*], Marianna Szczypka [1], Agnieszka Suszko-Pawłowska [1], Aleksandra Pawlak [1], Łukasz Bobak [2] and Bożena Obmińska-Mrukowicz [1]

1 Department of Pharmacology and Toxicology, Faculty of Veterinary Medicine, Wroclaw University of Environmental and Life Sciences, C. K. Norwida 31, 50-375 Wrocław, Poland; marianna.szczypka@upwr.edu.pl (M.S.); agnieszka.suszko@upwr.edu.pl (A.S.-P.); aleksandra.pawlak@upwr.edu.pl (A.P.); bozena.obminska-mrukowicz@upwr.edu.pl (B.O.-M.)

2 Department of Functional Food Products Development, Faculty of Biotechnology and Food Science, Wroclaw University of Environmental and Life Sciences, Chełmońskiego 37, 51-630 Wrocław, Poland; lukasz.bobak@upwr.edu.pl

* Correspondence: magdalena.lis@upwr.edu.pl

Abstract: Designed hen eggs enriched in DHA and EPA are an alternative source of essential phospholipids. This study assessed the effects of ovophospholipids on lymphocyte subsets in non-immunized mice and on the humoral immune response in sheep red blood cells (SRBC)-immunized mice. Ovophospholipids were administered orally for 14 days (once a day) at doses of 100, 10, and 1 mg/kg. Ovophospholipids increased the total lymphocyte count of in the lymphoid organs. At 10 and 1 mg/kg, ovophospholipids increased the subsets of $CD4^-CD8^-$ and $CD4^+CD8^+$ thymocytes but decreased the percentage of $CD4^+$ and $CD8^+$ thymocytes. A stimulating effect on splenocytes was particularly evident 24 h after administration of the 10 and 1 mg/kg doses. Ovophospholipids also elevated the absolute counts of $CD3^+$ and $CD19^+$ splenocytes. An increase in the absolute count of $CD3^+$, $CD4^+$, $CD8^+$, and $CD19^+$ lymphocytes of the mesenteric lymph nodes was observed 24 h after administration of the lowest dose. The increase in the percentage and absolute count of $CD19^+$ cells and in the absolute count of $CD3^+$ cells was still observed after 72 h. At all doses, ovophospholipids elevated the number of plaque-forming cells on day 4 and increased 2-mercaptoethanol-resistant antibody titer on day 7 after priming. In conclusion, ovophospholipids can modulate the immune response in mice.

Keywords: ovophospholipids; phospholipids; lymphocytes; humoral immune response

1. Introduction

Phospholipids belong to complex lipids that are one of the major components of cell membranes, playing an essential role in the proper functioning of the human and animal body. The richest natural sources of phospholipids are nervous tissue, liver, egg yolk, and the seeds of oil-producing plants, especially soybeans and rapeseed [1–4].

Currently, oil plants, particularly soya, are the main industrial source of phospholipids. However, the phospholipid composition of plant-derived sources differs from that of hen egg yolk. The oil plants, especially soya, contain about 2% of phospholipids [1,4]. Meanwhile, the yolk of a typical egg contains 33% of phospholipids in its dry matter, of which pure phosphatidylcholine (lecithin) accounts for 76% [1,3].

Omega-3 polyunsaturated fatty acids (n-3 PUFAs) (phospholipid components esterified in the phospholipid structure) play an important role in maintaining the human/animal body homeostasis, being involved in many physiological processes. Improper diet, rich

 https://doi.org/10.3390/molecules30112253

in saturated fatty acids and poor in n-3 PUFAs, with inappropriate n-6/n-3 PUFA ratio is, among others, a reason behind many the so-called "lifestyle diseases" [1]. The most relevant long-chain n-3 PUFAs are docosahexaenoic acid (DHA), eicosapentaenoic acid (EPA), and α-linolenic acid (ALA). The main sources of DHA and EPA are marine fish oil and algae. In phospholipids of plant origin, the only representative of n-3 PUFAs is ALA. In contrast, yolk phospholipids include a wider palette of n-3 PUFAs, such as ALA or DHA. It has been proven that the phospholipid content of egg yolk depends on genetic factors, the age and living conditions of laying hens, and, importantly, the type of feed they receive [5]. Therefore, it is possible to change the phospholipid profile of an egg yolk through introduction of some modifications in the hen diet, i.e., supplementation with ingredients rich in target fatty acids (peat preparations, rapeseed oil, linseed oil, sea algae) [1]. Such eggs, called designed eggs, may contain many more long-chain n-3 PUFAs (in comparison with ordinary eggs), also including EPA [1].

Taking into account the need to increase dietary intake of n-3 PUFAs (especially DHA and EPA) by humans and some limitations regarding edible products (sensory features—fish taste and smell, intolerance to soya protein) in which they are found, searching for their alternative sources is of special importance. Ovophospholipids isolated from designed eggs enriched in DHA and EPA seem a good solution.

The immunomodulatory action of DHA or EPA has been confirmed in many studies.

Regarding the impact of n-3 PUFAs on cytokine (IL-1β, IL-4, IL-6, IL-10, TNF-α, IFN-γ) synthesis, the results vary depending on the study. A stimulating effect of n3-PUFA on lymphocyte proliferation and cytokine production was observed by some authors [6], but not by others [7]. Downregulation of pathologically raised cytokine levels was also reported [8–10].

EPA and DHA reduced in vitro proliferation of concanavalin A (ConA)-stimulated T lymphocytes isolated from blood of both healthy and type I diabetic people, decreased IL-2 production, and increased IL-4 secretion by these cells [11]. Chapkin et al. [12] demonstrated ex vivo a suppressive effect of DHA on the proliferative response of purified murine T lymphocytes, following a direct stimulation of T cell receptor and coreceptor αCD3/αCD28. An in vivo study on an experimental autoimmune encephalomyelitis model showed significant inhibition of proliferation and IFN-γ and IL-17 production by $CD4^+$ T cells from the spleen and CNS, isolated from mice fed with DHA-enriched diet [13].

The effect of n-3 PUFAs on regulatory T cells (Treg) was also investigated. It was shown [14] that long-term administration of n-3 PUFAs to mice enhanced the percentage of hepatic Tregs as well as up-regulated the expression of IL-10, PPAR-γ (peroxisome proliferator activated receptor gamma), and TGF-β (transforming growth factor β). DHA, administered to mice, alleviated atopic dermatitis by inducing the differentiation of $CD4^+Foxp3^+$ Tregs [15]. Dendritic cells (DCs) cultured with DHA decreased T-cell proliferation and raised the proportion of T cells expressing Foxp3, indicating that DHA can promote induction of Tregs [16]. Splenic $CD4^+$ T cells isolated from C57BL/6 mice fed with diets enriched with DHA and/or EPA showed reduced polarization into inflammatory Th17 cells but not into Treg cells [17].

Gorjao et al. [6] showed that supplementation of DHA and EPA elevated phagocytic activity of neutrophils and monocytes, as well as the chemotactic response and production of reactive oxygen metabolites by neutrophils. On the other hand, Kew et al. [7] demonstrated no effect on the function (phagocytosis and the expression of adhesion molecules) of neutrophils and monocytes.

As shown in the studies cited above and others [18–26], the results regarding many aspects of the immune response are inconsistent and therefore inconclusive. For this reason, there is still a need for further investigation in this area.

The aim of this study was to determine the effect of ovophospholipids isolated from designed eggs enriched with n-3 PUFAs on lymphocyte subsets in the thymus, spleen, and mesenteric lymph nodes in non-immunized mice and on humoral immune response in SRBC-immunized mice, depending on the applied dose.

2. Results

2.1. Effects of Ovophospholipids on Lymphocyte Subsets

Ovophospholipids administered at a dose of 10 mg/kg increased the percentage of double-positive $CD4^+CD8^+$ thymocytes with corresponding decrease in the percentage of single-positive $CD4^+$ and $CD8^+$ thymic cells 24 h after their last administration. Seventy-two hours after administration of the last dose of 10 mg/kg, an increase was noticed in the total count of thymocytes and the percentage and absolute count of $CD4^+CD8^+$ thymocytes, accompanied by a decrease in the percentage of $CD4^+$ and $CD8^+$ thymic cells. The impact of a 1 mg/kg dose on the thymocytes was noticed especially 24 h after its last administration. Ovophospholipids enhanced the total count of the thymocytes as well as absolute count of $CD4^-CD8^-$ and $CD4^+$ thymic cells (but decreased their percentage) and the percentage and absolute count of $CD4^+CD8^+$ thymocytes. The increase in the percentage of $CD4^+CD8^+$ and decrease in the percentage of $CD4^+$ thymocytes 72 h after the last dose was observed. The only change noticed after administration of 100 mg/kg ovophospholipids was an increase in the percentage of $CD4^-CD8^-$ thymic cells that was observed 24 h after the last dose (Figure 1b–d). Ovophospholipids at the examined doses did not influence the thymus weight (Figure 1a).

Ovophospholipids exerted a stimulating effect on the splenic lymphocytes. The effect was observed especially after 24 h. At that time, ovophospholipids elevated the total count of the splenocytes in a dose-independent manner. A rise was noticed in the absolute count of the $CD3^+$ and $CD4^+$ splenic lymphocytes after the administration of 10 and 1 mg/kg doses of ovophospholipids. An increase in the percentage of $CD4^+$ splenocytes and the percentage and absolute count of $CD8^+$ cells in the presence of 1 mg/kg of ovophospholipids was also seen. Ovophospholipids elevated the absolute count of B lymphocytes at all examined doses. Seventy-two hours after the last dose of 10 mg/kg, a rise in total count but a decrease in the percentage of $CD3^+$ and $CD8^+$, and an increase in the absolute count of $CD19^+$ splenocytes were found (Figure 2b–d). Regardless of the dose, ovophospholipids did not change the spleen weight (Figure 2a).

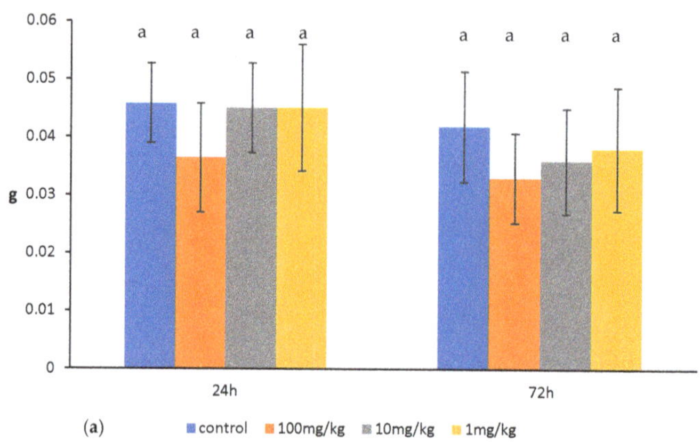

(a)

Figure 1. *Cont.*

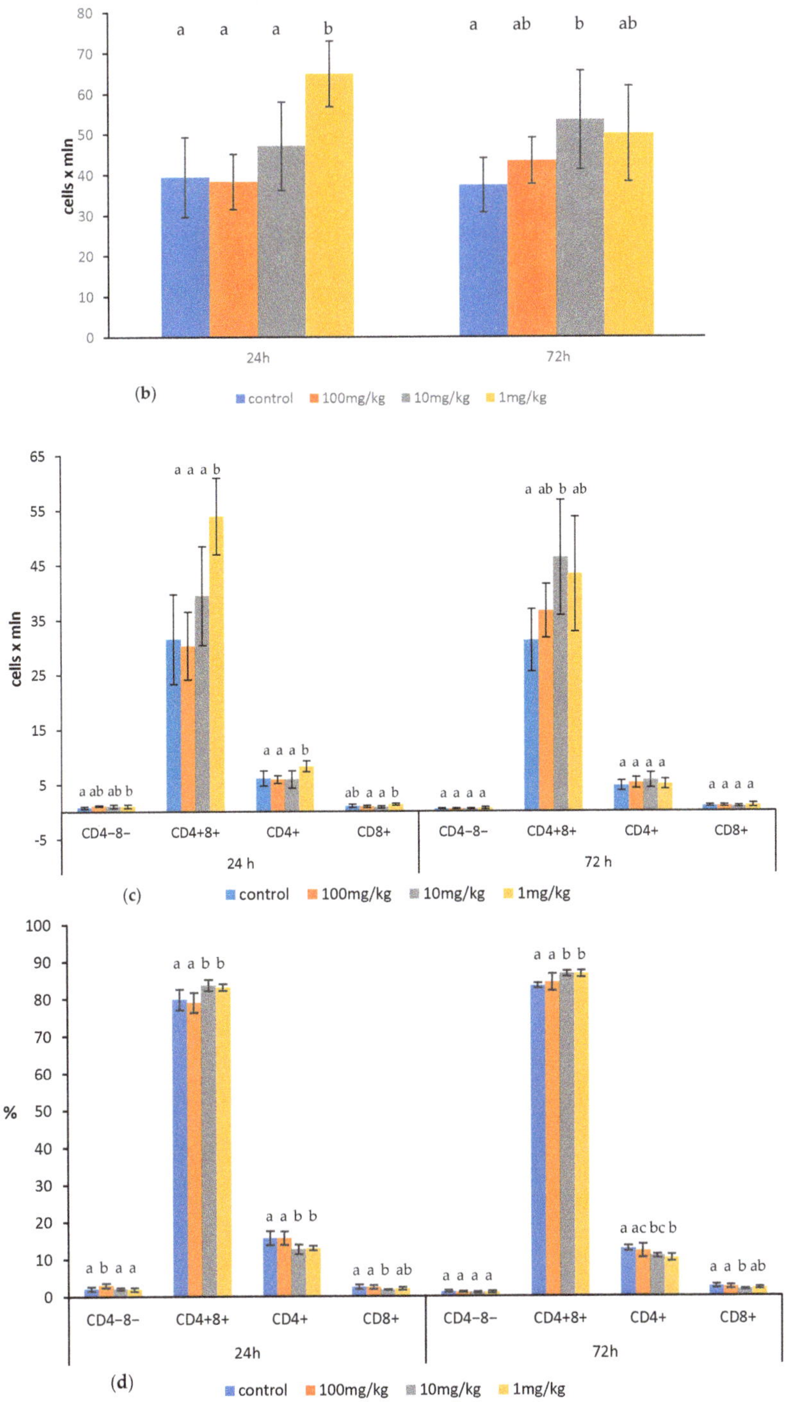

Figure 1. Thymus weight (**a**), total count of thymocytes (**b**), absolute count of thymocyte subpopulations (**c**), and the percentage of thymocyte subpopulations (**d**) in mice treated for 14 days (once a day) with ovophospholipids. The mean value ($n = 7$) and standard deviations are shown. Data with different superscript letters differ significantly ($p < 0.05$).

Ovophospholipids exerted a stimulating effect on the lymphocytes of the mesenteric lymph nodes. However, the effect was observed mostly for the lowest dose of 1 mg/kg. At that dose, ovophospholipids increased the total count of the lymphocytes of the mesenteric lymph nodes, which was observed 24 h (also at 10 mg/kg) and 72 h after the last administration. A rise in the absolute count of T lymphocytes ($CD3^+$) with both $CD4^+$ and $CD8^+$ subpopulations and B lymphocytes ($CD19^+$) was observed 24 h after the last administration. The effect on the absolute count of $CD3^+$ and $CD19^+$ lymphocytes was long-lasting, as it persisted 72 h after the last dose. Ovophospholipids administered at 10 and 1 mg/kg elevated also the percentage of $CD19^+$ cells 72 h after the last administration (Figure 3b–d). Ovophospholipids at the examined doses did not affect mesenteric lymph node weight (Figure 3a).

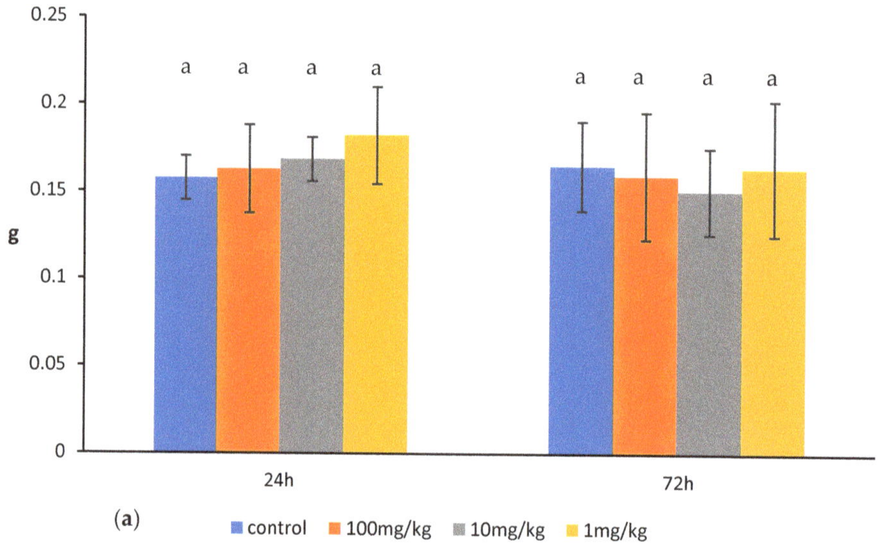

(**a**)

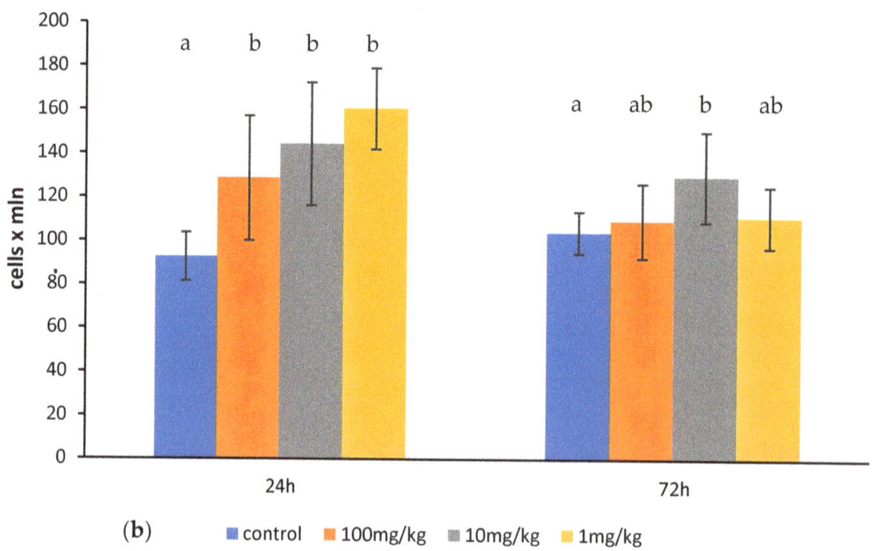

(**b**)

Figure 2. *Cont.*

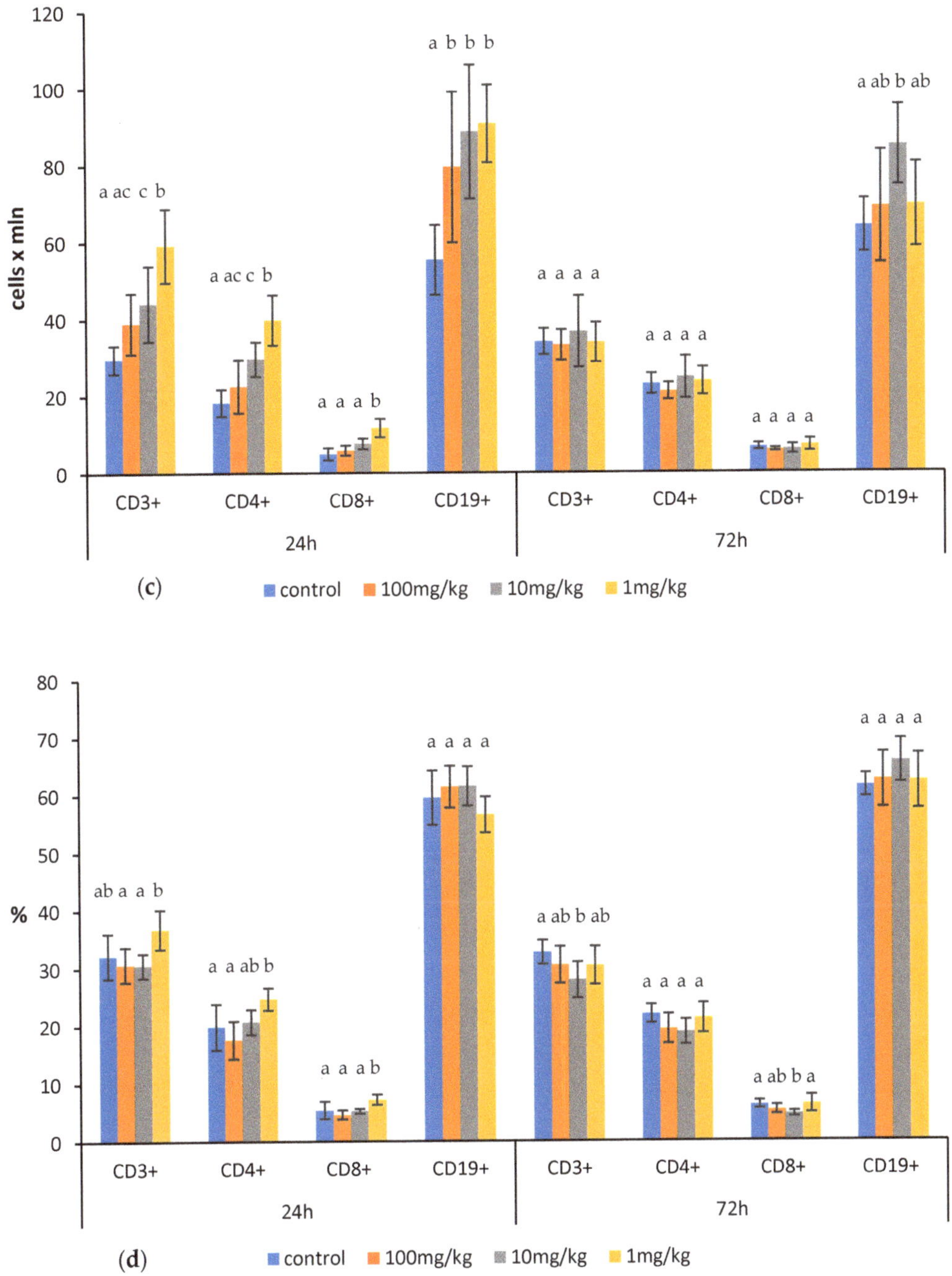

Figure 2. Spleen weight (**a**), total count of splenocytes (**b**), absolute count of splenocyte subpopulations (**c**), and the percentage of splenocyte subpopulations (**d**) in mice treated for 14 days (once a day) with ovophospholipids. The mean value (n = 7) and standard deviations are shown. Data with different superscript letters differ significantly (p < 0.05).

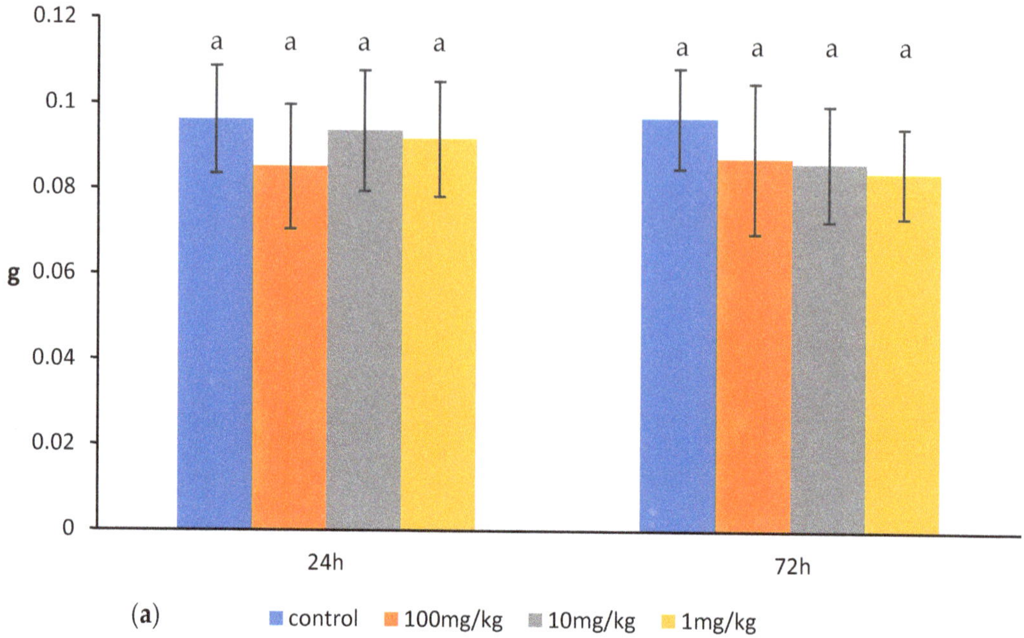

(**a**)

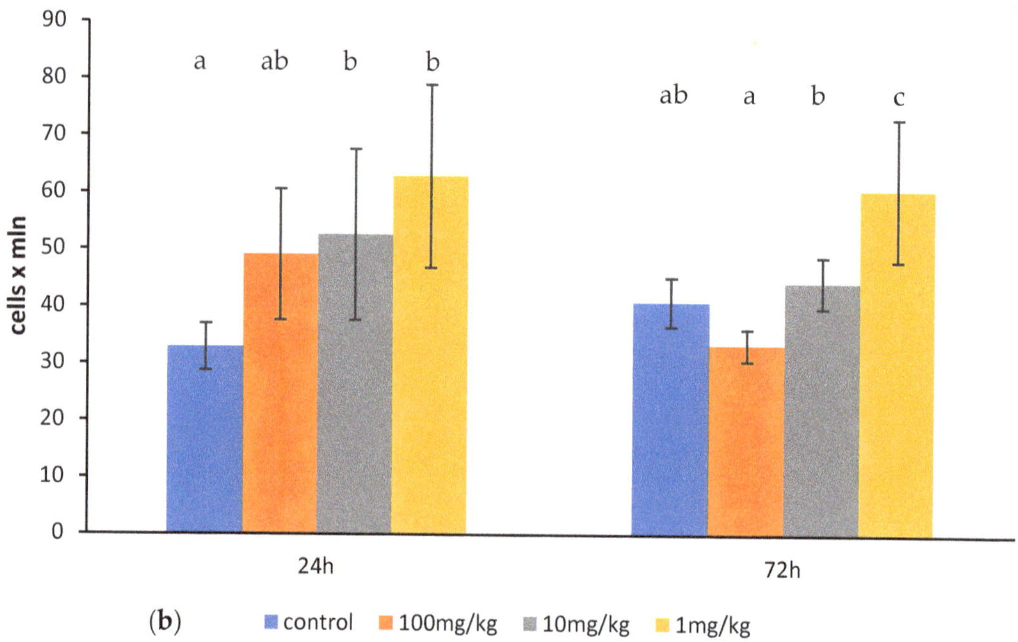

(**b**)

Figure 3. *Cont.*

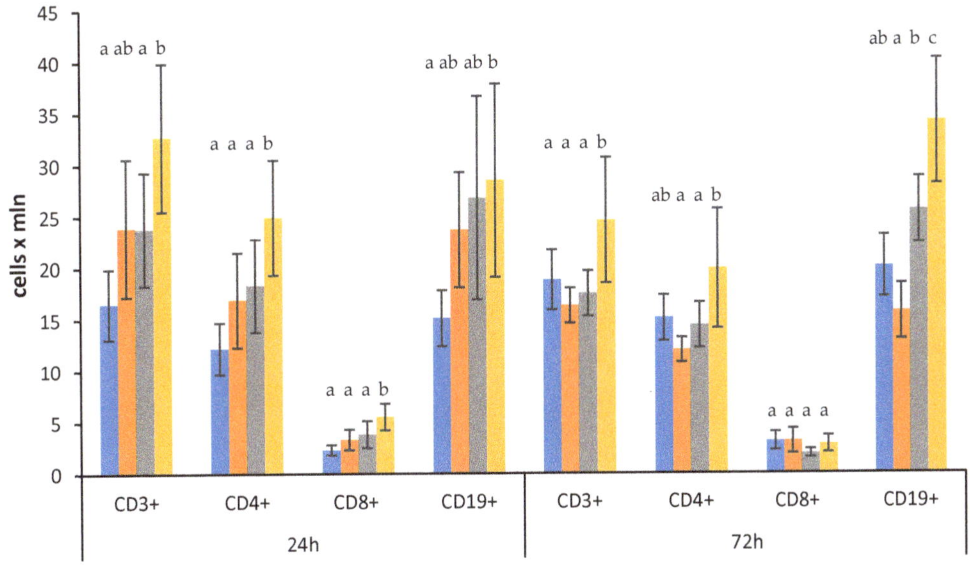

(c)

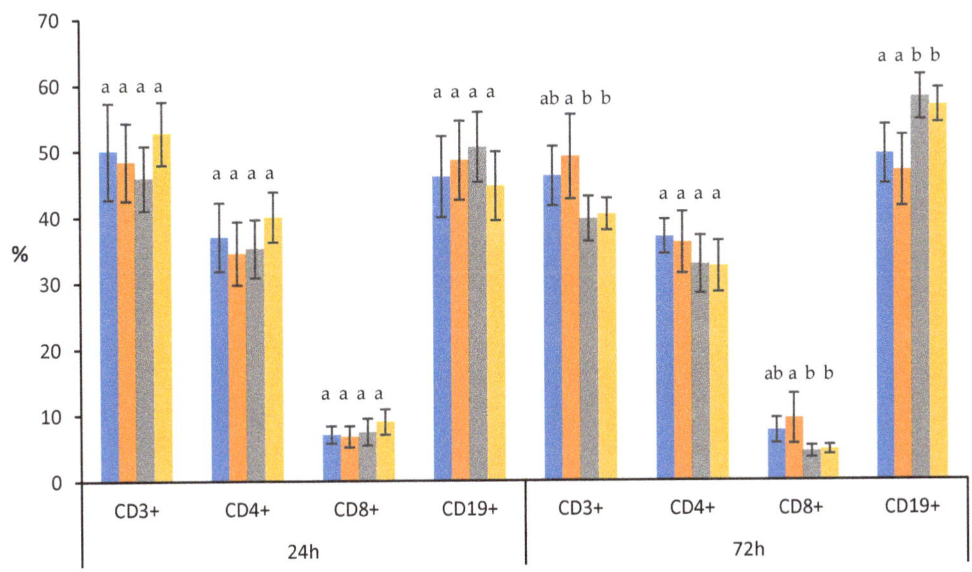

(d)

Figure 3. Mesenteric lymph node weight (**a**), total count of mesenteric lymph node lymphocytes (**b**), absolute count of mesenteric lymph node lymphocyte subpopulations (**c**), and the percentage of mesenteric lymph node lymphocyte subpopulations (**d**) in mice treated for 14 days (once a day) with ovophospholipids. The mean value ($n = 7$) and standard deviations are shown. Data with different superscript letters differ significantly ($p < 0.05$).

2.2. Effect of Ovophospholipids on TNF-α and IL-1β Levels in the Culture Supernatants of Peritoneal Macrophages Stimulated In Vitro with Lipopolysaccharide (LPS) from E. coli (055:B5)

An increase in TNF-α level was found for the ovophospholipid dose of 1 mg/kg 72 h after its last administration. However, an upward trend was also observed for other doses and also after 24 h (Figure 4a). Ovophospholipids at the examined doses did not affect IL-1β level (Figure 4b).

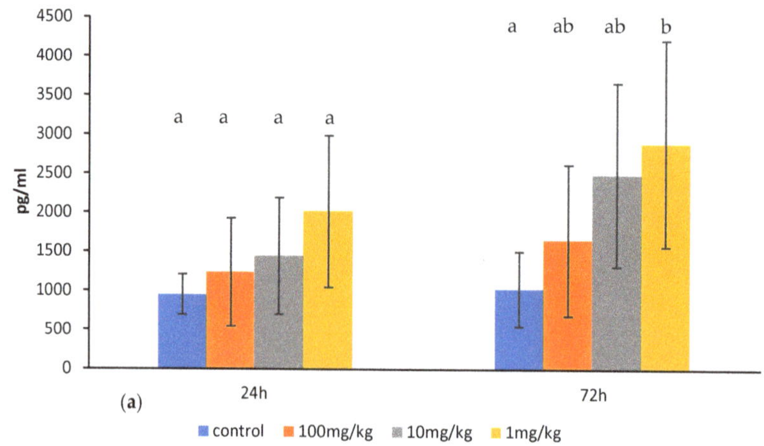

(**a**)

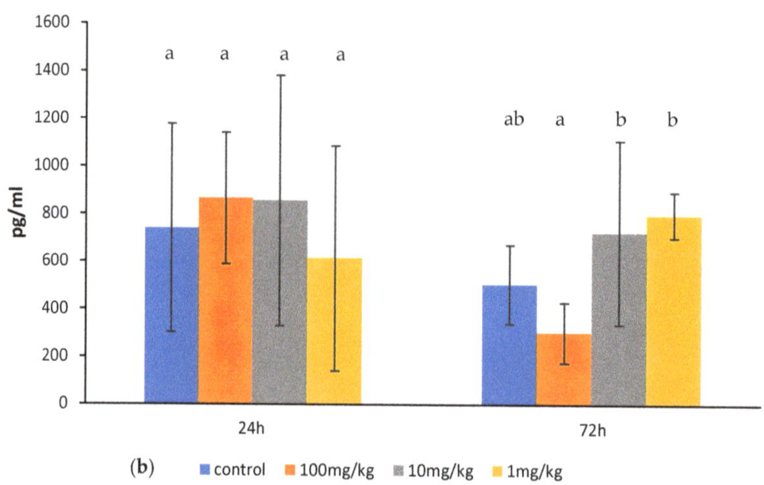

(**b**)

Figure 4. TNF-α (**a**) and IL-1β (**b**) levels in the culture supernatants of peritoneal macrophages obtained from mice treated with ovophospholipids for 14 days (once a day), stimulated in vitro with LPS. The mean value (n = 7) and standard deviations are shown. Data with different superscript letters differ significantly ($p < 0.05$).

2.3. Effect of Ovophospholipids on Humoral Immune Response

Ovophospholipids administered for 14 days (once a day) elevated the number of plaque-forming cells (PFCs) on day 4 after SRBC immunization. The effect was observed for all examined doses. An increase in total anti-SRBC hemagglutinin titer was found only for the dose of 1 mg/kg on day 4 after SRBC injection. However, a stimulating impact of ovophospholipids on 2-ME-resistant antibody titer was noticed for all three doses on day 7 after immunization (Figure 5a–c).

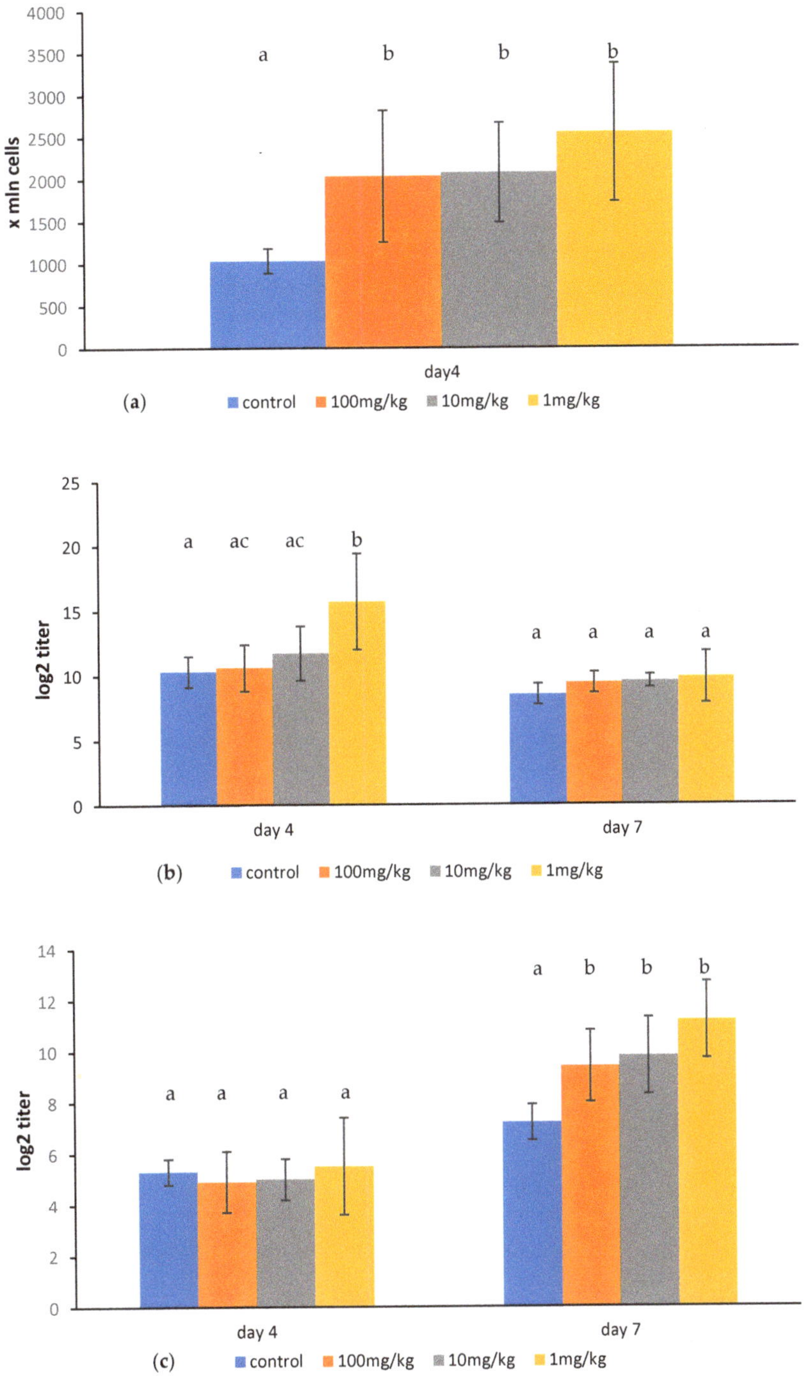

Figure 5. The number of PFCs: (**a**) total anti-SRBC hemagglutinin titer (**b**), and 2-ME-resistant anti-SRBC hemagglutinin titer (**c**) in SRBC-immunized mice treated for 14 days (once a day) with ovophospholipids. The mean value ($n = 7$) and standard deviations are shown. Data with different superscript letters differ significantly ($p < 0.05$).

3. Discussion

Studies on the biological activity of phospholipids and single fatty acids included in their composition have been conducted for many years. In the available literature, there are also numerous reports on the impact of different fatty acids on various aspects of the immune system. Ovophospholipids used in this study contain an enriched composition of fatty acids, especially n-3 PUFAs, i.e., DHA and EPA. In fact, no research has been published on the impact of ovophospholipids on the immune response. Therefore, in the discussion, we focused on the comparison of our results with the data from other authors regarding DHA/EPA or phospholipids of fish origin.

The impact of ovophospholipids on the lymphocytes in the thymus is ambiguous. An increase in the percentage and/or absolute count of immature $CD4^{+}CD8^{+}$ cells may suggest that ovophospholipids stimulate maturation of the thymic cells. However, the percentage of the mature $CD4^{+}$ and $CD8^{+}$ thymic cells was decreased. Taking into account that the population of T cells in the spleen and mesenteric lymph nodes increased, we may speculate that ovophospholipids accelerate migration of mature T cells from the thymus to the peripheral lymphoid organs.

The elevated total count of the thymus lymphocytes also observed in our study may be due to an increase in the number of immature thymocytes. In the available literature, there are almost no publications regarding the impact of fatty acids on thymocytes. The only study by Sasaki et al. [27] showed no effect on the number and percentage of thymocytes expressing $CD3^{+}$, $CD4^{+}$, and $CD8^{+}$ in mice fed a diet varying in the amount of DHA for 4 weeks.

We noticed a stimulating effect of ovophospholipids on T lymphocytes of the peripheral lymphoid organs (spleen and mesenteric lymph nodes). Regarding the splenocytes, it was observed in particular 24 h after administration of the lower doses, i.e., 10 and 1 mg/kg. However, it seems that the impact of ovophospholipids on the splenocytes was rather short-lasting, as 72 h after the last administration most changes were not perceived anymore. Regarding mesenteric lymph nodes, ovophospholipids increased the population of T cells especially at the dose of 1 mg/kg.

The influence of phospholipids/n-3 PUFAs included in fish oil or purified DHA/EPA on the count and function of T lymphocytes was described by other authors. Similarly to our results, Sasaki et al. [27] found a significant increase in the number of splenocytes in mice fed for 4 weeks with DHA-rich diet. However, the surface expression of $CD4^{+}$ and $CD8^{+}$ on splenic T cells decreased as the dietary DHA concentration increased (the expression of $CD3^{+}$ was unchanged). Analyzing the results of our team and those of Sasaki [27], we concluded that a certain regularity can be seen: the effect of phospholipids on the lymphocyte surface marker distribution strongly depends on the dose, and higher doses may affect the lymphocytes in different ways. In our study, the highest dose of ovophospholipids (100 mg/kg) had in fact no impact on T lymphocytes, contrary to the lower doses.

Other data [28] demonstrated that dietary fish oil enriched with DHA and administered for 12 weeks altered T lymphocyte populations and exacerbated colitis in mice. The percentage of $CD4^{+}CD3^{+}$ splenic T cells increased, but no differences were observed in the mesenteric lymph nodes. The percentage of $CD8^{+}CD3^{+}$ T lymphocytes was significantly reduced in both tissues. These results are in agreement with ours, as we also observed an increase in $CD4^{+}$ splenocytes 24 h after the last administration of ovophospholipids and a decrease in the percentage of $CD8^{+}$ splenocytes 72 h after the last administration.

A study by Paixão et al. [29] suggests that DHA and EPA had some anti-inflammatory activity and showed a beneficial effect on the immune system in newly diagnosed breast cancer patients. The anti-inflammatory effect was demonstrated by a constant level of serum high-sensitivity C-reactive protein (hsCRP) in DHA/EPA-treated patients, while in the placebo group, a significant increase in hsCRP was noticed. The immunomodulatory effect of the DHA/EPA administration was reflected in maintaining the percentage of peripheral blood CD4+ T cells, while in the placebo group, a significant reduction in the percentage of these cells was observed. The stimulating influence of ovophospholipids on $CD4^+$ T lymphocytes of the peripheral lymphoid organs (spleen and mesenteric lymph nodes) found in our research corresponds with the finding of Paixão et al. [29], i.e., a lack of decrease in CD4+ cells, which in fact can also be considered as a stimulating effect of n3-PUFA on CD4+ lymphocytes.

We demonstrated a stimulating effect of ovophospholipids on B lymphocytes of the spleen and mesenteric lymph nodes. Most changes were observed after the administration of ovophospholipids at the lower doses of 10 and 1 mg/kg. The ovophospholipids administered at all examined doses also stimulated the humoral immune response.

These outcomes correlate with other studies. Teague et al. [30] showed that n-3 PUFAs administered for 4 weeks elevated the percentage and frequency of splenic B-cell subsets in the absence or presence of antigen in mice. Using a murine model of obesity, the researchers [30,31] also demonstrated the effect of a high-fat diet enriched with DHA or EPA (administered for 5 or 10 weeks) on B cell activity. DHA and EPA differentially raised spleen weight, the frequency, and/or percentage of selected B-cell subsets. The most prominent effect was noticed for the frequency and/or percentage of $IgM^+IgD^-CD21^{low}CD23^-$ B splenocytes. The total serum IgM level was elevated after feeding the animals with DHA and EPA, and cecal IgA increased following the EPA administration [30,31].

Another in vivo study [32] showed that a diet containing DHA-enriched fish oil (mice fed for 5 weeks) significantly raised the percentage of B cells (B220 used as a pan-B cell marker) and the expression of functional surface markers in the mesenteric lymph nodes and the Peyer's Patches, as well as significantly elevated plasma levels of IL-5, IL-9, and cecal IgA.

IL-6 is involved in the maturation of B lymphocytes and stimulates B cells to produce immunoglobulins [33]. Gurzell et al. [32] reported that LPS-stimulated B cells from mice fed for 5 weeks with DHA-enriched fish oil significantly increased their CD40 expression and IL-6 production. Teague et al. [31] found that DHA or EPA (10-week supplementation) enhanced IL-6, TNFα, and IL-10 secretion by the murine B cells ex vivo. Thus, we can assume that the stimulating effect of ovophospholipids on B lymphocytes and humoral immune response is likely, at least in part, to be associated with their stimulating effect on the IL-6 production.

On the other hand, Weise et al. [34] showed in vitro that DHA inhibited, in a dose-dependent manner, the IgE production of human B cells by down-regulating both the CD40 and the IL-4 signaling pathway. The most prominent effect was observed for the highest concentration of DHA, i.e., 10 μM. The production of IgA was not altered, and the synthesis of IgG was only slightly reduced.

An explanation of this discrepancy in results may be the type of research (in vivo/ex vivo or in vitro). As found by Rockett et al. [35], the treatment of naïve B cells in vitro with 50 μM EPA or DHA for 48 h had no effect on the percentage of activated B cells, upregulation of cell surface molecules, and secretion of TNF-α, IFN-γ, and IL-10. Only the secretion of IL-6 was significantly suppressed. Ex vivo, when mice were fed n-3 PUFAs diet, there was still no effect on the percentage of B cells activated by LPS; however, this diet increased the B-cell CD69 surface expression and IL-6 and IFN-γ secretion [35].

We noticed a stimulating effect of the ovophospholipids administered at the dose of 1 mg/kg on the synthesis of TNF-α by murine peritoneal macrophages, and an upward trend was also observed for other doses. However, no changes were found in the level of IL-1β.

The influence of n3-PUFA on these cytokines was reported by other authors [6–8,31]. However, the results are inconsistent. Gorjao et al. [6] also demonstrated an increase in the synthesis of TNF-α by lymphocytes derived from male volunteers consuming DHA- and EPA- enriched fish oil. Contrary to that, Kew et al. [7] reported that supplementation of human diet with a DHA-rich oil had no effect on cytokine (i.a. TNF-α and IL-1β) production by peripheral blood mononuclear cells. Interestingly, Tan et al. [8] demonstrated that administration of EPA + DHA to aging adults with chronic venous leg ulcers significantly reduced high levels of circulating proinflammatory cytokines, i.e., IL-6, IL-1β, and TNF-α. Taking into account the findings presented above, we may conclude that the impact of n3-PUFA on the cytokines depends on many factors. The experimental protocol is one of the key determinants. We estimated the level of TNF-α and IL-1β produced by peritoneal macrophages stimulated in vitro with LPS while the other authors assessed these parameters in blood samples.

Stimulation of macrophages by LPS reflects infection and induction of inflammation in the body. TNF-α is one of the agents whose concentration increases in such situations, and one of its roles is the stimulation of cytotoxic activity of monocytes and macrophages as a response to, i.a., infection. Therefore, ovophospholipid-induced enhancement in TNF-α production by macrophages may contribute to more efficient response to infections. On the other hand, a rapid release of large amounts of TNF-α is highly unfavorable and can lead to respiratory and organ failure. Since we stimulated macrophages in vitro, further studies are needed to clearly assess the importance of the ovophospholipids in the TNF-α production.

Another fact worth discussing is that TNF-α induces the release of some cytokines, i.a., IL-6; and together with this cytokine may enhance proliferation and differentiation of B lymphocytes. Therefore, we cannot exclude the possibility that the stimulating effect of ovophospholipids on TNF-α synthesis may also indirectly contribute to the stimulating effect of ovophospholipids on B lymphocytes and humoral immune response.

Some differences between our findings and those of other authors may be attributed to several factors. One of the postulated mechanisms by which phospholipids influence immune cells is that PUFAs are incorporated into the cellular membranes and thus alter the lipid composition of the membrane microdomains and receptor signaling function [36]. Therefore, the composition of phospholipids, i.e., quantitative and qualitative content of individual fatty acids as well as their final administered dose/concentration are important factors determining the final result of the experiment. Moreover, differences in the time of exposure, which may also reflect the age and the metabolic profile of an animal, and the baseline immune status could influence the final effect. Other factors may include differences in experimental protocols and the type of experiment—in vitro versus ex vivo/in vivo study.

This work demonstrated that lower doses of ovophospholipids had more pronounced effect on the determined parameters. It is not surprising, as in our previous studies on other immunomodulating agents, we also found stronger immunomodulatory effects after the administration of lower experimental doses compared to higher ones [37,38].

In conclusion, our research showed that ovophospholipids exert a stimulating effect on the lymphocyte subsets and the humoral immune response in mice. Most changes were observed after the administration of the ovophospholipids at the lower doses of 10 and 1 mg/kg. Regarding T lymphocytes, the effect is rather short-lived, as most changes were observed only after 24 h following the administration of the last dose.

Stimulation of lymphocytes and immunoglobulin production are the pillars of the cellular and humoral immune response, respectively. Therefore, we may assume that the administration of ovophospholipids, resulting in an increase in lymphocyte subsets and antibody titers, may contribute to better resistance against infections or diseases. However, as there are many inconsistencies in the literature regarding the impact of fatty acids on the immune response, more experiments with ovophospholipids, taking into consideration different aspects of the immune system, should be carried out to assess their complex immunomodulatory potential and possible clinical indications.

4. Materials and Methods

4.1. Animals

The experiments were conducted on female Balb/c mice, aged 8–10 weeks, and with body weight of 18–20 g. The mice were purchased from the Breeding Centre of Laboratory Animals at the Institute of Occupational Medicine (Łódź, Poland). They were kept under conventional conditions and fed commercial food and water ad libitum. The study was conducted according to the requirements of the European Union, with the consent of the II Local Ethics Committee for Animal Experiments, Wrocław, Poland (permission number 12/2019).

4.2. Drugs and Treatments

Ovophospholipids were obtained in the project: "Innovative technologies of the production of biopreparations based on the new generation of eggs (OVOCURA)". Laying hens (Lohmann Brown line) were fed ad libitum with standard feed supplemented with fish oil (3%), dried algae (1.5%), Humokarbowit and Humobentofet humic preparations, and vitamin E (0.01%). The details of the method of ovophospholipid isolation were described in the Patent application No. 218452. The composition of the ovophospholipids is presented in Table 1.

Table 1. Fatty acid composition in ovophospholipids.

Acetone Insoluble Matter 75.68% **Phosphatidylcholine (Lecithin) 75.6%** **Phosphatidylethanolamine (Cephalin) 24.4%**	**Amount (%)**
Acids	
C14:0	0.53
C14:1	0.16
C16:0	25.51
C16:1	2.69
C17:0	0.19
C18:0	14.48
C18:1	27.09
C18:2; ω–6	13.43
C18:3; ω–3	3.32
C20:2; ω–6	0.16
C20:3; ω–6	0.30
C20:4; ω–6	1.99
C20:5; ω–3	0.92
C22:6; ω–3	9.24
Sum of ω–3 fatty acids	13.48
Sum of ω–6 fatty acids	15.88
ω–6/ω–3	1.18
Total saturated fatty acids (SFAs)	40.71
Total unsaturated fatty acids (UFAs)	59.29
Total MUFAs	29.94
Total PUFAs	29.35

Ovophospholipids were dissolved in aqueous starch solution and administered to mice orally (via a stomach tube) at the doses of 100, 10, and 1 mg/kg, for 14 days at 24 h intervals. The dose volume was 0.2 mL per mouse. The experiments in the control group were conducted simultaneously. The control mice received pure aqueous starch solution without the preparation. Each experimental and control group consisted of seven mice.

4.3. Measurements

The studies were performed according to two experimental protocols—in non-immunized mice and SRBC-immunized mice.

The following parameters were assessed in the non-immunized mice: (1) the weight of the thymi, spleens, and mesenteric lymph nodes; (2) the total number of lymphocytes in the thymus, spleen, and mesenteric lymph nodes; (3) the percentage and absolute count of lymphocyte subsets in the lymphatic organs, i.e., $CD4^-CD8^-$, $CD4^+CD8^+$, $CD4^+$, and $CD8^+$ in the thymus; $CD19^+$, $CD3^+$, $CD4^+$, and $CD8^+$ in the spleen and mesenteric lymph nodes; (4) synthesis of TNF-α and IL-1β in the culture supernatants of peritoneal macrophages stimulated in vitro with LPS from *E. coli* (055:B5). The parameters were assessed 24 h and 72 h after administration of the last dose of ovophospholipids. The absolute counts were calculated based on the total count of lymphocytes in individual lymphatic organs.

In the second experimental protocol, the mice were immunized with 4×10^8 SRBC per mouse (0.2 mL of 10% SRBC suspension), administered intraperitoneally 24 h after the last dose of ovophospholipids. Sheep blood was collected into Alsever's solution in sterile manner and kept at 4 °C for at least 3 days. The SRBC suspension in phosphate-buffered saline (PBS, Institute of Immunology and Experimental Therapy, Wrocław, Poland) was prepared ex tempore.

The following parameters in the SRBC-immunized mice were evaluated: (1) the number of PFCs in the spleen, and (2) anti-SRBC hemagglutinin titer in the serum. The number of PFCs was determined on day 4 after priming, while the number of anti-SRBC hemagglutinin titer was assessed on days 4 and 7 after immunization.

4.4. Determination of Total Count and Subsets of Lymphocytes in the Thymus, Spleen, and Mesenteric Lymph Nodes

The mice were anesthetized with halothane (Narcotan, Zentiva, Prague, Czech Republic) and killed by cervical dislocation. The thymuses, spleens, and mesenteric lymph nodes were weighed and placed into Petri dishes with sterile, ice-cold PBS. The suspended cells were obtained by passing the lymphatic organs through a nylon mesh into 1 mL of PBS. The number of lymphocytes in the thymus, spleen, and mesenteric lymph nodes was counted with a Thoma hemocytometer. The cell suspension was centrifuged (3000× *g*, 15 min, 4 °C) on a layer of Ficoll 400 (Pharmacia, Fine Chemicals AB, Uppsala, Sweden)/Urografin 76% (diatrizoate sodium and meglumine diatrizoate, Bayer Schering Pharma, Poland) in a 1:3 ratio, density of 1.076. Next, the lymphocytes were collected from the interphase and washed twice (375× *g*, 7 min, 4 °C) with ice-cold PBS supplemented with 1% bovine serum albumin (BSA; Sigma, Saint Louis, MO, USA). Lysis of erythrocytes present in the splenocyte suspensions was induced by incubation of the splenocytes with 0.84% ammonium chloride (POCH, Gliwice, Poland) for 5 min at 37 °C. After the second wash, the cells were resuspended in PBS with 1% BSA at 1×10^7 cells/mL. Viability of each cell suspension was assessed using the trypan blue dye exclusion assay. It was above 95%. Then, the thymocytes, splenocytes, and lymphocytes from the mesenteric lymph nodes resuspended in PBS containing 1% BSA were stained with the monoclonal Rat Anti-Mouse CD4:FITC/CD8:RPE dual-color reagent (AbD Serotec, Kidlington, UK) at a dilution rate recommended by the manufacturer. The lymphocytes from the spleen and mesenteric lymph nodes were stained additionally with the monoclonal Rat Anti-Mouse CD19:FITC/CD3:RPE dual-color reagent (AbD Serotec, Kidlington, UK) according to the manufacturer's instructions. The cells were incubated with the antibodies for 30 min at

4 °C and washed three times (375× *g*, 7 min, 4 °C) with ice-cold PBS. Fluorescence was analyzed with a flow cytometer (FACS Calibur; Becton-Dickinson Biosciences, San Jose, CA, USA). Distribution of the thymocyte, splenocyte, and lymphocyte of the mesenteric lymph node markers was analyzed with CellQuest 3.1 f. Pro software (Becton-Dickinson Biosciences, San Jose, CA, USA).

4.5. Determination of Synthesis of TNF-α and IL-1β in the Culture Supernatants of Peritoneal Macrophages Stimulated In Vitro with LPS from E. coli (055:B5)

Mice were anesthetized with halothane and killed by cervical dislocation. Peritoneal macrophages were harvested by lavage of the peritoneal cavity with sterile, ice-cold PBS supplemented with antibiotics: penicillin 10 U/mL and streptomycin 10 µg/mL (a stabilized Penicillin–Streptomycin solution, Sigma). The cells were centrifuged (375× *g*, 10 min, 4 °C). Then, the macrophages were suspended in RPMI-1640 medium (Institute of Immunology and Experimental Therapy, Wrocław, Poland) supplemented with 10% fetal bovine serum (FBS, Sigma), 10 mM HEPES (Sigma), 2 mM L-glutamine (Sigma), 10 U/mL of penicillin and 10 µg/mL of streptomycin. Viability of the macrophages was determined by the trypan blue dye exclusion assay, and it was 90–95%. Purity of the peritoneal cell suspension was estimated with the Pappenheim method. The macrophages accounted for 65–75% of the whole cell population. The macrophages were washed twice and adjusted to a concentration of 1.5×10^6 cells/mL. The cells were dispensed in a 96-well flat bottom plate (Nunc, Roskilde, Denmark) and incubated 3 h at 37 °C with 5% CO_2. After this time, the medium was replaced, and the incubation was continued for 18 h at the same conditions. Then, the medium was replaced again with the medium without FBS but with LPS from *E. coli*, serotype 055:B5 (Sigma) at a concentration of 2.5 µg/mL. The incubation was continued for further 24 h. Then, the supernatants were removed and stored at −80 °C.

Murine IL-1β and TNF-α levels in the culture supernatants of peritoneal macrophages were determined with commercial ELISA kits (Quantikine Mouse IL-1β and TNF-α Immunoassays, R&D Systems, Minneapolis, MN, USA) according to the manufacturer's protocols. The results were read on a spectrophotometric microplate reader (Elx800, BioTek, Winooski, VT, USA) at 450 nm with the wavelength correction of 570 with KC Junior software 1.4.

4.6. Determination of Plaque Forming Cells

The mice were euthanized by cervical dislocation after previous anesthesia with halothane. The spleens were removed and placed into ice-cold Hank's saline (Institute of Immunology and Experimental Therapy, Wrocław, Poland). The splenocytes were isolated according to the lymphocyte subsets' assay. After isolation, the cells were collected from the interphase and washed twice in Hank's saline (375× *g*, 7 min, 4 °C). Next, the cells were resuspended in Hank's saline to a concentration of 1×10^6 cells/mL. Viability of the splenocytes was determined by trypan blue dye exclusion assay, and it was above 95%. To assess the number of splenocytes producing hemolytic anti-SRBC antibodies (PFCs), a local hemolysis technique in an agar gel was used [39].

4.7. Determination of Serum Anti-SRBC Antibodies

Blood was collected from the retro-ocular arteries of the halothane-anesthetized mice and centrifuged for 15 min at 3500× *g*. Then, the sera were inactivated at 56 °C for 30 min. To determine the total (IgM + IgG) and 2-mercaptoethanol (2-ME)-resistant (IgG) serum hemagglutinin titers, an active hemagglutination test, carried out on microplates, was used [40]. The results were expressed as a value of $\log_2$.

4.8. Statistical Analysis

The data obtained in the study were analyzed statistically using a one-way analysis of variance (ANOVA), followed by Tukey's post hoc test for multiple comparisons. The differences were considered significant at $p < 0.05$.

Author Contributions: Conceptualization, B.O.-M.; methodology, B.O.-M., M.L., M.S. and A.S.-P.; investigation, B.O.-M., M.L., M.S., A.S.-P., A.P. and Ł.B.; data curation, M.L., M.S. and A.S.-P.; writing—original draft preparation, M.L. and M.S.; writing—review and editing, B.O.-M., M.L., M.S., A.S.-P. and Ł.B.; visualization, M.L.; supervision, B.O.-M., M.L., M.S. and A.S.-P.; project administration, B.O.-M.; funding acquisition, B.O.-M. All authors have read and agreed to the published version of the manuscript.

Funding: This research was performed as a part of the project "Innovative technologies of the production of biopreparations based on the new generation of eggs (OVOCURA)", co-financed by the European Regional Development Fund within the Innovative Economy Operational Programme, 2007–2013 (project No. POIG.01.03.01-00-133/08). The APC is financed by Wrocław University of Environmental and Life Sciences.

Institutional Review Board Statement: The study was conducted according to the requirements of the European Union, with the consent of the II Local Ethics Committee for Animal Experiments, Wrocław, Poland (permission number 12/2019).

Informed Consent Statement: Not applicable.

Data Availability Statement: The original contributions presented in this study are included in the article material. Further inquiries can be directed to the corresponding author.

Acknowledgments: The authors wish to thank Tadeusz Trziszka from the Institute of Agricultural Engineering, Faculty of Life Sciences and Technology, Wrocław University of Environmental and Life Sciences, Chełmońskiego 37, 51-630 Wrocław, Poland, who provided ovophospholipids for this study.

Conflicts of Interest: The authors declare no conflicts of interest.

References

1. Bubel, F.; Dobrzański, Z.; Bykowski, P.; Patkowska-Sokoła, B.; Trziszka, T. Enrichment of hen eggs with omega-3 polyunsaturated fatty acids-physiological and nutritional aspects. *Acta Sci. Pol. Med. Weterinaria* **2011**, *10*, 5–18.
2. Sun, N.; Chen, J.; Wang, D.; Lin, S. Advance in food-derived phospholipids: Sources, molecular species and structure as well as their biological activities. *Trends Food Sci. Technol.* **2018**, *80*, 199–211. [CrossRef]
3. Anton, M. Composition and Structure of Hen Egg Yolk. In *Bioactive Egg Compounds*; Huopalahti, R., López-Fandiño, R., Anton, M., Schade, R., Eds.; Springer: Berlin/Heidelberg, Germany, 2007; pp. 1–6.
4. Xu, D.; Ren, J.; Ali, B.; Jin, Y.; Jin, Z.; Xu, X. Water-in-oil soybean concentrated phospholipids hydrolysis based on the model of enzymatic deactivation and its application in bread. *Food Biosci.* **2021**, *44 Pt A*, 101412. [CrossRef]
5. Cherian, G. Egg quality and yolk polyunsaturated fatty acid status in relation to broiler breeder hen age and dietary n-3 oils. *Poult. Sci.* **2008**, *87*, 1131–1137. [CrossRef]
6. Gorjão, R.; Verlengia, R.; Lima, T.M.; Soriano, F.G.; Boaventura, M.F.; Kanunfre, C.C.; Peres, C.M.; Sampaio, S.C.; Otton, R.; Folador, A.; et al. Effect of docosahexaenoic acid-rich fish oil supplementation on human leukocyte function. *Clin. Nutr.* **2006**, *25*, 923–938. [CrossRef]
7. Kew, S.; Mesa, M.D.; Tricon, S.; Buckley, R.; Minihane, A.M.; Yaqoob, P. Effects of oils rich in eicosapentaenoic and docosahexaenoic acids on immune cell composition and function in healthy humans. *Am. J. Clin. Nutr.* **2004**, *79*, 674–681. [CrossRef] [PubMed]
8. Tan, A.; Sullenbarger, B.; Prakash, R.; McDaniel, J.C. Supplementation with eicosapentaenoic acid and docosahexaenoic acid reduces high levels of circulating proinflammatory cytokines in aging adults: A randomized, controlled study. *Prostaglandins Leukot. Essent. Fat. Acids* **2018**, *132*, 23–29. [CrossRef]
9. Olson, M.V.; Liu, Y.C.; Dangi, B.; Paul Zimmer, J.; Salem, N., Jr.; Nauroth, J.M. Docosahexaenoic acid reduces inflammation and joint destruction in mice with collagen-induced arthritis. *Inflamm. Res.* **2013**, *62*, 1003–1013. [CrossRef]
10. Che, H.; Li, H.; Song, L.; Dong, X.; Yang, X.; Zhang, T.; Wang, Y.; Xie, W. Orally Administered DHA-Enriched Phospholipids and DHA-Enriched Triglyceride Relieve Oxidative Stress, Improve Intestinal Barrier, Modulate Inflammatory Cytokine and Gut

Microbiota, and Meliorate Inflammatory Responses in the Brain in Dextran Sodium Sulfate Induced Colitis in Mice. *Mol. Nutr. Food Res.* **2021**, *65*, e2000986. [CrossRef]

11. Merzouk, S.A.; Saker, M.; Reguig, K.B.; Soulimane, N.; Merzouk, H.; Guermouche, B.; Berrouiguet, A.Y.; Hichami, A.; Narce, M.; Khan, N.A. N-3 polyunsaturated fatty acids modulate in-vitro T cell function in type I diabetic patients. *Lipids* **2008**, *43*, 485–497. [CrossRef]
12. Chapkin, R.S.; Arrington, J.L.; Apanasovich, T.V.; Carroll, R.J.; McMurray, D.N. Dietary n-3 PUFA affect TcR-mediated activation of purified murine T cells and accessory cell function in co-cultures. *Clin Exp Immunol.* **2002**, *130*, 12–18, Erratum in *Clin. Exp. Immunol.* **2002**, *130*, 557–558. [CrossRef] [PubMed]
13. Kong, W.; Yen, J.H.; Ganea, D. Docosahexaenoic acid prevents dendritic cell maturation, inhibits antigen-specific Th1/Th17 differentiation and suppresses experimental autoimmune encephalomyelitis. *Brain Behav. Immun.* **2011**, *25*, 872–882. [CrossRef]
14. Lian, M.; Luo, W.; Sui, Y.; Li, Z.; Hua, J. Dietary n-3 PUFA Protects Mice from Con A Induced Liver Injury by Modulating Regulatory T Cells and PPAR-γ Expression. *PLoS ONE* **2015**, *10*, e0132741. [CrossRef] [PubMed]
15. Han, S.C.; Koo, D.H.; Kang, N.J.; Yoon, W.J.; Kang, G.J.; Kang, H.K.; Yoo, E.S. Docosahexaenoic Acid Alleviates Atopic Dermatitis by Generating Tregs and IL-10/TGF-β-Modified Macrophages via a TGF-β-Dependent Mechanism. *J. Investig. Dermatol.* **2015**, *135*, 1556–1564. [CrossRef]
16. Carlsson, J.A.; Wold, A.E.; Sandberg, A.S.; Östman, S.M. The Polyunsaturated Fatty Acids Arachidonic Acid and Docosahexaenoic Acid Induce Mouse Dendritic Cells Maturation but Reduce T-Cell Responses In Vitro. *PLoS ONE* **2015**, *10*, e0143741. [CrossRef]
17. Monk, J.M.; Hou, T.Y.; Turk, H.F.; McMurray, D.N.; Chapkin, R.S. n3 PUFAs reduce mouse $CD4^+$ T-cell ex vivo polarization into Th17 cells. *J. Nutr.* **2013**, *143*, 1501–1508. [CrossRef]
18. Teague, H.; Rockett, B.D.; Harris, M.; Brown, D.A.; Shaikh, S.R. Dendritic cell activation, phagocytosis and CD69 expression on cognate T cells are suppressed by n-3 long-chain polyunsaturated fatty acids. *Immunology* **2013**, *139*, 386–394. [CrossRef] [PubMed]
19. Vedin, I.; Cederholm, T.; Freund Levi, Y.; Basun, H.; Garlind, A.; Faxén Irving, G.; Jönhagen, M.E.; Vessby, B.; Wahlund, L.O.; Palmblad, J. Effects of docosahexaenoic acid-rich n-3 fatty acid supplementation on cytokine release from blood mononuclear leukocytes: The OmegAD study. *Am. J. Clin. Nutr.* **2008**, *87*, 1616–1622. [CrossRef]
20. Rusnak, T.; Azarcoya-Barrera, J.; Makarowski, A.; Jacobs, R.L.; Richard, C. Plant- and Animal-Derived Dietary Sources of Phosphatidylcholine Have Differential Effects on Immune Function in The Context of A High-Fat Diet in Male Wistar Rats. *J. Nutr.* **2024**, *154*, 1936–1944. [CrossRef]
21. Yessoufou, A.; Plé, A.; Moutairou, K.; Hichami, A.; Khan, N.A. Docosahexaenoic acid reduces suppressive and migratory functions of CD4+CD25+ regulatory T-cells. *J. Lipid Res.* **2009**, *50*, 2377–2388. [CrossRef]
22. Wu, S.; Peng, H.; Li, S.; Huang, L.; Wang, X.; Li, Y.; Liu, Y.; Xiong, P.; Yang, Q.; Tian, K.; et al. The ω-3 Polyunsaturated Fatty Acid Docosahexaenoic Acid Enhances NK-Cell Antitumor Effector Functions. *Cancer Immunol. Res.* **2024**, *12*, 744–758. [CrossRef] [PubMed]
23. Gutiérrez, S.; Svahn, S.L.; Johansson, M.E. Effects of Omega-3 Fatty Acids on Immune Cells. *Int. J. Mol. Sci.* **2019**, *20*, 5028. [CrossRef] [PubMed]
24. Miles, E.A.; Calder, P.C. Influence of marine n-3 polyunsaturated fatty acids on immune function and a systematic review of their effects on clinical outcomes in rheumatoid arthritis. *Br. J. Nutr.* **2012**, *107* (Suppl. S2), S171–S184. [CrossRef]
25. Tomasdottir, V.; Thorleifsdottir, S.; Vikingsson, A.; Hardardottir, I.; Freysdottir, J. Dietary omega-3 fatty acids enhance the B1 but not the B2 cell immune response in mice with antigen-induced peritonitis. *J. Nutr. Biochem.* **2014**, *25*, 111–117. [CrossRef] [PubMed]
26. Juman, S.; Hashimoto, M.; Katakura, M.; Inoue, T.; Tanabe, Y.; Arita, M.; Miki, T.; Shido, O. Effects of long-term oral administration of arachidonic acid and docosahexaenoic acid on the immune functions of young rats. *Nutrients* **2013**, *5*, 1949–1961. [CrossRef]
27. Sasaki, T.; Kanke, Y.; Kudoh, K.; Misawa, Y.; Shimizu, J.; Takita, T. Effects of dietary docosahexaenoic acid on surface molecules involved in T cell proliferation. *Biochim. Biophys. Acta* **1999**, *1436*, 519–530. [CrossRef]
28. Woodworth, H.L.; McCaskey, S.J.; Duriancik, D.M.; Clinthorne, J.F.; Langohr, I.M.; Gardner, E.M.; Fenton, J.I. Dietary fish oil alters T lymphocyte cell populations and exacerbates disease in a mouse model of inflammatory colitis. *Cancer Res.* **2010**, *70*, 7960–7969. [CrossRef]
29. Paixão, E.M.D.S.; Oliveira, A.C.M.; Pizato, N.; Muniz-Junqueira, M.I.; Magalhães, K.G.; Nakano, E.Y.; Ito, M.K. The effects of EPA and DHA enriched fish oil on nutritional and immunological markers of treatment naïve breast cancer patients: A randomized double-blind controlled trial. *Nutr. J.* **2017**, *16*, 71. [CrossRef]
30. Teague, H.; Fhaner, C.J.; Harris, M.; Duriancik, D.M.; Reid, G.E.; Shaikh, S.R. n-3 PUFAs enhance the frequency of murine B-cell subsets and restore the impairment of antibody production to a T-independent antigen in obesity. *J. Lipid Res.* **2013**, *54*, 3130–3138. [CrossRef]
31. Teague, H.; Harris, M.; Fenton, J.; Lallemand, P.; Shewchuk, B.M.; Shaikh, S.R. Eicosapentaenoic and docosahexaenoic acid ethyl esters differentially enhance B-cell activity in murine obesity. *J. Lipid Res.* **2014**, *55*, 1420–1433. [CrossRef]

32. Gurzell, E.A.; Teague, H.; Harris, M.; Clinthorne, J.; Shaikh, S.R.; Fenton, J.I. DHA-enriched fish oil targets B cell lipid microdomains and enhances ex vivo and in vivo B cell function. *J. Leukoc. Biol.* **2013**, *93*, 463–470. [CrossRef] [PubMed]
33. Kaur, S.; Bansal, Y.; Kumar, R.; Bansal, G. A panoramic review of IL-6: Structure, pathophysiological roles and inhibitors. *Bioorg Med. Chem.* **2020**, *28*, 115327. [CrossRef] [PubMed]
34. Weise, C.; Hilt, K.; Milovanovic, M.; Ernst, D.; Rühl, R.; Worm, M. Inhibition of IgE production by docosahexaenoic acid is mediated by direct interference with STAT6 and NFκB pathway in human B cells. *J. Nutr. Biochem.* **2011**, *22*, 269–275. [CrossRef]
35. Rockett, B.D.; Salameh, M.; Carraway, K.; Morrison, K.; Shaikh, S.R. n-3 PUFA improves fatty acid composition, prevents palmitate-induced apoptosis, and differentially modifies B cell cytokine secretion in vitro and ex vivo. *J. Lipid Res.* **2010**, *51*, 1284–1297. [CrossRef] [PubMed]
36. Fan, Y.Y.; Fuentes, N.R.; Hou, T.Y.; Barhoumi, R.; Li, X.C.; Deutz, N.E.P.; Engelen, M.P.K.J.; McMurray, D.N.; Chapkin, R.S. Remodelling of primary human CD4+ T cell plasma membrane order by n-3 PUFA. *Br. J. Nutr.* **2018**, *119*, 163–175. [CrossRef]
37. Jine, Y.; Lis, M.; Szczypka, M.; Obmińska-Mrukowicz, B. Influence of betulinic acid on lymphocyte subsets and humoral immune response in mice. *Pol. J. Vet. Sci.* **2012**, *15*, 305–313. [CrossRef]
38. Lis, M.; Szczypka, M.; Suszko, A.; Obmińska-Mrukowicz, B. Influence of bestatin, an inhibitor of aminopeptidases, on T and B lymphocyte subsets in mice. *Pol. J. Vet. Sci.* **2011**, *14*, 393–403. [CrossRef]
39. Mishell, R.I.; Dutton, R.W. Immunization of dissociated spleen cell cultures from normal mice. *J. Exp. Med.* **1967**, *126*, 423–442. [CrossRef]
40. Hudson, L.; Hay, F.C. *Practical Immunology*; Blackwell Scientific Publications: Oxford, UK; London, UK; Edinburgh, UK; Boston, MA, USA; Melbourne, VIC, Australia, 1980.

MDPI AG
Grosspeteranlage 5
4052 Basel
Switzerland
Tel.: +41 61 683 77 34

Molecules Editorial Office
E-mail: molecules@mdpi.com
www.mdpi.com/journal/molecules

www.ingramcontent.com/pod-product-compliance
Lightning Source LLC
Chambersburg PA
CBHW040813250926
51850CB00007BA/1152
* 9 7 8 3 7 2 5 8 7 7 7 7 5 *